Disorders of the Anorectum and Pelvic Floor

Editors

DAVID J. MARON
STEVEN D. WEXNER

GASTROENTEROLOGY CLINICS OF NORTH AMERICA

www.gastro.theclinics.com

December 2013 • Volume 42 • Number 4

ELSEVIER

1600 John F. Kennedy Boulevard • Suite 1800 • Philadelphia, Pennsylvania, 19103-2899
http://www.theclinics.com

GASTROENTEROLOGY CLINICS OF NORTH AMERICA Volume 42, Number 4
December 2013 ISSN 0889-8553, ISBN-13: 978-0-323-26098-5

Editor: Kerry Holland

Gastroenterology Clinics of North America (ISSN 0889-8553) is published quarterly by Elsevier Inc., 360 Park Avenue South, New York, NY 10010-1710. Months of issue are March, June, September, and December. Business and Editorial Offices: 1600 John F. Kennedy Blvd., Suite 1800, Philadelphia, PA 19103-2899. Customer Service Office: 6277 Sea Harbor Drive, Orlando, FL 32887-4800. Periodicals postage paid at New York, NY and additional mailing offices. Subscription prices are $320.00 per year (US individuals), $160.00 per year (US students), $530.00 per year (US institutions), $350.00 per year (Canadian individuals), $651.00 per year (Canadian institutions), $445.00 per year (international individuals), $220.00 per year (international students), and $651.00 per year (international institutions). Foreign air speed delivery is included in all *Clinics* subscription prices. All prices are subject to change without notice. **POSTMASTER**: Send address changes to *Gastroenterology Clinics of North America*, Elsevier Health Sciences Division, Subscription Customer Service, 3251 Riverport Lane, Maryland Heights, MO 63043. Telephone: 1-800-654-2452 (U.S. and Canada); 314-447-8871 (outside U.S. and Canada). Fax: 314-447-8029. E-mail: journalscustomerservice-usa@elsevier.com (for print support); journalsonlinesupport-usa@elsevier.com (for online support).

Reprints. For copies of 100 or more, of articles in this publication, please contact the Commercial Reprints Department, Elsevier Inc., 360 Part Avenue South, New York, New York 10010-1710. Tel. 212-633-3874, Fax: 212-633-3820, E-mail: reprints@elsevier.com.

Gastroenterology Clinics of North America is also published in Italian by II Pensiero Scientifico Editore, Rome, Italy; and in Portuguese by Interlivros Edicoes Ltda., Rua Commandante Coelho 1085, 21250 Cordovil, Rio de Janeiro, Brazil.

Gastroenterology Clinics of North America is covered in *MEDLINE/PubMed (Index Medicus), Excerpta Medica, Current Contents/Clinical Medicine, Science Citation Index, ISI/BIOMED,* and *BIOSIS.*

Printed and bound by CPI Group (UK) Ltd, Croydon, CR0 4YY

Transferred to digital print 2012

Contributors

EDITORS

DAVID J. MARON, MD, MBA, FACS, FASCRS
Vice Chairman, Department of Colorectal Surgery, Director, Colorectal Surgery
Residency Program, Cleveland Clinic Florida, Weston; Assistant Clinical Professor of
Surgery, Florida Atlantic University College of Medicine, Boca Raton, Florida

STEVEN D. WEXNER, MD, PhD(Hon), FACS, FRCS, FRCS(Ed)
Director, Digestive Disease Center, Chairman, Department of Colorectal Surgery,
Cleveland Clinic Florida, Weston; Associate Dean for Academic Affairs, Florida
Atlantic University College of Medicine, Boca Raton; Affiliate Dean for Clinical Education,
Florida International University College of Medicine, Miami, Florida

AUTHORS

PABLO A. BEJARANO, MD
Director of Gastrointestinal Pathology, RT Institute of Pathology and Laboratory Medicine,
Cleveland Clinic Florida, Weston, Florida

MARIANA BERHO, MD
Chair, RT Institute of Pathology and Laboratory Medicine, Cleveland Clinic Florida,
Weston, Florida

JOSHUA I.S. BLEIER, MD, FACS, FASCRS
Assistant Professor of Surgery, Division of Colon and Rectal Surgery, Pennsylvania
Hospital/Hospital of the University of Pennsylvania, University of Pennsylvania,
Philadelphia, Pennsylvania

MARYLISE BOUTROS, MD
Assistant Professor, Department of Surgery, McGill University, Jewish General Hospital,
Montreal, Quebec, Canada

MOLLY M. CONE, MD, Assistant Professor, Department of Colon and Rectal Surgery,
Vanderbilt University Medical Center, Nashville, Tennessee

MEAGAN COSTEDIO, MD, FACS
Staff Surgeon, Department of Colorectal Surgery, Cleveland Clinic Foundation,
Cleveland, Ohio

GIOVANNA DA SILVA, MD, FACS
Colorectal Surgeon, Director of Clinical Research, Department of Colorectal Surgery,
Cleveland Clinic Florida, Weston; Associate Professor, Department of Surgery,
Charles E Schmidt College of Medicine at Florida Atlantic University, Boca Raton, Florida;
Associate Professor, Department of Surgery, ROSS University, Roseau, Commonwealth
of Dominica, West Indies

BRADLEY DAVIS, MD, FACS, FASCRS
Associate Professor, Department of Surgery, University of Cincinnati, Cincinnati, Ohio

CHARLES M. FRIEL, MD
Associate Professor, Department of Surgery, University of Virginia, Charlottesville, Virginia

JASON F. HALL, MD, MPH, FACS
Senior Surgeon, Department of Colon and Rectal Surgery, Lahey Clinic, Burlington;
Assistant Professor, Department of Surgery, Tufts University School of Medicine,
Boston, Massachusetts

QUINTON HATCH, MD
Department of Surgery, Madigan Army Medical Center, Fort Lewis, Washington

TRACI L. HEDRICK, MD
Assistant Professor, Department of Surgery, University of Virginia, Charlottesville, Virginia

BRIAN R. KANN, MD, FACS, FASCRS
Assistant Professor of Surgery, Division of Colon and Rectal Surgery, Penn Presbyterian
Medical Center, University of Pennsylvania, Philadelphia, Pennsylvania

JUSTIN A. MAYKEL, MD
Chief, Division of Colon and Rectal Surgery, Department of Surgery, University of
Massachusetts Medical School, Worcester, Massachusetts

YOSEF Y. NASSERI, MD
The Surgery Group of Los Angeles, Los Angeles, California

MARC C. OSBORNE, MD
Division of Colon and Rectal Surgery, Department of Surgery, University of Minnesota;
Colon and Rectal Surgery Associates, St Paul, Minnesota

BASHAR SAFAR, MBBS, MRCS
Assistant Professor, Department of Surgery, The Johns Hopkins Hospital, Baltimore,
Maryland

ANKIT SARIN, MD, MHA
Assistant Professor of Surgery, Division of Colon and Rectal Surgery, University of
California-San Francisco, San Francisco, California

SHERIEF SHAWKI, MD
Department of Colorectal Surgery, Cleveland Clinic Foundation, Cleveland, Ohio

ERICA B. SNEIDER, MD
General Surgery Chief Resident, Department of Surgery, University of Massachusetts
Medical School, Worcester, Massachusetts

PATRICK SOLAN, MD
Department of Surgery, University of Cincinnati, Cincinnati, Ohio

SCOTT R. STEELE, MD, FACS
Chief, Division of Colon and Rectal Surgery, Madigan Army Medical Center,
Fort Lewis, Washington

SHARON L. STEIN, MD
Associate Professor, Division of Colorectal Surgery, Department of Surgery, University
Hospitals Case Medical Center, Cleveland, Ohio

JULIE ANN M. VAN KOUGHNETT, MD, MEd, FRCSC
Clinical Associate, Department of Colorectal Surgery, Cleveland Clinic Florida, Weston, Florida

CHARLES B. WHITLOW, MD
Staff Surgeon, Department of Colon and Rectal Surgery, Ochsner Clinic Foundation, New Orleans, Louisiana

Contents

Preface: Disorders of the Anorectum and Pelvic Floor   xiii

David J. Maron and Steven D. Wexner

Dedication   xv

David J. Maron and Steven D. Wexner

Anorectal Anatomy and Imaging Techniques   701

Patrick Solan and Bradley Davis

> The rectum and anus are two anatomically complex organs with diverse pathologies. This article reviews the basic anatomy of the rectum and anus. In addition, it addresses the current radiographic techniques used to evaluate these structures, specifically ultrasound, magnetic resonance imaging, and defecography.

Anorectal Physiology and Testing   713

Julie Ann M. Van Koughnett and Giovanna da Silva

> A good understanding of anorectal physiology is essential for the diagnosis and appropriate treatment of various anorectal disorders, such as fecal incontinence, constipation, and pain. This article reviews the physiology of the anorectum and details the various investigations used to diagnose anorectal physiology disorders. These anatomic and functional tests include anal manometry, endoanal ultrasound, defecography, balloon expulsion test, magnetic resonance imaging, pudendal nerve terminal motor latency, electromyography, and colonic transit studies. Indications for investigations, steps in performing the tests, and interpretation of results are discussed.

Anal Fissure and Stenosis   729

Sherief Shawki and Meagan Costedio

> Anal fissure is a common anorectal disorder resulting in anal pain and bleeding. Fissures can either heal spontaneously and be classified as acute or persist for 6 or more weeks and be classified as chronic, ultimately necessitating treatment. Anal stenosis is a challenging problem most commonly resulting from trauma, such as excisional hemorrhoidectomy. This frustrating issue for the patient is equally as challenging to the surgeon. This article reviews these 2 anorectal disorders, covering their etiology, mechanism of disease, diagnosis, and algorithm of management.

Modern Management of Hemorrhoidal Disease   759

Jason F. Hall

> Complaints secondary to hemorrhoidal disease have been treated by health care providers for centuries. Most symptoms referable to hemorrhoidal disease can be managed nonoperatively. When symptoms do not respond to

medical therapy, procedural intervention is recommended. Surgical hemorrhoidectomy is usually reserved for patients who are refractory to or unable to tolerate office procedures. This article reviews the pathophysiology of hemorrhoidal disease and the most commonly used techniques for the nonoperative and operative palliation of hemorrhoidal complaints.

Anal Abscess and Fistula   773

Erica B. Sneider and Justin A. Maykel

Benign anorectal diseases, such as anal abscesses and fistula, are commonly seen by primary care physicians, gastroenterologists, emergency physicians, general surgeons, and colorectal surgeons. It is important to have a thorough understanding of the complexity of these 2 disease processes so as to provide appropriate and timely treatment. We review the pathophysiology, presentation, diagnosis, and treatment options for both anal abscesses and fistulas.

Chronic Pelvic Pain   785

Sharon L. Stein

Chronic pelvic pain is pain lasting longer than 6 months and is estimated to occur in 15% of women. Causes of pelvic pain include disorders of gynecologic, urologic, gastroenterologic, and musculoskeletal systems. The multidisciplinary nature of chronic pelvic pain may complicate diagnosis and treatment. Treatments vary by cause but may include medicinal, neuroablative, and surgical treatments.

Pruritus Ani: Diagnosis and Treatment   801

Yosef Y. Nasseri and Marc C. Osborne

Pruritus ani is a common condition with multiple causes. Primary causes are thought to be fecal soiling or food irritants. Secondary causes include malignancy, infections including sexually transmitted diseases, benign anorectal diseases, systemic diseases, and inflammatory conditions. A broad differential diagnosis must be considered. A reassessment of the diagnosis is required if symptoms or findings are not responsive to therapy. The pathophysiology of itching, an overview of primary and secondary causes, and various treatment options are reviewed.

Surgical Management of Fecal Incontinence   815

Joshua I.S. Bleier and Brian R. Kann

The surgical approach to treating fecal incontinence is complex. After optimal medical management has failed, surgery remains the best option for restoring function. Patient factors, such as prior surgery, anatomic derangements, and degree of incontinence, help inform the astute surgeon regarding the most appropriate option. Many varied approaches to surgical management are available, ranging from more conservative approaches, such as anal canal bulking agents and neuromodulation, to more aggressive approaches, including sphincter repair, anal cerclage techniques, and muscle transposition. Efficacy and morbidity of these approaches also range widely, and this article presents the data and operative considerations for these approaches.

Rectal Prolapse and Intussusception   837

Quinton Hatch and Scott R. Steele

 A video of robotic assisted rectopexy accompanies this article

Rectal prolapse continues to be problematic for both patients and surgeons alike, in part because of increased recurrence rates despite several well-described operations. Patients should be aware that although the prolapse will resolve with operative therapy, functional results may continue to be problematic. This article describes the recommended evaluation, role of adjunctive testing, and outcomes associated with both perineal and abdominal approaches.

Constipation and Pelvic Outlet Obstruction   863

Traci L. Hedrick and Charles M. Friel

 A video of defecography for rectocele diagnosis accompanies this article

Caring for patients with constipation and pelvic outlet obstruction can be challenging, requiring skill, patience, and empathy on the part of the medical professional. The mainstay of treatment is behavioral with surgery reserved for a select group of patients. The evaluation, diagnostic, and treatment modalities of both constipation and pelvic outlet with a focus on current advancements and technology are explored in depth.

Sexually Transmitted and Anorectal Infectious Diseases   877

Molly M. Cone and Charles B. Whitlow

Sexually transmitted diseases (STDs) are common and they can involve the anus and rectum in both men and women. In this article, the main bacterial and viral STDs that affect the anus and rectum are discussed, including their prevalence, presentation, and treatment.

Anal Squamous Intraepithelial Neoplasia   893

Pablo A. Bejarano, Marylise Boutros, and Mariana Berho

Diagnosis, follow up, and treatment of anal intraepithelial neoplasia are complex and not standardized. This may be partly caused by poor communication of biopsy and cytology findings between pathologists and clinicians as a result of a disparate and confusing terminology used to classify these lesions. This article focuses on general aspects of epidemiology and on clarifying the current terminology of intraepithelial squamous neoplasia, its relationship with human papilloma virus infection, and the current methods that exist to diagnose and treat this condition.

Management of Radiation Proctitis   913

Ankit Sarin and Bashar Safar

Radiation damage to the rectum following radiotherapy for pelvic malignancies can range from acute dose-limiting side effects to major morbidity affecting health-related quality of life. No standard guidelines exist for diagnosis and management of radiation proctitis. This article reviews the definitions, staging, and clinical features of radiation proctitis, and summarizes the modalities available for the treatment of acute and chronic radiation proctitis. Because of the paucity of well-controlled, blinded, randomized studies, it is not possible to fully assess the comparative efficacy of the different approaches to management. However, the evidence and rationale for use of the different strategies are presented.

Index   927

GASTROENTEROLOGY
CLINICS OF NORTH AMERICA

FORTHCOMING ISSUES

March 2014
GERD
Joel Richter, MD, *Editor*

June 2014
Eosinophilic Esophagitis
Ikuo Hirano, MD, *Editor*

September 2014
Upper GI Bleeding
Ian Gralnek, MD, *Editor*

RECENT ISSUES

September 2013
Colonoscopy and Polypectomy
Charles J. Kahi, MD, *Editor*

June 2013
Gastric Cancer
Steven F. Moss, MD, *Editor*

March 2013
Benign and Neoplastic Conditions of the
Esophagus
Nicholas J. Shaheen, MD, *Editor*

Preface
Disorders of the Anorectum and Pelvic Floor

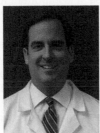
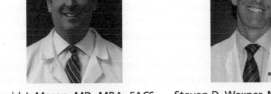

David J. Maron, MD, MBA, FACS,
FASCRS

Steven D. Wexner, MD, PhD(Hon),
FACS, FRCS, FRCS(Ed)

Editors

We are delighted to present you with this issue of *Gastroenterology Clinics of North America*. The issue is focused on diseases of the anorectum and pelvic floor and provides a thorough, comprehensive overview of the disorders, diagnoses, and applicable investigations for these areas. We have tried to select the topics that would be seen in a gastroenterologic practice. Some of these problems may be able to be treated medically, while others may need to be referred to a surgeon. The authorship of the articles has been undertaken by numerous highly expert colorectal surgeons. We have deliberately selected the "rising stars" within colorectal surgery, rather than relying on more senior authorship. All of the authors produced very high-quality insightful and clinically relevant articles.

A detailed knowledge of the anatomy and physiology of the pelvic floor is integral in understanding the pathophysiology of symptoms affecting the pelvic floor. The issue therefore begins with an excellent review of anorectal anatomy with an emphasis on imaging techniques, followed by an article detailing the sensorimotor and neurophysiologic function and assessment of disorders of the pelvic floor. Anorectal pain is a common presenting complaint, and it is necessary for the practicing physician to be able to accurately diagnose and treat conditions of the anus and rectum that result in pain. Included in this issue are detailed reviews of the literature regarding the medical and surgical treatment of anal fissure, as well as a discussion on the treatment of anal stenosis. Nonoperative and operative therapy of hemorrhoidal disease is presented, including newer techniques such as Doppler-guided hemorrhoidal artery ligation. Chronic pelvic pain can affect up to 15% of women and be particularly difficult to diagnose and treat, as causes, evaluation, and treatments may traverse multiple specialties.

Fecal incontinence is an embarrassing and socially paralyzing condition that affects up to 18% of the population and as many as half of all nursing home residents. Multiple

Gastroenterol Clin N Am 42 (2013) xiii–xiv
http://dx.doi.org/10.1016/j.gtc.2013.10.001
gastro.theclinics.com

treatment options are available, including newer modalities such as the use of radio-frequency energy and neuromodulation of the sacral nerve plexus and the tibial nerve. This issue also contains a comprehensive discussion of the cause and management of constipation, with an emphasis on the diagnosis and treatment of pelvic outlet obstruction. A superb review of rectal prolapse and intussusception includes a discussion of newer minimally invasive techniques for the treatment of these disorders.

Finally, as the practice of anoreceptive intercourse increases, it is important for the gastroenterologist to be able to recognize the presenting symptoms of sexually transmitted diseases of the anorectum and to be familiar with their treatments. Anal intraepithelial neoplasia (AIN) is a particularly worrisome sexually transmitted disease resulting from infection with the human papillomavirus, as there may be a relationship between AIN and the development of anal cancer. A comprehensive review of the literature including controversies regarding the diagnosis and treatment of AIN is included as well.

We wish to extend our appreciation to each and every one of our authors for their respective individual time and expertise, which have insured the production of a superlative educational volume. We are confident that you will find the information in these pages to be current, comprehensive, and highly clinically relevant.

David J. Maron, MD, MBA, FACS, FASCRS
Department of Colorectal Surgery
Colorectal Surgery Residency Program
Cleveland Clinic Florida, Weston
FL, USA

Steven D. Wexner, MD, PhD(Hon), FACS, FRCS, FRCS(Ed)
Digestive Disease Center
Department of Colorectal Surgery
Cleveland Clinic Florida, Weston
FL, USA

E-mail addresses:
MAROND@ccf.org (D.J. Maron)
WEXNERS@ccf.org (S.D. Wexner)

Dedication

To my wife, Kammy, for her constant understanding and unending love and emotional support. And to my sons, Connor, Christopher, and Luke, for making every day a new adventure.
  (D.J.M.)

To my parents, whose wisdom, support, and love enabled me to realize and fulfill my dreams.
  (S.D.W.)

David J. Maron, MD, MBA, FACS, FASCRS
Department of Colorectal Surgery
Colorectal Surgery Residency Program
Cleveland Clinic Florida, Weston
FL, USA

Steven D. Wexner, MD, PhD(Hon), FACS, FRCS, FRCS(Ed)
Digestive Disease Center
Department of Colorectal Surgery
Cleveland Clinic Florida, Weston
FL, USA

E-mail addresses:
MAROND@ccf.org (D.J. Maron)
WEXNERS@ccf.org (S.D. Wexner)

Gastroenterol Clin N Am 42 (2013) xv
http://dx.doi.org/10.1016/j.gtc.2013.10.002
0889-8553/13/$ – see front matter © 2013 Elsevier Inc. All rights reserved.

Anorectal Anatomy and Imaging Techniques

Patrick Solan, MD, Bradley Davis, MD*

KEYWORDS

- Anorectal anatomy • Endorectal ultrasound • Anorectal imaging • Defecography

KEY POINTS

- The rectum and anus are two anatomically complex organs with diverse pathologies.
- The focus of this article is a review of the basic anatomy of the rectum and anus.
- In addition, we also address the current radiographic techniques used to evaluate these structures, specifically ultrasound, MRI, and defecography.

EMBRYOLOGY

The embryo begins the third week of development as a bilayered germ disk. During week 3 the surface facing the yolk sac becomes the definitive endoderm; the surface facing the amniotic sac becomes the ectoderm. The middle layer is called mesoderm. The long axis and left-right axis of the embryo also are established at this time. The buccopharyngeal membrane marks the oral opening; the future openings of the urogenital and the digestive tracts become identifiable as the cloacal membrane. At 4 weeks of gestation, the alimentary tract is divided into three parts: (1) foregut, (2) midgut, and (3) hindgut. The primitive gut results from incorporation of the endoderm-lined yolk sac cavity into the embryo, following embryonic cephalocaudal and lateral folding. The endoderm gives rise to the epithelial lining of the gastrointestinal tract while muscle, connective tissue, and peritoneum originate from the splanchnic mesoderm.[1,2] Development progresses through the stages of physiologic herniation return to the abdomen, and fixation. The acquisition of length and formation of dedicated blood and lymphatic supplies takes place during this time. With folding of the embryo during the fourth week of development, the mesodermal layer splits. The portion that adheres to endoderm forms the visceral peritoneum, whereas the part that adheres to ectoderm forms the parietal peritoneum. The space between the two layers becomes the peritoneal cavity. Foregut-derived structures end at the second portion of the duodenum and rely on the celiac artery for blood supply. The midgut, extending

Department of Surgery, University of Cincinnati, 231 Albert Sabin Way, Cincinnati, OH 45267–0558, USA
* Corresponding author.
E-mail address: bradley.davis@uc.edu

Gastroenterol Clin N Am 42 (2013) 701–712
http://dx.doi.org/10.1016/j.gtc.2013.09.008
0889-8553/13/$ – see front matter © 2013 Elsevier Inc. All rights reserved.

gastro.theclinics.com

from the duodenal ampulla to the distal transverse colon, is based on the superior mesenteric artery.[3] The distal third of the transverse colon, descending colon, and rectum evolve from the hindgut fold and are supplied by the inferior mesenteric artery. Venous and lymphatic channels mirror their arterial counterparts and follow the same embryologic divisions. At the dentate line, endoderm-derived tissues fuse with the ectoderm-derived proctodeum, or ingrowth from the anal pit.[4] Two major theories exist to explain the differentiation of the hindgut into the urogenital (ventral) and anorectal (dorsal) part: the theory of the septation of the cloaca; and the theory of the migration of the rectum. In the initial stages of development the hindgut is in continuity with the midgut cranially; caudally, it is in direct contact with the ectoderm. As development progresses, the caudal part of the hindgut, the cloaca, differentiates into two separate organ systems: the urogenital tract and the anorectal tract. The normal development of these tracts depends on the proper differentiation of the cloaca by the urorectal septum. Anorectal separation from the urogenital structures occurs as a result of either a cranially orientated septum growing down to reach the cloacal membrane and fuse with it or from lateral folds encroaching on the lumen of the cloaca from either side and fusing in the middle, or from a combination of the two processes.[5]

RECTAL ANATOMY

The rectum is the terminal segment of the large intestine. It begins proximally at the rectosigmoid junction and extends approximately 12 to 15 cm where it terminates at the level of the levator ani. The rectosigmoid junction is identified intra-abdominally as the point where the distinct taenia coli of the colon splay onto the anterior surface of the rectum, with subsequent absence of distinct taenia coli on the rectum. Furthermore, the haustra (**Fig. 1**) that are prominent throughout the colon are no longer apparent at the proximal portion of the rectum.

Identifying the proximal and distal aspects of rectum becomes more difficult when viewed endoscopically. The most consistent landmarks are the valves of Houston. The valves of Houston are folds of rectum that do not contain all layers of the rectal wall and have no known physiologic function. Most commonly, there are three valves, but the number and location of these valves is variable. The uppermost valve is usually seen on the left lateral wall of the rectum at 8 to 16 cm from the anal verge. The middle

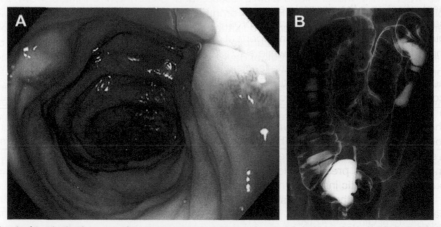

Fig. 1. (A, B) The haustra that are prominent throughout the colon are no longer apparent at the proximal portion of the rectum.

valve is located 7 to 12 cm from the anal verge and is on the right lateral wall of the rectum. Finally, the most distal fold is at 5 to 10 cm from the anal verge and is found on the left lateral rectal wall. Of the three valves, the middle valve is most consistent and is closely associated with the peritoneal reflection, and is also referred to as Kohl-rausch plica.[6,7]

The blood supply of the rectum comes mainly from the superior hemorrhoidal artery. The superior hemorrhoidal is a direct extension of the inferior mesenteric artery and perfuses the proximal two-thirds of the rectum. The middle hemorrhoidal artery is generally described as a branch of the internal iliac artery and travels anterolaterlaly, to supply the lower one-third of the rectum, but its course and origin are highly variable. The inferior hemorrhoidal artery supplies mainly the anus, but does perfuse the rectum by an extensive submucosal network of vessels.[8,9]

The venous drainage of the rectum mirrors that of the arterial supply. The superior rectal vein drains into the inferior mesenteric vein and subsequently the portal circulation. The middle rectal vein drains to the internal iliac vein, which then flows to the inferior vena cava, thereby bypassing the portal circulation.

Like the venous drainage, the lymphatic system mirrors the arterial supply. The upper two-thirds of the rectum drains along the superior hemorrhoidal artery to inferior mesenteric nodes and then para-aortic nodes. The lower one-third of rectum drains both superiorly along the superior hemorrhoidal distribution, and laterally, following the middle hemorrhoidal artery to a nodal basin along the internal iliac artery.[10]

The rectum is surrounded by an investing fascia propria that envelopes the rectum, perirectal fat, and a plexus of blood vessels. The tissues surrounding the rectum that are bound by the fascia propria are commonly referred to as the mesorectum. The mesorectum contains many perirectal lymph nodes that can harbor nodal metastases in rectal cancer. Given this, recognizing and preserving the fascia propria during a proctectomy for cancer is essential for performing an adequate cancer operation. Posterior to the rectum and fascia propria is the presacral fascia. This lining separates the rectum from the presacral venous plexus. Again, it is critical to identify and avoid injury to this fascial layer operatively, because injury to the underlying venous plexus can cause brisk bleeding that is often very difficult to control. As the presacral fascia descends further into the pelvis (S2-S4), it fuses with the posterior mesorectal fasica forming a reflection known as the rectosacral fascia, or Waldeyer fascia. Anteriorly, the peritoneum extends along about two-thirds of the rectum. Just caudal to the peritoneal reflection is the visceral pelvic fascia or Denonvilliers fascia. This fascial covering separates the mesorectum from the prostate and seminal vesicles in men, and the vagina in women. Again, this is an important anatomic landmark in proctectomy to avoid injury to important structures while also preserving an intact mesorectum.[11–14]

Lying in the plane between the fascia propria and the presacral fascia are the pelvic nerves. Innervation to the rectum is composed of sympathetic and parasympathetic components. The sympathetic nerves branch from the sympathetic trunk at L1-L3 and synapse at the preaoritc plexus. Some postsynaptic nerves travel directly to the upper rectum to supply sympathetic innervation. Other nerves travel distally and form the hypogastric plexus. This plexus extends laterally along the rectum and forms a second, more distal pelvic plexus. They continue on distally and course between the mesorectum and presacral plexus. Nerves from the hypogastric and pelvic plexus supply sympathetic innervation to the lower rectum.

The parasympathetic nerves originate from S2-S4 and exit the spinal canal by the sacral foramina and join the hypogastric and pelvic plexus. This group of parasympathetic nerves is also known as the nervi erigentes. These nerves then travel postsynaptically in a proximal direction to send parasympathetic innervation to the distal colon and upper rectum. They also travel directly to the lower rectum and anus. Both sympathetic and parasympathetic fibers travel anterior and form a plexus of nerves along Denonvilliers fascia, known as the periprostatic plexus in men. This group of nerves is much harder to identify and can be injured if the operative plane of dissection is too lateral.

The sympathetic and parasympathetic fibers coursing along the rectum are also responsible for innervation of the remainder of the pelvic organs, and thus essential for sexual function. In men, sympathetic innervation is responsible for emission of semen, whereas parasympathetic innervation is responsible for ejaculation. Given this, injury to proximal sympathetic nerves with preservation of the nervi erigentes results in retrograde ejaculation. As one travels distally, the nervi erigentes become threatened, particularly at the level of the lateral rectal stalks. Injury at this level leads to a loss of erectile function and ejaculation. Finally, dissection anterior to the rectum threatens the periprostatic plexus, with injury here also resulting in loss of erectile function and bladder dysfunction. In women, the role of specific nerves in sexual function is not well understood, but dysfunction resulting from nerve injury during pelvic dissection is well documented. Following pelvic dissection the most commonly reported symptoms of sexual dysfunction are dyspareunia and decreased lubrication during intercourse.[15–18]

ANAL ANATOMY

The anus is a short, yet complex structure at the terminal end of the gastrointestinal tract. It is grossly composed of the anal canal, anal verge, and anal margin. Surrounding these structures is a group of muscles that are essential for maintenance of fecal continence, and injuries to this intricate area can lead to devastating consequences.

The anal canal is anatomically defined as extending from the dentate line to the anal verge. Functionally, however, the accepted boundaries extend from the proximal aspect of the internal anal sphincter (IAS)/levator ani muscle to the anal verge, a length of approximately 4 cm. The anal canal includes the dentate line and is surrounded by the IAS and external anal sphincter (EAS).[19]

The dentate line represents an important landmark, because the blood supply and innervation of the anal canal transition at this point. Proximal to the dentate line, the anus is innervated by sympathetic and parasympathetic nerves, with no somatic pain fibers. However, distal to the dentate line, the anal canal has somatic innervation. The dentate line itself is identified by the anal valves. These valves are extensions of anal glands, with ducts carrying mucous from gland into valves. These ducts course outward from the anal valve, originating at anal glands either in the IAS or in the intersphincteric groove between the IAS and EAS. Knowledge of this anatomy is important because it helps to explain the location of perianal abscesses.

The anal verge is a narrow band of tissue that separates anal canal from perianal skin. It extends from the intersphincteric groove onto the skin surrounding the anus. It is covered with thin squamous epithelium that is easily identified because it lacks hair follicles (anoderm). The distinct border between anal verge and perianal skin, as identified by the appearance of hair follicles and keratinized epithelium, is the anal margin. This anatomic landmark is important to recognize, because it is frequently used as the external reference point for proximal lesions or pathology.

The muscles surrounding the anal canal provide for continence. They can be separated into the IAS, EAS, and the levator ani. Each plays an important role in maintaining continence, with injury to the muscle or nervous supply to each component causing varying degrees of problems.

The IAS is a direct extension of the inner circular muscle layer of the rectum. It extends distally just beyond the EAS and approximately 1 cm beyond the dentate line. The space between the IAS and EAS is the intersphincteric groove, and can be usually palpated on digital rectal examination. The IAS is smooth muscle, and subsequently innervated with sympathetic nerves from L5 and parasympathetic nerves from S2-S4, with a state of tonic contraction that contributes to baseline continence.[20]

The EAS is wrapped radially around the IAS, extending the length of the anal canal and terminating just proximal to the IAS. It is "suspended" around the anus, with the anococcygeal ligament anchoring it anteriorly to the perineal body and posteriorly to the coccyx. Although it has been divided into multiple units (deep vs superficial), it functions as a single muscular unit and is best thought of as such. Unlike the IAS, the EAS is composed of skeletal muscle and is innervated by branches of the pudendal nerve and the perineal branch of S4. The EAS is also in a constant state of tonic contraction, but also has a component of voluntary control. During episodes of threatened continence, the EAS can increase its contractile strength to avoid fecal or gaseous incontinence.

The levator ani, with the proximal aspect of the EAS, marks the proximal extent of the anal canal. It is a broad, thin sheet of three defined muscles that form the pelvic floor. The puborectalis muscle forms a sling around the anal canal, with anterior attachments on the pubis. It is found just cephalad to the EAS and intimately associated with the anal canal. Essentially, this sling pulls the anal canal anteriorly, forming the anorectal angle, another component of fecal continence. The other two muscles comprising the levator ani, the pubococcygeus and iliococcygeus, form the major component of the pelvic floor. The pubococcygeus fans out from posterior attachments to the anococcygeal raphe, with anterior attachments along the length of the pubis, forming the main anterior part of the pelvic floor. The posterior aspect of the pelvic floor is comprised of the coccygeus muscle that also extends from bony attachments to S3, S4, and the coccyx to the anococcygeal raphe.[21]

Although the muscular function of the IAS and EAS contribute to full continence, the sensory function of the anal canal also plays an important role. The upper anal canal has an abundance of nerve endings to help with sensation of stool and gas in the lower rectum. Furthermore, there are nervous plexuses that are responsible for sensation of pressure, touch, and temperature that also contribute to maintenance of continence. These nerves travel by the pudendal nerve to the central nervous system.

ANORECTAL IMAGING
Endorectal/Endoanal Ultrasound

Endorectal ultrasound (ERUS) has become a mainstay in evaluation of anorectal masses. It can be performed easily in the office setting with minimal patient discomfort. Using a proctoscope, the US probe is advanced into the rectum. The probe is housed in a balloon that is inflated with water until maximum apposition with the rectal wall is obtained. This provides for a medium through which the US waves are transduced. The transducer is usually 10 mHz, with lower-frequency transducers used to visualize structures further from the rectal mucosa.[22,23]

ERUS displays five distinct layers of the rectal wall (**Fig. 2**). The first layer is hyperechoic and represents the interface between balloon and rectal mucosa. This is followed by a hypoechoic layer, representing mucosa and muscularis mucosa. Layer three is a hyperechoic layer, representing the submucosa. Layer four is again hypoechoic because it is muscularis propria. The final layer is hyperechooic and is the interface between serosa and perirectal fat.[12–25]

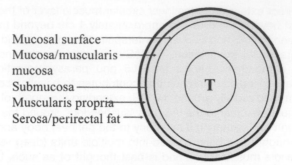

Mucosal surface
Mucosa/muscularis
mucosa
Submucosa
Muscularis propria
Serosa/perirectal fat

T

Fig. 2. ERUS displays five distinct layers of the rectal wall.

The most common application for ERUS is staging of rectal cancer (**Fig. 3**). Accurate staging is imperative in the treatment of rectal cancer, because depth of tumor invasion and nodal status both impact the treatment algorithm.[26–28] ERUS has become an important tool in determining the depth of invasion and nodal involvement of rectal cancers. Numerous studies have shown an overall accuracy of ERUS in determining T stage varying from 69% to 91%,[29] with overstaging being the most common error. Accuracy of N stage prediction is not as precise, with accuracy rates reported between 56% and 76%.[29] One major limitation to ERUS is the large interobserver variation in interpretation.[30]

Endoanal US can also provide a large amount of information in the office setting with minimal patient discomfort and risk. A cap is placed over the same probe used for ERUS, and this cap is filled with water to provide a transduction medium.[23] The US images allow for identification of the IAS (hypoechoic band deep to the mucosa/submucosa) and EAS (band of mixed echogenicity lying deep to the IAS). Because the EAS is composed of striated skeletal muscle and differs in appearance between genders, it is the most difficult structure to identify using endoanal US.[31,32] During interpretation of endoanal US, the anal canal is divided into thirds, with the upper third identified as the area of the puborectalis. The middle third is the area where the sphincter complex reaches maximal diameter. The lower third is the most distal aspect of the anal canal where the sphincter complex has thinned significantly.[23] Endoanal US is used mainly in the evaluation of fecal incontinence, because it readily detects sphincter complex defects (**Fig. 4**). However, it is also a valuable imaging tool

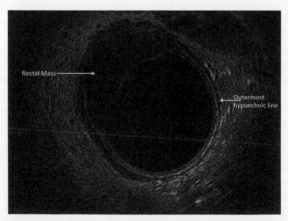

Rectal Mass

Outermost
hypoechoic line

Fig. 3. The most common application for ERUS is staging of rectal cancer.

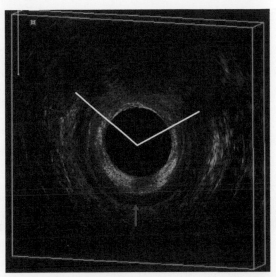

Fig. 4. Endoanal ultrasound is used mainly for evaluation of fecal incontinence because it readily detects sphincter complex defects. External sphincter (*blue arrow*), internal sphincter (*red arrow*), extent of defect (*yellow angle*).

in evaluation of anal masses, perianal Crohn disease, and fistula in ano. In particular, the addition of hydrogen peroxide contrast to an endoanal US can help delineate fistula tracts in greater detail.[32–40]

Magnetic Resonance Imaging

Magnetic resonance imaging (MRI) is quickly becoming a preferred imaging technique for disorders of the anorectum. This is mainly because of the ability of MRI to provide superior definition of soft tissue and the planes separating these structures. Furthermore, MRI does not use radiation and therefore does not carry the inherent risk that is associated with traditional x-ray or CT scans. Most MRIs are now done on a 1.5- or 3-T phased-array coil. A dilute barium mixture can be instilled into the rectum to provide for negative contrast on T2-weighted images, which allows for the best definition of soft tissue structure. Most centers now provide diffusion-weighted images that allow for adequate imaging of a neoplasm and lymph nodes without the use of intravenous contrast. The larger coil sizes and the techniques used in most modern MRIs have made the use of the endorectal coil obsolete.[41,42]

Similar to US, MRI is capable of identifying the distinct layers of the rectal wall. The mucosa and submucosa are best appreciated on T2-weighted images and appear hyperintense (**Fig. 5**). A hypointense layer is visualized outside of the submucosa, corresponding to the muscularis propria. Finally, a hyperintense layer surrounds the muscle, correlating to the mesorectal fat. It is the definition of these layers, especially the mesorectal fat, which has made the use of MRI more prevalent, especially as it pertains to rectal cancer imaging.[24,41]

Accurately predicting rectal cancer staging is of paramount importance in rectal cancer, because it influences treatment decisions and subsequent prognosis. Of particular importance is defining depth of invasion and nodal involvement, because this directs the decision for preoperative chemoradiotherapy.[26–28] Although US and MRI are generally comparable in staging T1 to T2 tumors, MRI has a distinct

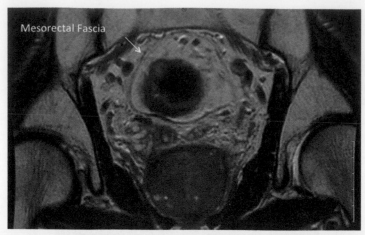

Fig. 5. The mucosa and submucosa are best appreciated on T2-weighted images and appear hyperintense.

advantage in staging of tumors of greater depth, given the inherent limitations of US. Additionally, MRI provides excellent definition of the border between muscularis propria and mesorectal fascia, allowing for accurate prediction of mesorectal fascial invasion and subsequent ability to achieve complete pathologic resection.[43–46] As the prevalence of phased-array MRI increases and costs decrease, MRI is beginning to supplant US as the preferred method of preoperative imaging in rectal cancer.

MRI is also useful in the evaluation of several perianal disorders. It can detect extension of an anal tumor into the IAS or EAS, thus influencing surgical decision making.[47] Its use in benign conditions is also prevalent. It can accurately identify fistula-in-ano and should be used in complicated cases to aid in operative and nonoperative management.[48–51] The role of MRI in evaluation of perianal Crohn disease is also expanding, aiding in the diagnosis of perianal fistulae and abscesses.[36,52,53] Finally, MRI can be used as an adjunct to endoanal US in the assessment of fecal incontinence.[54,55]

Defecography

The evaluation of pelvic floor disorders is often difficult and based on a confluence of history, physical examination, and radiographic findings. A mainstay in the evaluation of pelvic floor disorders is defecography, which assesses the functional aspect of defecation, and provides specific measurements of the anorectal angle, perineal descent, and puborectalis length. The patient is placed on a radiolucent commode and a barium paste of stool consistency is injected into the rectum. The use of vaginal barium paste and some oral thin barium can improve the diagnostic yield of defecography by highlighting the position of the vagina and small bowel during defecation (**Fig. 6**). Using fluoroscopy, the anorectal canal is evaluated at rest, during Valsalva with a closed sphincter, and during all phases of defecation.[56–58] The images and video allow for diagnosis of anatomic and functional disorders. Rectoceles are identified as outward herniations of the rectal wall through an area of weakness, usually anterior. Enteroceles are seen as a downward herniation of the small bowel into the pelvis through a large pelvic inlet and a deep cul de sac. Rectal intussusceptions and prolapse appear as an inward invagination on rectal mucosa with straining subsequent obstruction of the anal canal. Perineal descent syndrome is categorized by an excursion of the perineum by a distance greater than 3 cm from rest during defecation.

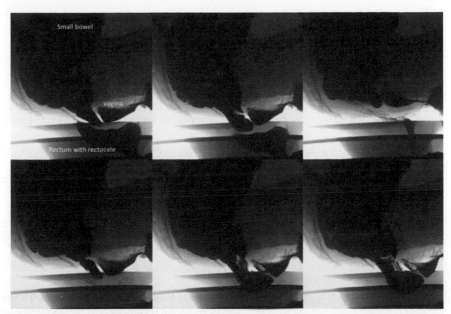

Fig. 6. The use of vaginal barium paste and some oral thin barium can improve the diagnostic yield of defecography by highlighting the position of the vagina and small bowel during defecation.

Finally, nonrelaxing puborectalis syndrome is categorized by contraction of the puborectalis muscle, causing a more acute anorectal angle during evacuation.[56,57,59]

Because many patients find traditional defecography embarrassing, dynamic MRI imaging has been proposed as an alternative. Although some studies suggest MRI can provide a viable alternative to cinedefecography,[60–63] MRI has inherent limitations. A recent comparison of MRI versus cinedefecography showed that MRI tended to underreport pelvic floor disorders, mainly because of incomplete evacuation.[64] This incomplete evacuation is attributed to patients lying in a supine position during MRI. Until there is widespread availability of open MRI to allow patients to sit while evacuating and more prospective trials validate the findings of MRI, traditional cinedefecography remains the gold standard imaging technique for evaluation of pelvic floor disorders.

REFERENCES

1. Snyder WH Jr. The embryology of the alimentary tract, with special emphasis on the colon and rectum. Surg Gynecol Obstet 1958;106(4):311–23 Epub 1958/04/01.
2. Hollinshead WH. Embryology and surgical anatomy of the colon. Dis Colon Rectum 1962;5:23–7 Epub 1962/01/01.
3. Schumpelick V, Dreuw B, Ophoff K, et al. Appendix and cecum. Embryology, anatomy, and surgical applications. Surg Clin North Am 2000;80(1):295–318 Epub 2000/02/24.
4. Dujovny N, Quiros RM, Saclarides TJ. Anorectal anatomy and embryology. Surg Oncol Clin N Am 2004;13(2):277–93 Epub 2004/05/13.
5. Stephens FD. Congenital malformations of the rectum and anus in female children. Aust N Z J Surg 1961;31:90–104 Epub 1961/11/01.

6. Abramson DJ. The valves of Houston in adults. Am J Surg 1978;136(3):334–6.
7. Shafik A, Doss S, Ali YA, et al. Transverse folds of rectum: anatomic study and clinical implications. Clin Anat 2001;14(3):196–203.
8. Siddharth P, Ravo B. Colorectal neurovasculature and anal sphincter. Surg Clin North Am 1988;68(6):1185–200.
9. Michels NA, Siddarth P, Kornblith PL, et al. The variant blood supply to the descending colon, rectosigmoid and rectum based on 400 dissections. Its importance in regional resections: a review of medical literature. Dis Colon Rectum 1965;8:251–78.
10. Heald RJ, Moran BJ. Embryology and anatomy of the rectum. Semin Surg Oncol 1998;15(2):66–71.
11. Lindsey I, Guy RJ, Warren BF, et al. Anatomy of Denonvilliers' fascia and pelvic nerves, impotence, and implications for the colorectal surgeon. Br J Surg 2000; 87(10):1288–99.
12. Chapuis P, Bokey L, Fahrer M, et al. Mobilization of the rectum: anatomic concepts and the bookshelf revisited. Dis Colon Rectum 2002;45(1):1–8 [discussion: 8–9].
13. Lin M, Chen W, Huang L, et al. The anatomic basis of total mesorectal excision. Am J Surg 2011;201(4):537–43.
14. Church JM, Raudkivi PJ, Hill GL. The surgical anatomy of the rectum: a review with particular relevance to the hazards of rectal mobilisation. Int J Colorectal Dis 1987;2(3):158–66.
15. Morpurgo E, Hall MC, Galandiuk S. A simple technique for identification and preservation of the hypogastric nerves during rectal surgery. Arch Surg 2004; 139(10):1106–9.
16. Böhm G, Kirschner-Hermanns R, Decius A, et al. Anorectal, bladder, and sexual function in females following colorectal surgery for carcinoma. Int J Colorectal Dis 2008;23(9):893–900.
17. Daniels IR, Woodward S, Taylor FG, et al. Female urogenital dysfunction following total mesorectal excision for rectal cancer. World J Surg Oncol 2006;4:6.
18. Platell CF, Thompson PJ, Makin GB. Sexual health in women following pelvic surgery for rectal cancer. Br J Surg 2004;91(4):465–8.
19. Thompson-Fawcett MW, Warren BF, Mortensen NJ. A new look at the anal transitional zone with reference to restorative proctocolectomy and the columnar cuff. Br J Surg 1998;85(11):1517–21.
20. Frenckner B, Ihre T. Influence of autonomic nerves on the internal and sphincter in man. Gut 1976;17(4):306–12.
21. Ayoub SF. The anterior fibres of the levator ani muscle in man. J Anat 1979; 128(Pt 3):571–80.
22. Schaffzin DM, Wong WD. Endorectal ultrasound in the preoperative evaluation of rectal cancer. Clin Colorectal Cancer 2004;4(2):124–32.
23. Nogueras J. Endorectal ultrasonography: technique, image interpretation and expanding indications in 1995. Semin Colon Rectal Surg 1995;6(2):70–7.
24. Liang TY, Anil G, Ang BW. Imaging paradigms in assessment of rectal carcinoma: loco-regional and distant staging. Cancer Imaging 2012;12:290–303.
25. St Ville EW, Jafri SZ, Madrazo BL, et al. Endorectal sonography in the evaluation of rectal and perirectal disease. AJR Am J Roentgenol 1991;157(3):503–8.
26. Anonymous. Improved survival with preoperative radiotherapy in resectable rectal cancer. Swedish Rectal Cancer Trial. N Engl J Med 1997;336(14): 980–7.

27. Mellgren A, Sirivongs P, Rothenberger DA, et al. Is local excision adequate therapy for early rectal cancer? Dis Colon Rectum 2000;43(8):1064–71 [discussion: 1071–4].

28. MacFarlane JK, Ryall RD, Heald RJ. Mesorectal excision for rectal cancer. Lancet 1993;341(8843):457–60.

29. Edelman BR, Weiser MR. Endorectal ultrasound: its role in the diagnosis and treatment of rectal cancer. Clin Colon Rectal Surg 2008;21(3):167–77.

30. Mor I, Hull T, Hammel J, et al. Rectal endosonography: just how good are we at its interpretation? Int J Colorectal Dis 2010;25(1):87–90.

31. Tjandra JJ, Milsom JW, Stolfi VM, et al. Endoluminal ultrasound defines anatomy of the anal canal and pelvic floor. Dis Colon Rectum 1992;35(5): 465–70.

32. Rottenberg GT, Williams AB. Endoanal ultrasound. Br J Radiol 2002;75(893): 482–8.

33. Yang YK, Wexner SD, Nogueras JJ. The role of anal ultrasound in the assessment of benign anorectal disease. Coloproctology 1993;5:260–4.

34. Bernstein MA, Nogueras JJ, Weiss EG, et al. The use of endoanal ultrasonography in identifying fistula-in-ano. Coloproctology 1997;19(2):72–6.

35. Lewis RT, Maron DJ. Anorectal Crohn's disease. Surg Clin North Am 2010;90(1): 83–97.

36. Singh B, McC Mortensen NJ, Jewell DP, et al. Perianal Crohn's disease. Br J Surg 2004;91(7):801–14.

37. Deen KI, Williams JG, Hutchinson R, et al. Fistulas in ano: endoanal ultrasonographic assessment assists decision making for surgery. Gut 1994;35(3): 391–4.

38. Deen KI, Kumar D, Williams JG, et al. Anal sphincter defects. Correlation between endoanal ultrasound and surgery. Ann Surg 1993;218(2):201–5.

39. Dobben AC, Terra MP, Slors JF, et al. External anal sphincter defects in patients with fecal incontinence: comparison of endoanal MR imaging and endoanal US. Radiology 2007;242(2):463–71.

40. Tsankov T, Tankova L, Deredjan H, et al. Contrast-enhanced endoanal and transperineal sonography in perianal fistulas. Hepatogastroenterology 2008; 55(81):13–6.

41. Dewhurst CE, Mortele KJ. Magnetic resonance imaging of rectal cancer. Radiol Clin North Am 2013;51(1):121–31.

42. Matsuoka H, Nakamura A, Masaki T, et al. Comparison between endorectal coil and pelvic phased-array coil magnetic resonance imaging in patients with anorectal tumor. Am J Surg 2003;185(4):328–32.

43. Brown G, Radcliffe AG, Newcombe RG, et al. Preoperative assessment of prognostic factors in rectal cancer using high-resolution magnetic resonance imaging. Br J Surg 2003;90(3):355–64.

44. Brown G, Kirkham A, Williams GT, et al. High-resolution MRI of the anatomy important in total mesorectal excision of the rectum. AJR Am J Roentgenol 2004;182(2):431–9.

45. MERCURY Study Group. Diagnostic accuracy of preoperative magnetic resonance imaging in predicting curative resection of rectal cancer: prospective observational study. BMJ 2006;333(7572):779.

46. Taylor FG, Quirke P, Heald RJ, et al, MERCURY Study Group. Preoperative high-resolution magnetic resonance imaging can identify good prognosis stage I, II, and III rectal cancer best managed by surgery alone: a prospective, multicenter, European study. Ann Surg 2011;253(4):711–9.

47. Holzer B, Urban M, Hölbling N, et al. Magnetic resonance imaging predicts sphincter invasion of low rectal cancer and influences selection of operation. Surgery 2003;133(6):656–61.
48. O'Malley RB, Al-Hawary MM, Kaza RK, et al. Rectal imaging: part 2, Perianal fistula evaluation on pelvic MRI–what the radiologist needs to know. AJR Am J Roentgenol 2012;199(1):W43–53.
49. Buchanan GN, Halligan S, Bartram CI, et al. Clinical examination, endosonography, and MR imaging in preoperative assessment of fistula in ano: comparison with outcome-based reference standard. Radiology 2004;233(3):674–81 Epub 2004 Oct 21.
50. Stoker J, Rociu E, Wiersma TG, et al. Imaging of anorectal disease. Br J Surg 2000;87(1):10–27.
51. Lunniss PJ, Armstrong P, Barker PG, et al. Magnetic resonance imaging of anal fistulae. Lancet 1992;340(8816):394–6.
52. Horsthuis K, Stoker J. MRI of perianal Crohn's disease. AJR Am J Roentgenol 2004;183(5):1309–15.
53. Horsthuis K, Lavini C, Bipat S, et al. Perianal Crohn disease: evaluation of dynamic contrast-enhanced MR imaging as an indicator of disease activity. Radiology 2009;251(2):380–7.
54. Dobben AC, Felt-Bersma RJ, ten Kate FJ, et al. Cross-sectional imaging of the anal sphincter in fecal incontinence. AJR Am J Roentgenol 2008;190(3):671–82.
55. Terra MP, Beets-Tan RG, van der Hulst VP, et al. MRI in evaluating atrophy of the external anal sphincter in patients with fecal incontinence. AJR Am J Roentgenol 2006;187(4):991–9.
56. Karasick S, Karasick D, Karasick SR. Functional disorders of the anus and rectum: findings on defecography. AJR Am J Roentgenol 1993;160(4):777–82.
57. Jorge JM, Habr-Gama A, Wexner SD. Clinical applications and techniques of cinedefecography. Am J Surg 2001;182(1):93–101.
58. Mahieu P, Pringot J, Bodart P. Defecography: I. Description of a new procedure and results in normal patients. Gastrointest Radiol 1984;9(3):247–51.
59. Bartolo DC, Bartram CI, Ekberg O, et al. Symposium. Proctography. Int J Colorectal Dis 1988;3(2):67–89.
60. Kruyt RH, Delemarre JB, Doornbos J, et al. Normal anorectum: dynamic MR imaging anatomy. Radiology 1991;179(1):159–63.
61. Hetzer FH, Andreisek G, Tsagari C, et al. MR defecography in patients with fecal incontinence: imaging findings and their effect on surgical management. Radiology 2006;240(2):449–57.
62. Reiner CS, Tutuian R, Solopova AE, et al. MR defecography in patients with dyssynergic defecation: spectrum of imaging findings and diagnostic value. Br J Radiol 2011;84(998):136–44.
63. Lamb GM, de Jode MG, Gould SW, et al. Upright dynamic MR defaecating proctography in an open configuration MR system. Br J Radiol 2000;73(866):152–5.
64. Pilkington SA, Nugent KP, Brenner J, et al. Barium proctography vs magnetic resonance proctography for pelvic floor disorders: a comparative study. Colorectal Dis 2012;14(10):1224–30.

Anorectal Physiology and Testing

Julie Ann M. Van Koughnett, MD, MEd, FRCSC[a],
Giovanna da Silva, MD[a,b,c],*

KEYWORDS

- Anorectal physiology • Endoanal ultrasound • Manometry • Defecography
- Electromyography

KEY POINTS

- Anorectal physiology involves muscle and nervous coordination to ensure controlled and timely bowel movements.
- The understanding of anorectal physiology is essential so that the physician may order appropriate testing to elicit the most useful information to guide the diagnosis and treatment of anorectal disorders, such as fecal incontinence, constipation, and pain.
- Digital rectal examination should be performed to gain information about a patient's anorectal physiology and to guide investigations.
- Anal manometry, endoanal ultrasound, defecography, balloon expulsion test, magnetic resonance imaging, colonic transit studies, pudendal nerve terminal motor latency studies, and electromyography are commonly used in testing anorectal physiology and are ordered as appropriate based on the patients' symptoms.

INTRODUCTION

The processes of defecation and maintenance of fecal continence are complex, involving both voluntary and involuntary muscular activity. The pudendal and sacral nerves provide important sensory and motor information. The rectum functions as a distensible reservoir to permit time control over the evacuation of stool. All of these activities and anatomic units must act in concert for effective defecation. When there is dysfunction, various disorders may result. These disorders include fecal incontinence, constipation, obstructed defecation, pelvic pain, and the symptoms of ineffective defecation, such as incomplete evacuation or clustered frequent bowel movements.

These disorders have major impacts on the daily life of patients. Patients may, for example, be unable to work because of pain or avoid social activities because of fecal

Disclosures: None for either author.
[a] Department of Colorectal Surgery, Cleveland Clinic Florida, 2950 Cleveland Clinic Boulevard, Weston, FL 33331, USA; [b] Department of Surgery, Charles E Schmidt College of Medicine at Florida Atlantic University, 777 Glades Road, Building 71, Boca Raton, FL 33431, USA; [c] Department of Surgery, ROSS University, PO Box 266, Roseau, Commonwealth of Dominica, West Indies
* Corresponding author. Department of Colorectal Surgery, Cleveland Clinic Florida, 2950 Cleveland Clinic Boulevard, Weston, FL 33331.
E-mail address: dasilvg@ccf.org

Gastroenterol Clin N Am 42 (2013) 713–728
http://dx.doi.org/10.1016/j.gtc.2013.08.001
0889-8553/13/$ – see front matter © 2013 Elsevier Inc. All rights reserved.

incontinence. The morbidities of these conditions are wide reaching, and the proper treatment may have just as powerful of an effect on patients' lives. Anorectal testing is used to discern the most effective potential treatments for an individual patient. The anorectal investigations described in this article are not all available in every institution. Specialized equipment is needed for nearly all of the tests, as are educated health care professionals to both perform the tests and interpret the results. For a fully comprehensive anorectal physiology program, expertise may be used from colorectal surgery, gastroenterology, radiology, and neurology. Although much of the anorectal physiology testing may be office based, an equipped radiology department is needed for tests, such as defecography and magnetic resonance imaging (MRI).

Anorectal testing can be divided into anatomic and functional tests, with some overlap. The anatomic tests include endoanal ultrasound, defecography, and MRI. Functional tests include anal manometry, balloon expulsion test, defecography, dynamic MRI, colonic transit studies, pudendal nerve terminal motor latency study, and electromyography. Each test is described later.

ANORECTAL PHYSIOLOGY

Anorectal physiology is complex. It involves the pelvic floor muscles, motor and sensory neural pathways and is intimately related to the colon physiology. Maintenance of continence depends largely on the pelvic floor musculature, which reacts to signals related to stool consistency and overall bowel motility.[1]

Sensory Physiology

The anal canal receives sensory input from the S2, S3, and S4 nerve roots; composing the pudendal nerve. Although the rectum is only sensitive to stretch, the anus is sensitive to temperature, touch, and pain. These sensations may help a person to assess when it is inconvenient to evacuate stool from an environmental perspective. This area of sensation represents the anal canal, which is kept closed at rest mainly by the internal sphincter muscle.

When the rectum senses stool or flatus, the sensory mechanism allows the rectum to be compliant and stretch to accommodate stool. This sensation should not be a painful sensory response and, in fact, will alleviate the discomfort of the sensation of urgency. Once rectal distension has reached a threshold of compliance, anal canal sensory reflexes result in relaxation and evacuation of stool. The relationship between rectal sensation and anal canal sensation exists but is not essential to maintain continence. For example, most patients with colonic or ileal pouches are able to maintain continence despite not having a rectum to signal to the anal canal.[2,3]

Motor Physiology

The main muscles to consider in anal physiology, namely, the maintenance of continence and effective defecation, are the internal sphincter, external sphincter, and puborectalis muscles. The sphincters are not paired to each other and have distinct functions. The internal anal sphincter is an involuntary muscle. It is innervated by the hypogastric and pelvic plexi and contributes to more than 50% of the resting anal tone. It plays a vital role in continence.[4] At rest, a basal tone of the internal sphincter is maintained by slow, constant waves of contraction.[1] During defecation, the internal sphincter involuntarily relaxes to allow for the evacuation of stool.

The external anal sphincter contributes 30% of the resting tone, with hemorrhoidal tissue contributing the remaining 15%. It contains mainly striated type I fibers muscle, which allows the maintenance of a baseline tone at rest. It is innervated by the pudendal nerve. A baseline level of tone is maintained at rest. Voluntary contraction may be performed to increase tone and hold in flatus or stool and can last up to 1 minute before the muscle fatigues. During evacuation, voluntary relaxation of the external anal sphincter occurs to permit the passage of stool and flatus.

The puborectalis is a striated muscle that inserts into the pubis and acts as a sling for the rectum. This sling effect creates the anorectal angle at rest, which helps to limit the volume of stool passing into the distal rectum and anal canal. During defecation, the puborectalis relaxes and lengthens, allowing the rectum to straighten and stool to move into the distal rectum and anal canal for evacuation. If paradoxic contraction or nonrelaxation occurs, patients may experience pain, constipation, and incomplete evacuation. Along with the internal and external anal sphincters, the puborectalis is an identifiable anatomic landmark when performing endoanal ultrasound.

There are numerous anorectal reflexes. These reflexes are summarized in **Table 1**.

ANORECTAL TESTING

The tools used to investigate anorectal disorders include both anatomic and functional testing. Not every test is necessary for each patient or each disorder. Investigations should be ordered based on the following:

- Complete history and physical examination
- Digital rectal examination

Table 1
Anorectal reflexes

Name	Reflex	Notes
Rectoanal Inhibitory reflex	Internal anal sphincter muscle relaxation caused by rectal distension	• Internal anal sphincter muscle relaxation caused by rectal distension • Provides contact of the anal canal with flatus and stool, allowing the person to discriminate and pass flatus selectively without soiling of stool • Absent in Hirschsprung disease • May be transiently or permanently lost after proctectomy[5]
Cutaneous anal sphincter reflex	Contraction of the distal external sphincter muscle with touch or pain stimulus of anal skin	• Fatigues within seconds • Absent in cauda equina spinal injuries
Bulbocavernosus reflex	Contraction of external anal sphincter muscle with squeezing the glans penis or clitoris or pulling on urethral catheter	• Absent in S2 to S4 injuries • Early reflex to recover following spinal shock
Cough-anal reflex	Contraction of the external anal sphincter muscle in response to coughing or sniffing	• Provides continence during sudden increase in abdominal pressure, such as with coughing, sneezing, or laughing • Absent in sacral nerve or cauda equina injuries

- Review of previous investigations and consultations
- Stool diary when appropriate

General indications for each of the anorectal tests discussed in this article are summarized in **Table 2**.

Digital Rectal Examination

Although not an anorectal physiology *test* or *investigation*, special mention must be given to the utility of a digital rectal examination. It is an essential portion of the physical examination for an anorectal problem. The components of a digital rectal examination are listed in **Box 1**. Digital rectal examination should be performed in a systematic fashion to gather the most useful information. Patients should be placed ideally in a prone kneeling position on an examination table that may be raised and tilted to permit the best view of the anorectum. If this is not available, patients should be positioned in the lateral decubitus position.

Table 2
Anorectal physiology tests and their indications

Test	Potential Indications
Anal manometry	Fecal incontinence Constipation Hirschsprung Anal fissure Anal pain
Endoanal ultrasound	Fecal incontinence Constipation Sphincter defect Anal Fistula Anal pain
Defecography	Constipation Fecal incontinence Obstructed defecation Pelvic descent Suspected prolapse Suspected rectocele Anal pain
MRI	Constipation Fecal incontinence Obstructed defecation Pelvic descent, multiple compartments Sphincter defect Suspected rectocele Anal pain
Balloon expulsion test	Obstructed defecation Constipation
Pudendal nerve terminal motor latency	Fecal incontinence Constipation Suspected nerve injury
Electromyography	Fecal incontinence Suspected nerve injury Constipation
Colonic transit study	Constipation Obstructed defecation

Box 1
Components of a digital rectal examination

- Inspection
- Digital examination
- Anoscopy

The digital rectal examination should begin with inspection of the perianal skin for rashes, skin changes, scars, external skin tags, fissure, and evidence of active infection, such as induration or drainage. While inspecting, patients should be instructed to squeeze the sphincter muscles. A perianal wink should be visualized. Perianal sensation can be tested using a pinprick method when indicated. Patients should be instructed that a lubricated finger will be inserted into the anus. Initial contact with the perianal skin should produce a visible involuntary reflex. Digital examination should be performed to the full length of the finger if tolerated by the patients. The clinician should feel for bulky internal hemorrhoids, prostate, ulceration, and mass. With the finger inserted, resting and squeeze tone should be tested by asking patients to squeeze and relax the anal sphincters. Paradoxic contraction may be assessed by having patients valsalva while the finger is inserted and noting the presence of abnormal sphincter contraction around the finger. Anoscopy may be performed if indicated. This examination allows for the visualization of the anal canal and hemorrhoid columns. Occult blood testing may be performed if there is a concern for rectal bleeding by using fecal material from the gloved finger.

The digital rectal examination may help diagnose anorectal disorders and guide other anorectal testing. In women with constipation and incomplete evacuation, clinical examination with digital rectal examination revealed hypertonic sphincters or rectoceles in 40% of cases.[6] Digital rectal examination, when compared with physiology tests, is accurate in the assessment of sphincter function but should not be used to solely diagnose sphincter defects.[7] The overall sensitivity and specificity of digital rectal examination in evaluating normal resting and squeeze tone has been shown to be more than 75% and is accurate in detecting rectoceles.[8,9] It should always be the starting point for the assessment of anorectal physiology and function.

Anal Manometry

Manometry is a functional test that assesses the tone and function of the anal sphincter muscles. It is performed in the office or physiology laboratory with awake patients. Manometry is useful in the assessment of both fecal incontinence and constipation because it provides a measure of the effectiveness of the anorectal musculature, the rectoanal inhibitory reflex, sensation, and compliance of the rectum. Variations in technique are used to assess these functions, namely, the pull-through or stationary techniques. Newer variations using 3-dimensional measurements and high-resolution technologies are being developed to improve the utility of manometric results.[10,11] The authors' preference is the pull-through technique.

When using anal manometry in one's practice, it is important to note that normal values vary between patient groups. Women have lower resting and squeeze pressures when compared with men.[12–14] Younger women have resting and squeeze pressure that approach those of men, especially nulliparous young women.[12,13] Accurate and useful results depend on having a trained operator for the equipment and consideration of patient age and gender.

To perform an anal manometry, patients are positioned in the left decubitus position. Digital rectal examination is performed to ensure there is no obstruction before inserting the catheter. A manometry probe with a deflated latex balloon at the tip is calibrated to the machine at the level of the anus. The probe is inserted to a distance of 6 to 10 cm and held at that level using a mechanical arm and left in place for 30 seconds before attaining any measurements. Resting and squeeze pressures are measured 3 times each, and mean pressures are calculated. Each squeeze pressure is measured for a sustained squeeze period of 30 seconds. A small volume of water is instilled into the balloon for the measurement of first sensation, typically between 20 and 60 mL of water. Compliance is measured by instilling further water into the balloon until not tolerated by patients, with normal compliance being between 100 and 200 mL of water. The water is then removed. A small volume of air, about 20 mL, is instilled into the balloon over 1 to 2 seconds to elicit a rectoanal inhibitory reflex by a characteristic manometric curve seen on the screen. If the reflex is absent, the process is repeated using 10 mL of more air each time up to the volume of first sensation to see if the reflex is present. **Fig. 1** shows the pressure curve of a normal rectoanal inhibitory reflex.

The results of anal manometry may be used to guide further testing or treatment. Some examples are the following:

- Isolated absence of rectoanal inhibitory reflex may suggest the need for surgical biopsy if Hirschsprung disease is suspected.
- Low resting tone may suggest the need for endoanal ultrasound if the history suggests possible sphincter damage or defect.
- Low resting and squeeze tone may guide patients toward biofeedback strengthening in patients who are incontinent.
- Resting and squeeze tone may be assessed before colostomy reversal in patients with prior rectal trauma.
- High compliance may suggest outlet obstruction in patients who are constipated.

Endoanal Ultrasound

Endoanal ultrasound is an anatomic test used to visualize the anal canal and surrounding structures. Along with endorectal ultrasound, ultrasonographic techniques are now widely used to evaluate rectal lesions, including large polyps and rectal cancer, for depth of invasion and also for complex anal fistulas to document internal communication.[15,16] From a physiology perspective, ultrasound is used to visualize the internal and external anal sphincters. Ideally, a 10-MHz probe is used to provide the best picture, and 3-dimensional imaging allows for various cross sections of the anal canal to be examined.[17] If not available, a 2-dimensional system will still allow for axial imaging of the anal canal and anal sphincters.

Only properly trained clinicians should perform endoanal ultrasound to ensure accurate results, which are user dependent. Patients are first positioned in the lateral decubitus position with the anus positioned at the very edge of the bed to allow for movement of the probe by the operator. Digital rectal examination is performed to rule out a distal obstruction. The lubricated probe is inserted blindly through the anus to the level of the distal rectum. Of note, a rigid proctoscope is not used for endoanal ultrasound, although it is used as part of endorectal ultrasound. With the probe centered, the layers of the anal canal are examined (**Fig. 2**).[17] In the upper anal canal, the puborectalis muscle can be seen posteriorly and laterally as a slinglike stricture. Images should be taken in the upper, middle, and lower anal canal. Sphincter defects are characterized as a segmental defect in the circular ring of a sphincter muscle, and the degree and location of the defect should be measured and recorded.

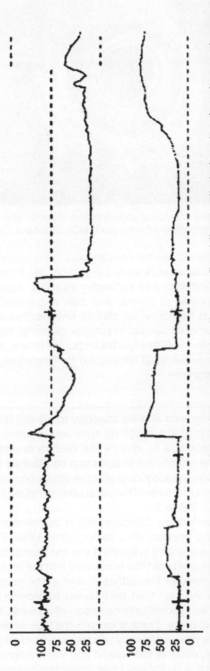

Fig. 1. Normal rectoanal inhibitory reflex during anal manometry. After the balloon is inflated (*bottom line*), there is a sharp increase in pressure followed by lowering of the anal pressure, signaling sphincter relaxation (*upper line*). (*From* Vrees MD, Weiss EG. The evaluation of constipation. Clin Colon Rectal Surg 2005;18(2):69; with permission.)

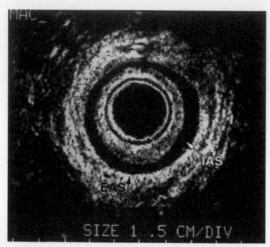

Fig. 2. Ultrasound image of the anal canal showing the internal anal sphincter (IAS) and external anal sphincter (EAS). (*Courtesy of* Tracy Hull, MD, Cleveland Clinic, Cleveland, OH.)

Results of endoanal ultrasound can be used to plan the surgical approach to fecal incontinence. If the surgeon has not personally performed the ultrasound, essentials to look for in the report include thinning of sphincter muscles, documented sphincter defect, location of defect, degree of defect, and bulk of perineal body. Ultrasound may detect sphincter defects not found on clinical examination alone.[18] Early work confirmed the utility of endoanal ultrasound in surgical planning, finding good correlation between ultrasonographic and histologic findings.[19,20] Newer developments have used dynamic endoanal or transperineal ultrasound for functional assessment of the anorectum, similar to defecography.[21]

Defecography

Defecography uses still radiographs and fluoroscopy to assess both anorectal anatomy and function. It is performed in a radiology suite and requires patients to administer enemas before the procedure to ensure the rectum is empty. Following the instillation of contrast into the rectum, the images can be attained in the lateral decubitus or sitting position, though the authors prefer the sitting position on a radiolucent commode because it more approximates the usual position of defecation. Indications for defecography are listed in **Table 2**.

The authors' method of performing defecography is as follows: patients are positioned in the lateral decubitus position on a radiographic table. For women, 25 mL of meglumine diatrizoate (Gastrografin) is injected into the vagina to outline this structure during defecation. A lubricated catheter is inserted into the rectum. Fifty to 100 mL of liquid barium is injected through the catheter, and a still radiograph is taken to confirm filling of the rectum. Air may then be injected to provide mucosal contrast. Thickened barium paste is then injected until contrast refluxes into the sigmoid or until patients do not tolerate further paste. The authors mix the barium paste with water and dry infant cereal mix to create the consistency of loose stool before it is injected. While holding in the paste contrast, patients then stand and the radiographic table is repositioned to the vertical position. A radiolucent commode is placed in front of the radiographic table, and patients sit in the usual position. Lateral radiographs are then taken, 3 while squeezing and 3 while relaxing. Patients then evacuate using their normal defecation maneuvers under fluoroscopy.

Interpretation of the defecography images and fluoroscopy video requires measurement of various anatomic lines and angles. The components of a defecography report are listed in **Box 2**.[22] **Table 3** outlines the normal parameters of defecography, and **Fig. 3** shows lateral views attained during defecography. Clearly, many anatomic and functional diagnoses can be made using defecography. Results may guide treatment, whether biofeedback or surgical intervention. As summarized previously, defecography can be performed in about 10 minutes, with basic radiologic equipment and contrast media, making it a desirable investigation for many anorectal disorders.[23] Reproducibility of results and interobserver agreement can be variable, though, for certain parameters, such as rectal emptying.[24] More recently, MRI defecography has replaced cinedefecography in many centers. MRI is discussed in a later section of this article.

Balloon Expulsion Test

The balloon expulsion test may be performed as part of anal manometry or as an isolated investigation. Its main use is in patients with constipation to attempt to differentiate between obstructed defecation or outlet-type constipation and functional constipation. Manometry or defecography will not be diagnostic in all patients, and the balloon expulsion test may help clarify results.[25] However, it is rarely the sole diagnostic test used and should be used in conjunction with other anorectal physiology studies in patients who are constipated.[26]

The balloon expulsion test may be performed during manometry or in the sitting position. During manometry, patients are kept in the lateral decubitus position; at the end of the manometry procedure, the balloon at the end of the probe is inserted into the rectum and between 50 and 150 mL of water is instilled. Patients are asked to strain and evacuate the balloon. Varying volumes of water may be instilled if patients cannot initially evacuate the balloon. For the sitting technique, patients are initially placed in the lateral decubitus position and a detachable balloon is inserted into the rectum, inflated with 50 to 150 mL of water, and detached from the catheter. Patients are then permitted to sit on a commode in a private bathroom and are asked to strain and evacuate the balloon.[27]

The result of the balloon expulsion test is binary and, thus, easy to interpret. However, the volume of water instilled into the balloon, the position of patients during the attempted evacuation, and time allowed for patients to evacuate are not standardized between studies and physiology laboratories.[26] Aside from the investigation of possible obstructed defecation in patients who are constipated, it need not be used in standard anorectal physiology testing.

Box 2
Components of defecography

- Puborectalis length at rest and straining anorectal angle at rest and straining
- Perineal descent with straining
- Rectocele
- Sigmoidocele
- Intussusception or prolapse
- Degree of opening of anal canal with evacuation
- Degree of emptying of rectocele with evacuation
- Complete or incomplete rectal emptying with evacuation

Table 3 Normal findings of defecography	
Finding	**Normal Range**
Puborectalis length	Rest: 14–16 cm Squeeze: 12–15 cm Push: 15–18 cm
Anorectal angle	Rest: 70°–140° Squeeze: 75°–90° Push: 100°–180°
Perineal descent	Rest: less than 3 cm Push: less than 3 cm change from rest
Puborectalis notch	Push: blunted notch
Rectocele	Less than 2 cm Complete emptying with push
Prolapse	Absent
Anal canal	Push: complete opening
Rectal emptying	10–12 seconds Complete

Data from Sands DR, Wexner SD. Setting up a colorectal physiology lab. In: Corman ML, editor. Corman's colon and rectal surgery. 6th edition. Philadelphia: Lippincott Williams and Wilkins; 2013. p. 150–77.

MRI

The use of MRI in the setting of anorectal physiology and testing was initially as an anatomic test. MRI is able to show the anatomy of the pelvic floor musculature, including the puborectalis and external and internal sphincters, which are often of interest in anorectal disorders. Both endoanal coil and phased array external coils have been used, with the external coil becoming more common because of the improved patient comfort during the investigation. MRI may be performed in a standard fashion for anatomic purposes or combined with dynamic images or MRI defecography. The indications for MRI in anorectal testing are outlined in **Table 2**.

MRI may provide advantages over other anorectal testing for the investigation of particular situations. MRI may be better than endoanal ultrasound at detecting external sphincter defects.[28] MRI allows for investigation of all pelvic compartments at one time and in relation to each other and so is better able to assess the interactions between multiple compartments.[29] Dynamic MRI is a single test that combines clear anatomic views of the anorectum with defecography functional results, which may be appealing to patients requiring multiple anorectal tests for diagnosis.[30,31] The disadvantages of MRI are the expense of the procedure, prolonged time, and decreased detection of rectal intussusceptions compared with standard defecography (which are rarely clinically significant). In addition, it requires a dedicated radiologist with experience in reading dynamic MRI.

Pudendal Nerve Terminal Motor Latency

The pudendal nerves innervate the external anal sphincter bilaterally. Patients with various anorectal disorders may have abnormal conduction of the pudendal nerves. Bilateral nerve conduction abnormalities are required to produce clinical significance.[32] Pudendal nerve terminal motor latency (PNTML) is the time required from the stimulation of the pudendal nerve to the contraction of the sphincter.

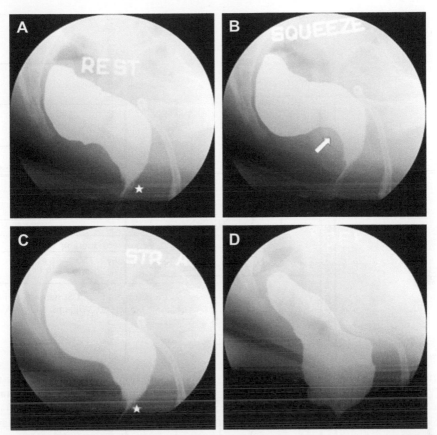

Fig. 3. Defecography images at rest (*A*) and during squeeze (*B*), strain (*C*), and evacuation (*D*), with the notch formed by the puborectalis (*arrow*) and the anorectal junction (*asterisk*) marked. (*From* Kim AY. How to interpret a functional or motility test–defecography. J Neurogastroenterol Motil © 2011;17:418; with permission.)

The process of performing a PNTML study is quick and requires a fingerstall device with implanted electrodes that are worn on the gloved index finger of the examiner. A rectal enema is administered before the test to reduce resistance. Patients are placed in the lateral decubitus position. An electrode gel is placed on the fingerstall device on the examiner's finger. The finger is inserted, and the coccyx is palpated. At the level of the coccyx, the finger is rotated laterally to one side. As short impulses are delivered through the electrodes, the finger is rotated until the site of maximal response is found on that side. A response is seen as contraction of the external anal sphincter around the examiner's finger. PNTML is measured at the site of maximal response 3 times and averaged. The finger is rotated to the other side, and the process is repeated.

Normal values of PNTML are about 2 milliseconds. Latency may be increased in the setting of incontinence or chronic rectal prolapse.[33] Typical PNTML tracings are shown in **Fig. 4**. Prolonged PNTML may help guide decision making regarding the potential treatments and their effectiveness for patients with fecal incontinence. The test is limited, however, by relatively low sensitivity, specificity, and operator dependence;

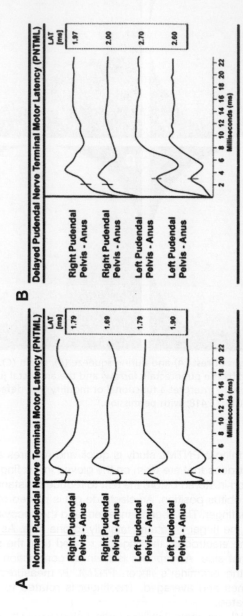

Fig. 4. Normal (*A*) and prolonged (*B*) PNTML tracings. (*From* Papaconstantinou HT. Evaluation of anal incontinence: minimal approach, maximal effectiveness. Clin Colon Rectal Surg 2005;18:9–16; with permission.)

results should be used only as part of the information used to guide treatment decisions.[34,35]

Electromyography

Similar to PNTML studies, electromyography (EMG) is used to assess the contraction of the external anal sphincter. EMG measures depolarization strength (not latency time), and the activity of both the external anal sphincter and puborectalis is captured. The main indication for EMG is fecal incontinence, although it is performed less commonly in this setting with the increased use of endoanal ultrasound.[22] EMG is also commonly used as part of ongoing muscle retraining during biofeedback therapy.[36] The response to treatment is assessed, and EMG may be used during the therapy sessions themselves. EMG can also be applied to the assessment of constipation.

There are various ways of performing EMG, including needle, surface, and anal plug. The choice of technique depends on indication and clinical preference. Needle EMG may be painful for some, although it is most often tolerated very well. Patients are usually placed in the lateral decubitus position. Surface electrodes are placed about the anus if indicated. Needle electrodes may consist of single-fiber electrode or concentric needle electrodes and are placed if indicated. An anal plug electrode is placed if indicated. Depending on the modality chosen, EMG activity may be recorded at rest and with squeeze and push efforts.

Normal findings on EMG are as follows:

- Amplitude of motor unit contraction is up to 2 mV
- Voluntary contraction potential lasts 5.0 to 7.5 milliseconds
- During defecation, EMG activity should be almost zero

Amplitude will be decreased in patients with nerve injury or stretch. EMG activity may be high during defecation in patients with paradoxic puborectalis contraction and difficult evacuation. Thus, EMG may provide some very practical answers in anorectal problems to help guide treatment planning.

Colonic Transit Studies

Within the realm of anorectal physiology testing, a colonic transit study is indicated for the workup of constipation when one wishes to distinguish between slow transit constipation and outlet-type constipation or obstructed defecation. Gastric emptying studies and small bowel transit studies may also be indicated in certain patients when global dysmotility is a considered diagnosis, but these are considered on a case-specific basis. Patients must be willing to stop all laxatives for 5 days during the procedure. Other than stopping laxatives, the test is very well tolerated with little interruption of daily activities. No enemas or bowel preparation is needed. Patients swallow a capsule containing radiopaque markers, commonly 24 markers per capsule. A health care professional should witness patients swallowing the capsule. A flat plate abdominal radiograph is taken to document the location and passage of the markers at various times, depending on center-specific protocols.[37] Common protocols include radiographs on day 5 only, days 1 and 5, or on days 1, 3, and 5.

A normal colonic transit study equates to the passage of at least 80% of the markers, or 19 of the 24 markers, at 5 days. Ninety-five percent of normal patients will pass 80% of the markers within 120 hours.[38,39] Five or fewer markers present after 5 days indicates normal colonic transit. More than 5 markers scattered throughout the colon suggests colonic inertia or hypomotility. More than 5 markers clustered in the rectum suggest outlet-type obstructed constipation.

SUMMARY

Anorectal physiology functions to maintain continence and allow for effective evacuation in a socially acceptable time and place. Disorders of anorectal physiology can have a profound effect on a person's life. The disruption of normal motor, sensory, or reflexive activities of the anal canal can result in complex problems, which pose challenges to the clinician. Various anatomic and functional tests are available to make an accurate diagnosis and discern between various medical and surgical treatment options. Not all anorectal physiology tests are needed in each situation. The clinician must be thoughtful and prudent when considering the numerous investigations. When used effectively, along with a complete history and physical examination, anorectal physiology tests can provide valuable information on the motor, sensory, and neurologic status of the anorectum and guide treatment decisions accordingly.

REFERENCES

1. Karulf RE. Anorectal physiology. In: Beck DE, Roberts PL, Saclarides TJ, et al, editors. The ASCRS textbook of colon and rectal surgery. 2nd edition. New York: Springer; 2011. p. 41–61.
2. Michelassi F, Lee J, Rubin M, et al. Long-term functional results after ileal pouch anal restorative proctocolectomy for ulcerative colitis: a prospective observational study. Ann Surg 2003;238:433–41.
3. de Zeeuw S, Ahmed Ali U, Donders RA, et al. Update of complications and functional outcome of the ileo-pouch anal anastomosis: overview of evidence and meta-analysis of 96 observational studies. Int J Colorectal Dis 2012;27:843–53.
4. Zbar AP, Khaikin M. Should we care about the internal anal sphincter? Dis Colon Rectum 2012;55:105–8.
5. van Duijvendijk P, Slors F, Taat CW, et al. A prospective evaluation of anorectal function after total mesorectal excision in patients with a rectal carcinoma. Surgery 2003;133:56–65.
6. Lam TJ, Felt-Bersma RJ. Clinical examination remains more important than anorectal function tests to identify treatable conditions in women with constipation. Int Urogynecol J 2013;24:67–72.
7. Dobben AC, Terra MP, Deutekom M, et al. Anal inspection and digital rectal examination compared to anorectal physiology tests and endoanal ultrasonography in evaluating fecal incontinence. Int J Colorectal Dis 2007;22:783–90.
8. Rao SS, Meduri K. What is necessary to diagnose constipation? Best Pract Res Clin Gastroenterol 2011;25:127–40.
9. Tantiphlachiva K, Rao P, Attaluri A, et al. Digital rectal examination is a useful tool for identifying patients with dyssynergia. Am J Gastroenterol 2010;8:955–60.
10. Li Y, Yang X, Xu C, et al. Normal values and pressure morphology for three-dimensional high-resolution anorectal manometry of asymptomatic adults: a study in 110 subjects. Int J Colorectal Dis 2013;28(8):1161–8.
11. Jones MP, Post J, Crowell MD. High-resolution manometry in the evaluation of anorectal disorders: a simultaneous comparison with water-perfused manometry. Am J Gastroenterol 2007;102:850–5.
12. Schuld J, Kollmar O, Schlutter C. Normative values in anorectal manometry using microtip technology: a cohort study in 172 subjects. Int J Colorectal Dis 2012;27:1199–205.

13. Cali RL, Blatchford GJ, Perry RE, et al. Normal variation in anorectal manometry. Dis Colon Rectum 1992;35:1161–4.
14. Chaliha C, Sultan AH, Emmanuel AV. Normal ranges for anorectal manometry and sensation in women of reproductive age. Colorectal Dis 2006;9:839–44.
15. Schaffzin DM, Wong WD. Endorectal ultrasound in the preoperative evaluation of rectal cancer. Clin Colorectal Cancer 2004;4:124–32.
16. Ratto C, Grillo E, Parello A, et al. Endoanal ultrasound-guided surgery for anal fistula. Endoscopy 2005;37:722–8.
17. Tjandra JJ, Milsom JW, Stolfi VM, et al. Endoluminal ultrasound defines anatomy of the anal canal and pelvic floor. Dis Colon Rectum 1992;35:465–70.
18. Stoker J, Halligan S, Bartram CI. Pelvic floor imaging. Radiology 2001;218:621–41.
19. Sultan AH, Nicholls RJ, Kamm MA, et al. Anal endosonography and correlation with in vitro and in vivo anatomy. Br J Surg 1993;80:508–11.
20. Sultan AH, Kamm MA, Talbot IC. Anal endosonography for identifying external sphincter defects confirmed histologically. Br J Surg 1994;81:463–5.
21. Vitton V, Vignally P, Barthet M, et al. Dynamic anal endosonography and MRI defecography in diagnosis of pelvic floor disorders: comparison with conventional defecography. Dis Colon Rectum 2011;54:1398–404.
22. Sands DR, Wexner SD. Setting up a colorectal physiology lab. In: Corman ML, editor. Corman's colon and rectal surgery. 6th edition. Philadelphia: Lippincott Williams and Wilkins; 2013. p. 150–77.
23. Jorge JM, Habr-Gama A, Wexner SD. Clinical applications and techniques in cinedefecography. Am J Surg 2001;182:93–101.
24. Klauser AG, Ting KH, Mangel E, et al. Interobserver agreement in defecography. Dis Colon Rectum 1994;37:1310–6.
25. Minguez M, Herreros B, Sanchiz V, et al. Predictive value of the balloon expulsion test for excluding the diagnosis of pelvic floor dyssynergia in constipation. Gastroenterology 2004;126:57–62.
26. Bove A, Pucciani F, Bellini M, et al. Consensus statement AIGO/SICCR: diagnosis and treatment of chronic constipation and obstructed defecation (part I: diagnosis). World J Gastroenterol 2012;18:1555–64.
27. Beck DE. A simplified balloon expulsion test. Dis Colon Rectum 1992;35:597–8.
28. Terra M, Beets-Tan R, van der Hulst V, et al. MRI in evaluating atrophy of the external anal sphincter in patients with fecal incontinence. Am J Roentgenol 2006;187:991–9.
29. Rentsch M, Paetzel C, Lenhart M, et al. Dynamic magnetic resonance imaging defecography: a diagnostic alternative in the assessment of pelvic floor disorders in proctology. Dis Colon Rectum 2001;44:999–1007.
30. Fletcher JG, Busse RF, Riederer SJ, et al. Magnetic resonance imaging of anatomic and dynamic defects of the pelvic floor in defecatory disorders. Am J Gastroenterol 2003;98:399–411.
31. Bharucha AE. Update of tests of colon and rectal structure and function. J Clin Gastroenterol 2006;40:96–103.
32. Ricciardi R, Mellgren AF, Madoff RD, et al. The utility of pudendal nerve terminal motor latencies in idiopathic incontinence. Dis Colon Rectum 2006;49:852–7.
33. Wexner SD, Marchetti F, Salanga VD, et al. Neurophysiologic assessment of the anal sphincters. Dis Colon Rectum 1991;34:606–12.
34. Hill J, Hosker G, Kiff E. Pudendal nerve terminal motor latency measurements: what they do and do not tell us. Br J Surg 2002;89(10):1268–9.
35. Madoff RD, Parker SC, Varma MG, et al. Faecal incontinence in adults. Lancet 2004;364:621–32.

36. Boselli AS, Pinna F, Cecchini S, et al. Biofeedback therapy plus anal electrostimulation for fecal incontinence: prognostic factors and effects on anorectal physiology. World J Surg 2010;34:815–21.

37. Alame AM, Bahna H. Evaluation of constipation. Clin Colon Rectal Surg 2012;25: 5–11.

38. Evans RC, Kamm MA, Hinton JM, et al. The normal range and a simple diagram for recording whole gut transit time. Int J Colorectal Dis 1992;7:15–7.

39. Kim ER, Rhee PL. How to interpret a functional or motility test – colon transit study. J Neurogastroenterol Motil 2012;18:94–9.

Anal Fissure and Stenosis

Sherief Shawki, MD, Meagan Costedio, MD*

KEYWORDS

- Anal fissure • Anal stenosis • Anorectal flap procedures
- Lateral internal sphincterotomy

KEY POINTS

- Anal fissure is arbitrarily classified as acute and chronic fissure, with the cutoff being non-healing for 6 weeks or more.
- Whereas most acute fissures heal spontaneously, chronic anal fissures require treatment.
- The foundation of treatment relies on reversing internal sphincter hypertonia, thereby improving blood perfusion and promoting healing.
- Treatment options include:
  ○ Nonsurgical: ointments (nitroglycerin, diltiazem, nifedipine)
  ○ Chemodenervation: type A botulinum toxin
  ○ Surgical: lateral internal sphincterotomy
- Algorithm of treatment usually starts with ointments or chemodenervation. Given the possibility of anal continence compromise, surgery is used as a last resort for refractory, non-healing fissures in patients with hypertonic sphincters.
- Mucosal advancement flaps are a viable surgical option for low-pressure fissures, or those at high risk for postoperative incontinence.
- The most common cause of anal stenosis is overzealous hemorrhoidectomy.
- Anal stenosis is classified based on the level, degree, and area of anal canal involved.
- Management of anal stenosis is challenging, and should be conducted by an experienced surgeon who is familiar with the disease.
- Management is tailored based on etiology and the level, degree, and area involved in stenosis.

INTRODUCTION: BACKGROUND, ETIOLOGY, AND PATHOPHYSIOLOGY
Anatomic and Physiologic Background

The functional anal canal starts at the anorectal ring and extends 3 to 4 cm to the anal verge. Proximally it is lined with columnar cells, which transition to squamous cells approximately 1 to 1.5 cm proximal to the dentate line; hence the term anal transition

Department of Colorectal Surgery, Cleveland Clinic Foundation, 9500 Euclid Avenue, Cleveland, OH 44195, USA
* Corresponding author.
E-mail address: costedm@ccf.org

Gastroenterol Clin N Am 42 (2013) 729–758
http://dx.doi.org/10.1016/j.gtc.2013.09.007
0889-8553/13/$ – see front matter © 2013 Elsevier Inc. All rights reserved.

zone. Distal to the dentate line the multilayered squamous cell lining is rich with somatic nerves. Unlike skin, this area lacks sebaceous and skin glands and hair follicles, and is commonly referred to as the anoderm.

The anal canal lies at an angle with the rectum, owing to the effect of the sling-like puborectalis muscle around the rectum. The internal anal sphincter (IAS) is a thickened continuation of the longitudinal smooth muscle layer of the rectum. At rest the IAS is continuously contracted; is responsible for resting anal pressure, and causes passive continence. On defecation, the puborectalis muscle relaxes, resulting in straightening of the anorectal angle. The IAS relaxes, via the rectoanal inhibitory reflex, and the delicate pliable anoderm stretches and dilates to accommodate the passage of a column of stool.[1,2]

Physiology of IAS Muscle Contraction

The IAS comprises smooth muscle fibers that are continuously contracted and regulated by the autonomic and enteric nervous systems. Contraction is mediated via an increase in cytoplasmic calcium. Conversely, a decrease in cytoplasmic calcium would result in relaxation.[3–5]

β-Adrenoceptor stimulation induces the return of cytosolic calcium to the sarcoplasmic reticulum via cyclic adenosine monophosphate, which leads to muscle relaxation. Similarly, relaxation is induced by nonadrenergic, noncholinergic nitric oxide (NO), which is mediated via cyclic guanosine monophosphate (cGMP).[5,6] Alternatively, blocking direct influx of extracellular calcium through the membranes of calcium channels would achieve the same results; α-adrenoceptor stimulation leads to the release of calcium from the sarcoplasmic reticulum, resulting in contraction.[5]

Epidemiology

Fissure in ano is a longitudinal or elliptical tear in the mucosal lining of the anal canal distal to the dentate line.[7] At this location, the anoderm lining is composed of multiple layers of squamous epithelium and is richly innervated with pain fibers.[8] Anal fissures (AFs) result in significant morbidity and reduction of quality of life in otherwise healthy young individuals.[9]

Although fissures are more commonly encountered in a young age group, with equal ratio among both genders, they can also affect extremes of age.[10] The exact incidence is unknown,[11] likely because many patients with acute fissures do not seek medical advice, and improve without treatment.[12] However, it has been suggested that the lifetime incidence is 11%.[13]

Fissures are usually single, and lie in the posterior midline in 80% to 90% of cases. Anterior midline AFs are most commonly found in women.[14] About 3% to 10% of AFs occur in the postpartum period, and these are often in the anterior midline.[10,15–20]

Primary AFs are idiopathic, usually anterior or posterior, and are not caused by underlying disease. Secondary fissures often occur in the lateral positions and are associated with other disease processes.[14] Multiple fissures should raise suspicion of other causes such as inflammatory bowel disease (mainly Crohn disease), human immunodeficiency virus, syphilis, tuberculosis, cancer, or leukemia. Alternatively, fissures refractory to treatment should prompt examination under anesthesia and biopsy to rule out malignancy.[21]

Primary fissures tend to occur more commonly in young age groups of both genders.[19] Those fissures occurring in persons older than 65 years are more likely to be a secondary, so testing to rule out inciting pathology should be performed.[22] AFs are arbitrarily classified as acute AF (AAF) and chronic AF (CAF) based on the duration of the disease process, with the cutoff being 6 weeks of persistent symptoms.[23]

Etiology

Although AF is a commonly encountered anal problem, the exact etiology is poorly defined. The following mechanisms are thought to cause this condition.[10,14]

Constipation and low-fiber diet

Trauma by passage of hard stool is thought to be an initiating factor. However, it has been reported that constipation occurs in only 1 in 4 patients; furthermore, in about 4% to 7% of instances fissure will follow bouts of diarrhea.[10,13,23,24] Nevertheless, a low-fiber diet seems to be associated with an increased risk of developing a fissure.[25]

Trauma during pregnancy

Up to 10% of chronic AFs occur postpartum,[16] thought to be secondary to shearing forces from the fetus on the anal canal. Alternatively, the anal canal mucosa loses pliability and becomes tethered to underlying tissues, rendering it more susceptible to trauma while stretching during defecation. This type of AF tends not to be associated with high resting anal pressures.[10]

Internal anal sphincter hypertonicity/spasm

As mentioned earlier, mean resting anal pressure (MRAP) is maintained by continuous contraction of the IAS. This contraction is mediated by α-adrenergic pathways as well as inherent myogenic tone.[1,4] Once thought to be secondary to anal pain, high internal sphincter tonicity is now envisioned as a plausible cause of chronic AF. There has been evidence relating AF to high MRAP secondary to spasm of the IAS. Postmortem angiographic studies demonstrate relatively low perfusion at the posterior commissure of anal canal, where 90% of fissures are found.[26] Doppler laser flowmetric study of the anodermal blood flow confirms the same findings.[27] In healthy volunteers, the resting anal canal pressure is about 80 to 100 mm Hg, almost approaching the intra-arterial systolic pressure of the inferior rectal artery. Hypertonia of the IAS would impede blood flow, creating an area of relative ischemia and resulting in superficial ischemic ulcer (ie, AF).[28,29] This correlation between abnormally high anal pressure and decreased anal blood flow is the foundation of AF treatment.

SYMPTOMS

Typically, AF presents with painful defecation described as a tearing sensation. Pain may persist a few minutes to hours following defecation, and can be accompanied by the passing of a modest amount of bright red blood that is usually separate from the stool. Larger amounts of blood could be a sign of another abnormality, such as hemorrhoids, as these 2 conditions may coexist. Blood mixed with stool should prompt further evaluation to rule out coexistent pathologic conditions.[10,21]

EXAMINATION

On examination, patients are usually apprehensive and use their gluteal muscles as protection to avoid pain. Once relaxed, and with gentle separation of the buttocks, the tear can be visualized in the distal anal canal. The combination of pain and spasm often precludes digital rectal examination, and there is no need to subject the patient to a painful digital examination if the history and inspection confirm the diagnosis.[21] If the diagnosis is in question, an examination under anesthesia is a less traumatic option by which to perform a thorough examination and obtain tissue samples.

AAF is usually superficial, and has the appearance of a tear with well-delineated mucosal edges and a granulating base. Findings associated with chronicity include fibrotic rolled skin edges, sentinel tags, a hypertrophied anal papilla, visible transverse fibers of IAS at base of fissure, and duration of symptoms of at least 6 to 8 weeks.[22,30,31]

TREATMENT
Acute Anal Fissures

AAFs are usually of short duration and more than 50% will heal spontaneously. The majority respond to a high-fiber diet and water intake to produce large bulky stool, resulting in physiologic anal dilation. Occasionally laxatives may be needed to soften the hard stool to avoid traumatic defecation. Warm sitz baths (up to 49 C as tolerable, 2–3 times a day, and/or after each bowel movement for 10–15 minutes) can help with symptomatic relief.[32]

Topical hydrocortisone and anesthetic creams are less effective in relieving the symptoms of AAF. However, in one study 3 weeks of topical hydrocortisone resulted in healing rates comparable to those of fiber and sitz baths.[33]

Chronic Anal Fissures

After 6 to 8 weeks without healing, fissures are classified as chronic. Only 10% of fissures that become chronic will spontaneously heal, meaning the majority will require some sort of treatment.[10]

Management of CAF aims at treating the triad of anal pain, spasm, and ischemia by breaking the cycle of hypertonia-/spasm-induced ischemia. The goal is to lower the IAS pressure to improve perfusion while preserving continence.

Lateral internal sphincterotomy (LIS) (**Fig. 1**) results in overwhelming cure rates upward of 98%, which has made surgery the mainstay therapy for CAF. However, early reports on this irreversible procedure showed concerns with regard to compromised anal continence in up to 30%. This finding prompted clinicians to seek medical alternatives that would reduce anal pressure without jeopardizing continence.[34]

Different medical therapies have been tried, including NO donors (glyceryl trinitrate [GTN], isosorbide dinitrate), calcium-channel blockers (CCB), which cause the depletion of intracellular calcium, chemodenervation with botulinum neurotoxin A (BTX), muscarinic receptor stimulants, α-adrenergic receptor antagonists, and β-adrenergic receptor agonists.

MEDICAL MANAGEMENT
Nitric Oxide Donors

In both exogenous and endogenous forms, NO is a nonadrenergic, noncholinergic neurotransmitter that induces relaxation of the IAS.

NO stimulates guanylate cyclase, leading to formation of cGMP, which in turn activates protein kinases that ultimately dephosphorylate myosin light chains, resulting in muscle-fiber relaxation.[5] A lack of NO synthase activity has been demonstrated in portions of IAS muscle fibers obtained from patients with AF.[35] Soon after the inception of its role in relaxation of the internal sphincter, topical GTN was shown to impose a significant decrease in MRAP and improvement in blood flow to the fissure.[36,37] Subsequently, several studies have evaluated the efficacy of GTN in treating AF (**Table 1**).[38–51]

Overall, healing rates with a dose of 0.2% applied twice a day ranged from as low as 18%[39] to as high as 85%.[43] As noted in **Table 1**, lower rates are observed in studies with duration of treatment of 6 weeks. In randomized controlled trials (RCTs) with duration of therapy of 6 to 8 weeks, the average healing rate was 50% to 68%. The rate of

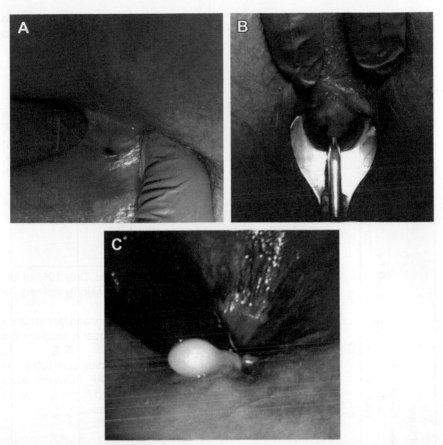

Fig. 1. A patient in prone position undergoing lateral sphincterotomy for chronic nonhealing anal fissure. (*A*) Posterior midline anal fissure. (*B*) Fissure and papilla is seen inside the anal canal. (*C*) Endoscopic view of papilla.

noncompliance ranged from 8% to 18%, related primarily to nitrate-induced headache.[52] Gagliardi and colleagues[50] evaluated optimal treatment duration using 0.4% topical GTN twice daily. Healing increased significantly in the first 6 weeks of therapy. However, they found no gained benefit on extension of the duration of therapy from 6 weeks to 12 weeks. Similarly, Lund and Scholefield[43] demonstrated an increase in healing rates from 36% to 85% from 4 to 6 weeks of treatment, respectively.

The most common side effect of topical GTN is headache, occurring in 20% to 90% of patients. It is usually transitory, and subsides within 15 minutes. Headache may be managed by educating patients before treatment, starting with a lower dose and escalating over 4 to 5 days, using finger cots for application to minimize the absorptive area, applying ointment in the recumbent position, and staying in this position for about 15 minutes after application.[8,53] Nevertheless, in approximately 10% to 15% of patients, headache is disabling and results in discontinuation of treatment.[50,54,55]

It has been demonstrated that CAF may heal faster with higher dosages/concentrations of NO donor ointments; however, this effect does not translate into superior healing rates in the long term. In addition, the higher-dosed NO donors increase the incidence of headaches and orthostatic hypotension, which may influence

Table 1
Studies of glyceryl trinitrate (GTN) ointment in patients with anal fissure

Authors,Ref./Year	Type of Study	Aim/Comparison	N	Dose	Duration of Treatment (wk)	Healing (%)	Headache (%)	F/U (mo)	Recurrence (%)	Comments
Gorfine,[38] 1995	P	GTN in AAF	15	0.5% qid	8	80	33	—	—	Efficient in AAF. Significant relief within minutes, lasting 2–6 h. HA self-limited
Lund et al,[39] 1996	P	Outcomes	21	0.2% bid	4 / 6	11 / 18	19	—	—	Three of 4 recurrences (75%) healed with another course
Lund et al,[40] 1997	RCT	GTN / Placebo	38 / 39	0.2% bid	8	68 / 8	58 / 18	12	8	Rapid relief; two-thirds avoid surgery; Recurrence treated with another course; Only 1 with HA withdrew
Bacher et al,[41] 1997	RCT	GTN vs Lidocaine	20 / 15	0.2% tid / 2%	4	80 / 40	—	—	—	CAF healing rates were 62% and 20%, respectively
Oettle,[42] 1997	RCT	GTN vs / IS	12 / 12	0.5 mg tid	2–4	83 / 100	—	Median 22	—	GTN healers had fast relief; GTN may reduce need for IS
Lund & Scholefield,[43] 1997	P	Outcomes	39	0.2% bid	4 / 6	36 / 85	20	—	13	Healing rate increased significantly at 6 wk. 4 of 5 recurrences healed with another course

Study	Type	Comparison	n	Dose	Duration					Comments
Kennedy et al,[44] 1999	RCT	GTN vs Placebo	24 / 19	0.2% bid	4	46 / 16	29 / 20	Mean 28	62	IAS pressure increased after completion of treatment; 40% of recurrences healed with another course; 60% long-term healing rate
Carapeti et al,[45] 1999	RCT dose finding	GTN vs ↑ Dose GTN Placebo	23 / 23 / 22	0.2% tid / — / 0.2%–0.6% tid	8	65 / 70 / 32	65 / 78 / 27	Median 9	33 / 25 / 43	Good alternative for 2 out of 3 patients. Escalating dose did not result in earlier healing. High recurrence. High HA
Altomare et al,[46] 2000	RCT role in AF	GTN vs Placebo	59 / 60	0.2%/12 h	4+	49 / 51	39 / 6	—	19	GTN: significant increase in anodermal blood flow. Cannot substitute IS
Zuberi et al,[47] 2000	RCT	Topical vs Patch Is	18 / 19 / 12	0.2% tid	8	67 / 63 / 92	72 / 63 / —	—	—	GTN patch is equally effective as GTN
Pitt et al,[48] 2001	P	Predictors of failure	64	0.2% bid	Until healing or IS	41	64	15	46	Sentinel pile adversely affects outcome. 15% with HA withdrew
Skinner et al,[49] 2001	P	Outcomes	51	0.2% qid	4	34	18	—	—	IS remains treatment of choice. 18% HA withdrew
Bailey et al,[11] 2002	RCT	GTN dose/ frequency. 8 groups	304	0, 0.1, 0.2, 0.4% (0–1.5 mg) bid and tid	8	Equal healing 59%	—	—	—	Reduced pain with 0.2 and 0.4% bid and tid

(continued on next page)

Table 1
(continued)

Authors,[Ref.] Year	Type of Study	Aim/ Comparison	N	Dose	Duration of Treatment (wk)	Healing (%)	Headache (%)	F/U (mo)	Recurrence (%)	Comments
Scholefield et al,[12] 2003	RCT dose response	181	49 47 37 —	0.1 0.2 0.4 All bid	8	47 40 54 37	20 42 90 12	—	—	Increased healing in placebo reflects problem in definition of chronicity
Gagliardi et al,[50] 2010	RCT optimal duration of treatment	74 79	74 79	0.4% bid	6 12	55 53	23	—	—	Overall healing 58%. Healing increased significantly around 6 wk. 8% withdrew due to HA
Perez-Legaz et al,[51] 2012	RCT	Endoanal Perianal	26 26	0.4% bid	8	23 54	—	6	—	Healing at 6 mo: 77% and 62%. Disabling HA in 15% of perianal group

Abbreviations: AAF, acute anal fissure; bid, twice daily; CAF, chronic anal fissure; F/U, follow-up; GTN, glyceryl trinitrate; HA, headache; IAS, internal anal sphincter; IS, internal sphincterotomy; P, prospective; qid, 4 times daily; RCT, randomized controlled trial; tid, 3 times daily.

compliance.[46,54] The effect of GTN on the IAS is reversible, and lacks a long-term effect on MRAP with subsequent increase in anal pressure on discontinuation. This drawback explains the incidence of relapse, which is as high as 30%. Again, higher rates were observed in studies with duration of therapy of less than 6 weeks.[44] Graziano and colleagues[56] correlated the recurrence to persistent hypertonia, and reported that CAFs were more likely to recur in the presence of a sentinel tag.[48] However, a significant amount of relapsing fissures healed with a repeat course of GTN, which further increased the overall rate of healing to 70%.[39,43]

Calcium-Channel Blockers

CCBs act by inhibiting voltage-dependent calcium channels located in the plasma membrane of electrically excitable muscle cells. Blocking these channels leads to a decrease in sarcoplasmic calcium ion concentration. The decrease in calcium interferes with calcium-mediated signal transduction and phosphorylation, ultimately decreasing contraction and resulting in the relaxation of muscle fibers.[5]

CCBs, often used in the treatment of cardiovascular disease, are also an effective treatment used to relax the lower esophageal sphincter in esophageal achalasia. The same concept was applied in treating CAF when diltiazem (DTZ) 2% topical gel was used to reduce IAS pressure, which achieved a healing rate of 67%.[57] **Table 2** highlights multiple studies evaluating the efficacy and safety of DTZ and nifedipine (NFDP).[57–73]

Approximately 50% of patents who failed previous treatment with topical 0.2% GTN healed their CAF after topical 2% DTZ, avoiding sphincterotomy in about70% of patients. The main side effects noted were perianal itching, soreness, or rash, occurring in about 10%, but this was generally well tolerated and did not compromise patient compliance.[61] Oral DTZ also has the ability to heal CAF; however, the healing rate was less than that of topical DTZ (38% vs 65%).[58]

A cohort of 112 patients with CAF was evaluated for long-term results after treatment with 2% DTZ cream twice daily. Whereas short-term results (68% healing rate) were similar to those previously reported,[40,45,47] over the 2-years period of follow-up retreatment was required (medical or surgical) in 59% of patients. Recurrence needs to be considered when counseling patients initially. A recent systematic review of 7 RCTs evaluating the effectiveness of DTZ versus GTN concluded that both are equally effective in managing CAF but with fewer headaches and recurrences associated with DTZ, favoring its use as the first line of treatment.[74] A similar report including only 2 RCTs failed to demonstrate any difference between treatments.[75]

Nifedipine

Nifedipine, 20 mg sublingually, was shown to decrease anal resting pressure significantly, by 30%.[76] The same dose orally achieved similar results among healthy volunteers (8 subjects) and patients with CAF (15 patients). Nine patients (60%) healed their fissures after 8 weeks. Although no episodes of postural hypotension or incontinence occurred, flushing and headaches were reported in 10 and 4 patients, respectively.[68] The same oral regimen was compared with 0.2% topical GTN, with equivalent healing rates but fewer side effects.[77]

Treatment with 0.2% topical nifedipine twice daily for 3 weeks was associated with a 95% healing rate and a 30% decrease in resting anal pressure, without major side effects.[78] Similar healing was obtained in patients with CAF using 0.3% NFDP in conjunction with 1.5% lidocaine ointment twice daily, as opposed to only a 16% healing rate when using 1.5% lidocaine and 1% hydrocortisone ointment. No systemic side effects were observed. Three fissures recurred within 1 year of follow-up, and

Table 2
Studies of calcium-channel blockers in patients with anal fissure

Authors,Ref. Year	Type of Study	Aim/ Comparison	N	Dose	Duration of Treatment (wk)	Healing (%)	Side Effects (%)	F/U (mo)	Recurrence (%)	Comments
Carapeti et al,[57] 2000	P	DTZ GTN	15 15	2% 0.1%	8 tid	67 60	— —	— —	— —	Similar healing to GTN, ↓ difference in MRAP between responders and nonresponders side effects. No
Jonas et al,[58] 2001	RCT	Topical PO	26 24	2% bid 60 mg	8	65 38	0 33	— —	— —	No significant ↓ in BP. Retains healing ability but ↓ healing rate, and more side effects
Das Gupta et al,[59] 2002	P	DTZ gel	23	2%	6–8 tid	48	0	3	0	Similar healing rates, ↓ side effects. Healed 75% (6/8) of patients who previously failed GTN
Kocher et al,[60] 2002	RCT	DTZ GTN	31 29	2% 0.2%	6–8 bid	77 86	42 72	—	—	Similar healing rates. Significant ↓ side effects and HA
Griffin et al,[61] 2002	Cohort	DTZ after failing GTN	46	2%	8 bid	48	—	—	—	Heals and further avoids surgery in about 50% in those failed on GTN
Jonas et al,[62] 2002	P	DTZ outcomes	39	2%	8 bid	49	10	—	—	27 of 39 failed previous GTN with 44% healing. 10% side effects, mainly perianal itching
Bielecki & Kolodziejczak,[63] 2003	RCT	DTZ GTN	22 21	2% 0.5%	8 bid	86 85	0 33	—	—	Equally effective. ↓ side effects
Shrivastava et al,[64] 2007	RCT	DTZ GTN Placebo	31 30 30	2% 0.2 —	Bid till healing	80 73 33	0 67 0	—	12 32 50	Both are effective modalities. DTZ ↑ healing, delayed recurrence (5.5 vs 3.5 mo)

Study	Type	Drug	N	Dose		Healing %				Comments
Sanei et al,[65] 2009	RCT	DTZ / GTN	51 / 51	2% / 0.2%	12 bid	66 / 55	—	—	—	DTZ significant reduction of symptoms. GTN faster healing
Jawaid et al,[66] 2009	RCT	DTZ / GTN	40 / 40	2% / 0.2%	8 tid	77 / 82	32 / 72	—	—	Equally effective, DTZ may be first line due to ↓ side effects
Ala et al,[67] 2012	RCT	DTZ / GTN	36 / 25	2% / 0.2%	8 bd	91 / 60	0 / 100	—	—	Superior healing rate. ↓ side effects
Nifedipine										
Cook et al,[68] 1999	P	PO NFDP / Volunteers	15 / 8	20 mg bid	8	91 / 15	100	—	—	Early ↓ in BP, resolved by 4th wk. ↓ in MRAP. 10 patients had flushing and 5 had HA
Perrotti et al,[69] 2002	RCT	NFDP + Lido / Lido + HC	55 / 55	0.3% + 1.5% / 1.5% + 1%	6 bid	94 / 16	—	18	6	Efficient combination. ↓ side effects. ↓ MRAP. Repeat course leads to further healing
Ansaloni et al,[70] 2002	P	PO NFDP	21	6 mg daily	4	90	33/2 wk	2	—	No changes in BP. Promising alternative. RCT and Long-term results needed
Ezri & Susmallian,[71] 2003	RCT	NFDP / GTN	26 / 26	0.5% / 0.2%	8 bid	89 / 58	5 / 40	3 / 4.5	42 / 31	More effective. ↓ HA. Frequent recurrence in both groups
Agaoglu et al,[72] 2003	P	NFDP / Volunteers	10 / 10	20 mg bid	8	50	10	—	—	No significant drop in BP. An alternative. Significant ↓ in MRAP
Golfam et al,[73] 2010	RCT	NFDP / Lidocaine	60 / 50	0.5% / 2%	4	70 / 12	—	12	26	Significant healing and pain control rates. ↑ Recurrence

Abbreviations: ↓, decrease; ↑, increase; bid, twice daily; BP, blood pressure; DTZ, diltiazem; F/U, follow-up; GTN, glyceryl trinitrate; HA, headache; HC, hydrocortisone; IS, internal sphincterotomy; Lido, lidocaine; MRAP, mean resting anal pressure; NFDP, nifedipine; PO, oral; P, prospective; qid, 4 times daily; RCT, randomized controlled trial; tid, 3 times daily.

2 healed with a second course.[69] When topical NFDP 0.2% was compared with topical GTN 0.2% over a 6-month period, healing rates were higher (89% vs 58%), and side effects in terms of headaches and flushing were decreased (5% vs 40%). Recurrence rates were relatively high among the groups, 42% and 31%, after a mean of 12 and 18 weeks, respectively.[71]

In another study, 23 of 27 patients (85%) healed their acute anal fissure (AAF) after completing 8 weeks of 0.5% NFDP ointment in conjunction with a high-fiber diet. Another 2 patients healed after 4 additional weeks with the same therapy. Only 2 patients reported moderate headache within the study period. After a mean follow-up of 23 months, 4 fissures recurred (16%), all of which were successfully treated with another 4-week course. The investigators concluded that topical NFDP 0.5% offers a high healing rate in acute AF, and may prevent evolution to chronicity.[79]

Botulinum Neurotoxin A

Role and mechanism of action

BTX is an endopeptidase that blocks acetylcholine release at the neuromuscular gap of α motor neurons, γ neurons in muscle spindles, and all parasympathetic and cholinergic postganglionic sympathetic neurons. BTX does not block synthesis or storage of acetylcholine, but rather its delivery, by interfering with vesicle transport.[5] Once injected into the neuromuscular junction, paralysis occurs within hours. This effect will persist for 3 to 4 months until axonal regeneration occurs with formation of new nerve terminals.[10]

The exact mechanism of action of BTX on smooth muscles is unclear. Unlike external anal sphincter (skeletal) muscle fibers, IAS (smooth) muscle fibers lack neuromuscular synapses. Despite this, injection of BTX into both the internal and external anal sphincter seems to be associated with sphincter relaxation and improvement of microcirculation.[80,81]

Gui and colleagues[82] prospectively injected a total of 15 U of BTX into the IAS (2 injections laterally and 1 posteriorly). At 2 months, evaluation 7 of 15 had healed their AF. At 3 months, 1 patient had relapsed and 1 experienced 1 day of incontinence to flatus, confirming the efficacy of BTX in treating CAF. An RCT followed, comparing BTX with placebo. At 2 months, 11 of the 15 patients in the treatment group had healed. The 4 patients (27%) who did not heal received a rescue dose of BTX (25 U), and subsequently all healed their fissures.[83] Many studies have evaluated the safety and efficacy of BTX, some of which are presented in **Table 3**.[84–95]

Massoud and colleagues[87] observed a 60% cure rate within 6 months, and recommend BTX as the first step in treating CAF. Long duration of symptoms (>12 months), presence of sentinel tag, and/or fissure-base fibrosis were all factors associated with a higher relapse rate.[86,89] The investigators recommend LIS as the first choice of therapy for this patient group. During 3 years of follow-up, the 5% of patients who experienced incontinence were all older than 50 years. The investigators recommended offering such older patients BTX to minimize the risk of incontinence associated with surgical sphincterotomy in this high-risk group.

De Nardi and colleagues[91] reported equivalent healing rates (57% BTX vs 66% GTN); however, the healing rate at 3 years dropped to 33% and 40%, respectively. A recent systematic review of studies using BTX revealed a recurrence rate ranging from 0% to 52%.[96] Minguez and colleagues[97] followed 53 patients for 42 months whose fissures healed with BTX. The late recurrence rate of 41.5% was associated with anterior location of the AF, long duration of the disease, need for reinjection or higher doses to achieve healing, and a lower posttreatment reduction of maximum squeeze pressure. Brisinda and colleagues[93] randomized 100 patients into 2 groups.

Group 1 received BTX in the form of either 30 U BTX or 90 U Dysport. Group 2 received GTN 0.2% 3 times daily for 8 weeks. Whereas the healing rate was 70% in group 2, group 1 had a healing rate of more than 90%, which concurred with results of their earlier study.[90] Sixteen nonhealing fissures in both groups (4 BTX and 12 GTN) underwent cross-over therapy, and all healed. Seven fissures relapsed in the GTN group, and all healed after treatment with BTX. However, in another study, 9 out of 17 patients (53%) treated with BTX in an RCT required LIS within 6 months.[88]

AF refractory to a single medical modality treatment may benefit from alternative therapy. When fissurectomy and BTX injection was offered to 30 patients with medically resistant fissures, 19 failed GTN and 11 failed both GTN and BTX. At a median of 16 weeks' follow-up, 93% healed their fissures, and the remaining unhealed 7% experienced improvement in their symptoms.[98] The investigators recommend this combination because it achieves a high healing rate and avoids further aggressive surgical procedures. This combined method was used to treat 46 continent women with CAF. Although short-term results were encouraging (healing rate of 85%), 16 of 32 patients had a recurrence at a follow-up of 22 months.[99] Another combination of BTX and GTN was compared with BTX alone in an RCT recruiting patients with medically resistant fissures. Despite the lack of significant differences, there was a higher trend in the combination group toward healing (47% vs 27%), symptomatic improvement (87% vs 67%), and avoidance of surgery (27% vs 47%).[100]

Thirty patients who failed isosorbide dinitrate (ISDN) previously were randomly assigned to receive either ISDN (2.5 mg 3 times daily for 3 months) + 20 U BTX injected into the IAS, or BTX alone. Healing rates were 66% for ISDN + BTX versus 20% for BTX at 6 weeks, 73% versus 73% at 8 weeks, and 60% versus 66% at 12 weeks. In this study, ISDN application induced a greater reduction in MRAP following BTX injection rather than when BTX was used alone.[101] A BTX dosage study found better healing results in a group of patients receiving 20 U and in a subgroup of patients who initially did not heal their fissure and were retreated with 25 U. This result was in contrast to that for patients who received 15 U followed by 20 U. Mean follow-up was 24 weeks, without adverse effects including continence disturbance.[102]

Chemodenervation (30 U BTX or 90 U Dysport) was used in 80 patients who failed LIS. At 2 months' evaluation, 74% had healed their fissures. Ten percent of patients experienced transient incontinence to flatus that resolved spontaneously. The 21 patients who failed initially received 50 U BTX or 150 U Dysport, and all healed. Eleven of these patients experienced incontinence to flatus, which again transiently and spontaneously resolved. Overall follow-up was 58 months and demonstrated no recurrences.[103]

As shown in **Table 3**, the site of BTX injection varied among studies. One study showed that injecting on both sides of the anterior midline was associated with higher healing rates (88% vs 60%) and a greater decrease in MRAP as opposed to injection on both sides of the posterior midline.

Application

BTX can be applied in the outpatient clinic in the left lateral position or, more favorably, in the operating room in the lithotomy position. The operating room can be helpful for evaluating and ruling out other diseases.

Complications secondary to injection include perianal pain, hematoma, thrombosis, and infection. Postoperative complications include incontinence, which is temporary. Some circumstances prohibit the use of BTX, such as hypersensitivity to BTX, pregnancy, myasthenia, Lambert-Eaton syndrome, and amyotrophic lateral sclerosis;

Table 3
Studies of safety and efficacy of BTX when compared with lateral internal sphincterotomy, nitric oxide donors, and calcium–channel blockers

Authors,[Ref.] Year	Study	N	Dose/Site	Healing Rate (%)	Incontinence (%)	F/U (mo)	Recurrence (%)	Comments
BTX vs LIS								
Mentes et al,[84] 2003	RCT	61 BTX 50 LIS	0.3 U/kg IAS/anterior both sides	74 98	0 16	12	13 4	BTX: acceptable healing rate. May require a repeat injection FI: transient and minor
Giral et al,[85] 2004	P	10 BTX 11 LIS	20 U Intersphincteric	70 82	0 0	14	0 0	Equally effective
Arroyo et al,[86] 2005	RCT	40 BTX 40 LIS	25 U IAS	45 90	0 5	36	—	Duration of symptoms and sentinel pile leads to recurrence FI in patients >50 y
Massoud et al,[87] 2005	RCT	25 BTX 25 LIS	25 U IAS	60 100	—	6	20 7	BTX effective alternative 60% chance of cure
Iswariah et al,[88] 2005	RCT	17 BTX 21 LIS	20 U IAS/fissure both sides	41 86	0 0	26	53 9	9 BTX; 53% required surgery within 6 mo
Nasr et al,[89] 2010	RCT	40 BTX 40 LIS	20 IAS/fissure both sides	62 90	0 5	18 wk	40 12	BTX outpatient LIS incontinence 15%–5% minor

BTX vs NO donor/CCB

Study	Type	Group	Regimen	Healing %	Recurrence %	F/U	FI %	Comment
Brisinda et al,[90] 1999	RCT	25 BTX / 25 GTN	20 U/IAS both sides ant / 0.2% tid, 6 wk	96 / 60	0 / 0	15	0 / 0	Both effective alternatives / GTN: 20% had HA
De Nardi et al,[91] 2006	RCT	15 BTX / 15 GTN	20 U/IAS both sides ant / 0.2% tid 8 wk	57 / 66	0 / 0	36–46	33 / 33	Healing at 3 y ↓ >20%
Fruehauf et al,[92] 2006	RCT	25 BTX / 25 GTN	30 U, 10 fissure both sides, 10 dorsal to fissure / 0.2% bid	—	—	—	—	GTN more effective
Brisinda et al,[93] 2007	RCT	50 BTX / 50 GTN	30 U BTX or 90 U Dysport both sides ant / 0.2% tid 8 wk	92 / 70	5 / 34	20 / 12	0 / 14	Both are good alternatives / BTX more effective
Festen et al,[94] 2009	RCT	37 BTX / 36 ISDN	20 U/IAS both sides art + placebo ointment / 1% ISDN + placebo injection	38 / 58	5 / 0	6.7	13 / 25	No advantages over NO donor / ISDN: 33% HA
Samim et al,[95] 2012	RCT	60 BTX / 74 DTZ	20 U left/right lateral, intersphincteric groove / 2%	43 / 43	5 / 8	39	11 / 17	Both comparable

Abbreviations: ↓, decrease; ant, anteriorly; BTX, botulinum neurotoxin A; CCB, calcium-channel blockers; DTZ, diltiazem; F/U, follow-up; FI, fecal incontinence; GTN, glyceryl trinitrate; IAS, internal anal sphincter; ISDN, isosorbice dinitrate; LIS, lateral internal sphincterotomy; NO, nitric oxide; P, prospective; RCT, randomized controlled trial; tid, 3 times daily.

and concomitant use of aminoglycosides because of a potential enhancement of action of the BTX.[96]

SURGICAL TREATMENT OF ANAL FISSURE

The treatment of CAF typically starts with pharmacologic agents as outlined earlier. Failure to heal or persistence of symptoms after at least 6 to 8 weeks of medical management warrants surgical intervention. The surgical approach relies on the same concepts used for medical management, reversing hypertonia and improving mucosal perfusion. The current options include manual anal dilation, sphincterotomy, and endoanal advancement flap.

Anal Dilation

The patient is taken to the operating room for manual stretching of the anal sphincter, ideally in a controlled fashion. Stretching is performed by inserting up to 4 fingers into the anal canal for 4 minutes.[17,104] Healing rates among acute and chronic AF varies from 40% to 70%, and recurrence rates range from 2% to 55%. While effective, this procedure is associated with the potential risk of sphincter damage, with reports of incontinence to flatus and soiling upward of 40%, and a 16% fecal incontinence rate. Other complications include bleeding at the fissure site, perianal bruising, and infection.[105–107] Because of this high complication rate, the procedure is rarely performed.

Lateral Internal Sphincterotomy

Initially, internal sphincterotomy was performed at the site of AF. The IAS fibers were divided at the base of the fissure, usually in the posterior midline; however, this led to a guttering of the residual midline scar and a "keyhole" deformity in 28% of patients, resulting in improper closure at the anal verge with associated trapping of feces and resultant soiling.[20] A technique was developed to score the IAS away from the fissure, namely, LIS. This technique can be used in either closed or open fashion, and avoids delayed healing and keyhole deformities. **Table 4** lists published outcomes of internal sphincterotomy.[108–119]

Healing rates after LIS are very effective, ranging from 90% to 100%, although post–internal sphincterotomy continence disturbances range from 0% to 47%.[120] Whereas some previous reports favored closed internal sphincterotomy over an open technique for reasons of less continence disturbance,[113] others found no significant difference in terms of healing rates or morbidity.[109,118]

Khubchandani and Reed[110] found a significantly higher proportion of patients with continence disturbance after internal sphincterotomy performed on patients older than 40 years.

Pernikoff and colleagues[112] reviewed 500 patients who underwent internal sphincterotomy and found overall disturbance incontinence of 8%, emphasizing that careful patient selection, meticulous preoperative history of continence problems, and meticulous surgical technique are imperative for improved outcomes.

Mucosal Advancement Flaps for Fissure

Advancement flaps may play a vital role in the previously discussed patient groups who are at risk of experiencing incontinence. A V-Y flap may be used to close a fissure site after fissurectomy. This approach includes excising the fibrotic rolled mucosal and skin edges, surrounding scar tissue, and sentinel tag, if present, and curetting the granulating base before securing the flap. In high-risk patients with hypertonia, advancement flap with simultaneous BTX injection is also an option. In one study,[121] all patients were healed at 30 days. After mean follow-up of 24 months there was an 8% recurrence rate, with no significant change in continence status from baseline, and no stenosis, keyhole deformity, or flap necrosis.[121] Similarly, using a rectangular dermal advancement flap in comparison with LIS, Hancke and colleagues[122] demonstrated similar healing rates and fewer incontinence incidents over long-term follow-up (70–94 months). A retrospective review comparing results of anal advancement flap with those of LIS for AF showed healing rates of 96% versus 88%, demonstrating the effectiveness of an advancement flap in treating CAF.[123]

ANAL STENOSIS

Anal stenosis occurs when the physiologic capacity of the anal canal is lost and the pliable tissues are replaced with scarred fibrotic tissue at the anoderm, which can include the IAS. Although stenosis can be localized to any portion of the anal canal, it is not uncommon to encounter stenoses involving its entire length.[124] Anal stenosis is classified as congenital, primary, and secondary. Congenital and primary causes are related to developmental and involutional processes, but the most common causes of stenosis are secondary in nature, primarily related to surgical trauma.

Post-hemorrhoidectomy anal stricture is the most common cause of anal stenosis, with a postoperative incidence from 1.5% to 4%[125]; this accounts for 90% of cases of anal stenosis.[126] Other causes include excision of perianal lesions, fistulectomy, fulguration of condyloma, rectal surgery with low anastomosis (ileal pouch, coloanal), radiotherapy, trauma, inflammatory bowel disease, chronic laxative use, sexually transmitted diseases, chronic suppurative diseases, and chronic diarrhea.

Anal canal stenosis is classified based on severity, level of the stricture, and degree of involvement of the anal canal. **Table 5** summarizes these classifications.[127]

Diagnosis

Patients present often with difficult evacuation and narrow caliber of stools. Other symptomatology may include constipation, painful defecation, and bleeding. Occasionally, patents present with incontinence secondary to overflow constipation. A concurrent ectropion will add seepage to the presentation. It is imperative to rule out primary causes of stenosis.

Examination

It is extremely important to delineate and characterize the stricture, and to provide appropriate management. Occasionally this will necessitate examination under anesthesia, especially in patients with severe or painful strictures.[124,126]

Nonoperative Management

Initially, conservative management is indicated in mild stenosis, especially stenosis low in the anal canal. Treatment includes fiber supplementation, stool softeners, and gradual anal dilation. Should the addition of stool softeners and bulk-forming agents fail, daily digital or mechanical anal dilations may be incorporated into management. Typically the first dilation occurs in the operative room, followed by daily self-digital or mechanical dilation at home.[128] This method is particularly helpful in patients with Crohn disease and those with previous radiotherapy, for whom any major surgical procedure may have potential healing complications secondary to the nature of the offending disease.[129]

Table 4
Studies demonstrating the efficacy and complication rate of lateral internal sphincterotomy

Authors,[Ref.] Year	Type of Study	Aim/Objective	N	Healing (%)	Incontinence (%)			Recurrence (%)	Comments
					Flatus	Stool	Soiling		
Gordon & Vasilevsky,[108] 1985	R	LIS, local anesthetic	133	—	2	1	NA	2	Outpatient procedure
Lewis et al,[109] 1988	R	Closed vs Open IS	247 103	94	16 20 (overall FI)		NA	6	No difference in techniques
Khubchandani & Reed,[110] 1989	Survey	Sequelae of IS	829	98	35	5	22	2	Fissurectomy unnecessary Incontinence higher if age >40 y No difference in location of sphincterotomy
Melange et al,[111] 1992	P	Outcomes, postop. midline IS	76	100	17	11	9	0	No correlation between manometry and pre- and postoperative symptoms
Pernikoff et al,[112] 1994	R	Outcome, partial LIS	500	99	3	1	4	3	Less incontinence. Patient selection, absence of preoperative continence problems results in better outcomes

									Comments
Garcia-Aguilar et al,[113] 1996	R	Open vs Closed IS	324 225	96 94	30 23	12 3	27 16	11 12	Significant incontinence complication. Closed IS has less impairment. Average F/U 10 mo longer in open
Littlejohn & Newstead,[114] 1997	R	Tailored LIS	287	99	2	0	1	1.4	Tailored IS efficacious with fewer incontinence events
Hananel & Gordon,[115] 1997	R	Outcomes of LIS	265	95	0.4	0.4	0.4	1.1	Acceptable complication rate
Nyam & Pemberton,[116] 1999	Survey	Long-term outcomes of LIS	487	96	6	1	8	8	Incontinence is minor and transient, but permanent in small group
Argov & Levandovsky,[117] 2000	R	Outcomes LIS	2108	96	1.5	—	—	1	Safe, acceptable outcomes
Wiley et al,[118] 2004	RCT	Closed vs Open	36 40	97 95	2.7	1.4 2.8	—	—	Incontinence after IS not insignificant. No difference among techniques
Garg et al,[119] 2013	Review	Long-term continence	4512	90–100	9	0.8	6	0–30	F/U 24–124 mo Overall continence disturbance 14%

Abbreviations: F/U, follow-up; FI, fecal incontinence; IS, internal sphincterotomy; LIS, lateral internal sphincterotomy; NA, not applicable; P, prospective; R, retrospective.

Table 5
Classifications used when assessing anal stenosis

Variable	Definition
Severity of stenosis	
Mild	Allows a well-lubricated index finger/medium Hill-Ferguson retractor
Moderate	Forceful insertion of a well-lubricated index finger/medium Hill-Ferguson retractor
Severe	Resistance to pass little finger or small Hill-Ferguson retractor
Level of stenosis	
Low	Distal to 0.5 cm below dentate line
Middle	A zone 0.5 cm distal and proximal to dentate line
High	Proximal to 0.5 cm above dentate line
Extent of anal canal involvement	
Localized	Confined to one level, and/or one quadrant of the anal canal
Diffuse	Involves more than one level of anal canal
Circumferential	Involves whole circumference of anal canal

Operative Management

General and important technical considerations

Operative treatment is indicated in the treatment of moderate to severe anal stenoses, and refractory cases of mild stenosis. The concept is to release the fibrotic scar, by either excision or incision, with a margin of healthy tissue. Subsequently, the goal is to mobilize either rectal mucosa or perianal skin (neo-anoderm) to bring healthy tissue to the area to achieve tension-free coverage of the defect. This approach theoretically restores the excessive loss of anoderm, with the goal of regaining pliability and capacity of the anal canal to stretch. Flaps can be classified as follows.[129]

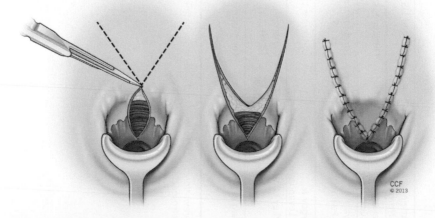

Fig. 2. V-Y advancement flap.

Advancement flaps (sliding flaps) A rectal mucosal or anal skin flap is raised while maintaining vascularity and continuity with the surrounding tissues and is subsequently advanced, and placed across the anoderm after the scar has been released. These flaps obtain blood supply via submucosal or subdermal vascular plexuses, respectively. Examples include mucosal advancement flap and the V-Y flap (**Fig. 2**).

Island flaps (adjacent tissue transfer flaps) The flap is designed and disconnected from the surrounding tissues, maintaining its blood supply from subcutaneous perforators arising from underlying muscle(s). Examples include diamond and house (**Fig. 3**), U-flap, and rectangular flaps.

Rotational flaps Large tissue flaps are raised, often bilaterally, while maintaining continuity with surrounding tissues, then rotated around the anus. Blood supply is from both subcutaneous and subdermal plexuses. Examples include the S-rotational flap (**Fig. 4**).

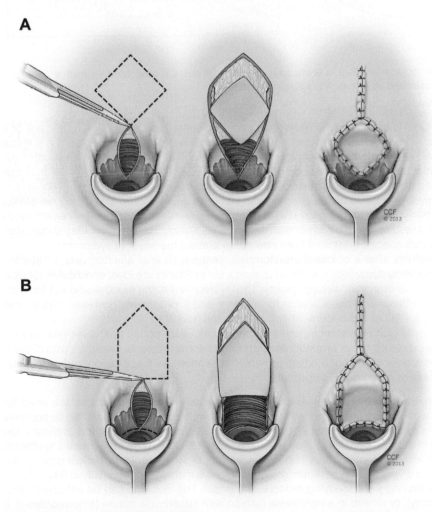

Fig. 3. (*A*) Diamond flap. (*B*) House flap.

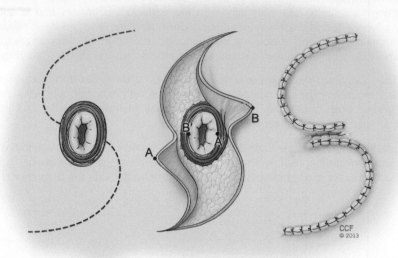

Fig. 4. Rotational S-flap. A is dissected free from A' and B is dissected free from B'. B is then approximated to A' and A is approximated to B'.

Special situations

Strictures in patients with inflammatory bowel disease (commonly Crohn disease) or a history of pelvic radiation have a high potential of healing complications. If a surgical procedure is undertaken such as a flap, and postoperative nonhealing complicates the situation, fecal diversion may be necessary to salvage the situation. It is imperative that these patients understand these aspects of the postoperative course during preoperative counseling. Patients with asymptomatic stenoses secondary to underlying neoplasia, infection, inflammatory bowel disease, or other diseases should have an examination under anesthesia with biopsy and culture. After pathologic confirmation, they should start diagnosis-specific treatment in an attempt to prevent the onset of symptoms.

Strictures after a coloanal anastomosis, ileal-pouch anal anastomosis, or stapled hemorrhoidectomy with short mild to moderate strictures are ideal candidates for dilation, stricturotomy, or stricturoplasty. The involvement of the mucosa and not the anoderm in these situations seems to confer a better prognosis; however, should this technique fail an advancement flap may be the next step.

Patients with persistent stricture following colo-/ileal-pouch anal anastomosis may require more complex procedures. Options include a transanal resection with circumferential colonic or pouch advancement, transabdominal mobilization and redo anastomosis, or a combined approach.[130]

Stricturotomy, stricture release, and stricturoplasty These procedures are used for mild to moderate short anorectal strictures. Simple stricture release may temporarily relieve symptoms, but usually the scar tissue will reform. This method is most often used in association with dilation when the patient is at high risk for general anesthesia, a surgical intervention (flap) is contraindicated, or when avoiding radical procedures such as diversion or proctectomy. The stricture is incised longitudinally in 3 to 4 quadrants, leaving the underlying musculature intact. The incisions can be left open (stricturotomy), or closed in a transverse fashion with absorbable suture (stricturoplasty). If this technique fails, an advancement flap is a good second option.[131]

Table 6
Different types of flaps and their best utilization

Feature of Stricture	Advancement Flap/Blood Supply		Island Flap/Blood Supply					Rotational Flap/Blood Supply
	Mucosal	Submucosal or Subdermal	Subcutaneous Vessels/Perforators from Underlying Muscles					Subdermal and Subcutaneous
		V-Y	V-Y	Rectangular	U	Diamond	House	S
Level of stricture								
Low	—	X	—	—	—	X	X	—
Middle	X	—	X	X	X	X	X	—
High	X	—	X	X	X	—	X	X
Severity of stricture								
Mild	—	X	X	—	—	—	X	—
Moderate	—	—	X	X	X	X	X	—
Severe	—	—	X	X	X	X	X	X
Extent of stricture								
Localized	X	X	X	X	X	X	X	—
Circumferential	—	—	—	—	X	X	X	X
Diffuse	—	—	—	—	—	—	X	X
Associated ectropion	—	X	X	X	X	X	X	X
Recurrent stricture	—	—	—	—	—	X	X	X

Sphincterotomy It is not uncommon to find that the cicatrized tissue involves the IAS, prompting single or multiple "partial" tailored internal sphincterotomy(ies) with concurrent chosen procedure or flap. This approach is usually beneficial in mild, low stenoses.[129] Others prefer not to perform sphincterotomy to avoid a possible compromising fecal continence mechanism.[131] Duieb and colleagues[132] suggested an algorithmic approach including 3 different flaps. Their approach starts with incising the stenosis longitudinally, creating a diamond defect. If there is a muscular component, they incise superficial fibers from IAS. Subsequently they attempt a mucosal advancement flap and primarily close the defect. If there is tension in the closure, a V-Y flap is attempted. If tension persists, the V-Y flap would become a diamond island flap. In severe stenoses, 2 flaps at opposite sides are performed. All of their patients had some level of improvement without long-term complication. **Table 6** summarizes the most appropriate procedure for the designated category of stenosis.

REFERENCES

1. Shawki S, Sands DR. Anorectal physiology. In: Sands LR, Sands DR, editors. Ambulatory colorectal surgery. 1st edition. New York: Informa Healthcare; 2008. p. 21–44.
2. Gordon PH. Anatomy and Physiology of the Anorectum. In: Fazio VW, Church JM, Delaney CP, editors. Current therapy in colon and rectal surgery. 2nd edition. Philadelphia: Mosby, Elsevier; 2005. p. 1–9.
3. Frenckner B, Euler CV. Influence of pudendal block on the function of the anal sphincters. Gut 1975;16:482–9.
4. Lestar B, Penninckx F, Kerremans R. The composition of anal basal pressure. An in vivo and in vitro study in man. Int J Colorectal Dis 1989;4:118–22.
5. Madalinski M, Kalinowski L. Novel options for the pharmacological treatment of chronic anal fissure—role of botulin toxin. Curr Clin Pharmacol 2009;4:47–52.
6. Bhardwaj R, Vaizey CJ, Boulos PB, et al. Neuromyogenic properties of the internal anal sphincter: therapeutic rationale for anal fissures. Gut 2000;46:861–8.
7. Corning C, Weiss EG. Anal fissure. In: Cameron JL, Cameron AM, editors. Current surgical therapy. 10th edition. Philadelphia: Saunders, Elsevier; 2011. p. 230–2.
8. Altomare DF, Binda GA, Canuti S, et al. The management of patients with primary chronic anal fissure: a position paper. Tech Coloproctol 2011;15:135–41.
9. Sailer M, Bussen D, Debus ES, et al. Quality of life in patients with benign anorectal disorders. Br J Surg 1998;85:1716–9.
10. Jonas M, Scholefield JH. Anal fissure. Gastroenterol Clin North Am 2001;30:167–81.
11. Bailey HR, Beck DE, Billingham RP, et al. A study to determine the nitroglycerin ointment dose and dosing interval that best promote the healing of chronic anal fissures. Dis Colon Rectum 2002;45:1192–9.
12. Scholefield JH, Bock JU, Marla B, et al. A dose finding study with 0.1%, 0.2%, and 0.4% glyceryl trinitrate ointment in patients with chronic anal fissures. Gut 2003;52:264–9.
13. Lock MR, Thomson JP. Fissure-in-ano: the initial management and prognosis. Br J Surg 1977;64:355–8.
14. Costedio M, Cataldo PA. Anal fissures. In: Cameron JL, editor. Current surgical therapy. 9th edition. Philadelphia: Elsevier; 2008. p. 268–71.
15. Graham-Stewart CW, Greenwood RK, Lloyd-Davies RW. A review of 50 patients with fissure in ano. Surg Gynecol Obstet 1961;113:445–8.

16. Martin JD. Postpartum anal fissure. Lancet 1953;1:271–3.
17. Goligher JC. Surgery of the anus, rectum and colon. 3rd edition. London: Ballier and Tindall; 1975.
18. Lund JN, Scholefield JH. Aetiology and treatment of anal fissure. Br J Surg 1996; 83:1335–44.
19. Hananel N, Gordon PH. Re-examination of clinical manifestations and response to therapy of fissure-in-ano. Dis Colon Rectum 1997;40:229–33.
20. Notaras MJ. Anal fissure and stenosis. Surg Clin North Am 1988;68:1427–40.
21. Dykes SL, Madoff RD. Benign anorectal: anal fissure. In: Wolf BG, Fleshman JW, Beck DE, et al, editors. The ASCRS textbook of colon and rectal surgery. New York: Springer; 2007. p. 203–18.
22. American Gastroenterological Association. American Gastroenterological Association medical position statement: diagnosis and care of patients with anal fissure. Gastroenterology 2003;124:233–4.
23. Keighley M, Williams N. Surgery of the anus, rectum, and colon. London: WB Saunders; 1993.
24. Mazier WP. Hemorrhoids, fissures, and pruritus ani. Surg Clin North Am 1994;74: 1277–92.
25. Jensen SL. Diet and other risk factors for fissure-in-ano. Prospective case control study. Dis Colon Rectum 1988;31:770–3.
26. Klosterhalfen B, Vogel P, Rixen H, et al. Topography of the inferior rectal artery: a possible cause of chronic, primary anal fissure. Dis Colon Rectum 1989;32: 43–52.
27. Schouten WR, Briel JW, Auwerda JJ. Relationship between anal pressure and anodermal blood flow. The vascular pathogenesis of anal fissures. Dis Colon Rectum 1994;37:664 9.
28. Schouten WR, Briel JW, Auwerda JJ, et al. Anal fissure: new concepts in pathogenesis and treatment. Scand J Gastroenterol Suppl 1996;218:78–81.
29. Schouten WR, Briel JW, Auwerda JJ, et al. Ischaemic nature of anal fissure. Br J Surg 1996;83:63–5.
30. Cross KL, Massey EJ, Fowler AL, et al. The management of anal fissure: ACPGBI position statement. Colorectal Dis 2008;10(Suppl 3):1–7.
31. Lindsey I, Jones OM, Cunningham C, et al. Chronic anal fissure. Br J Surg 2004; 91:270–9.
32. Schubert MC, Sridhar S, Schade RR, et al. What every gastroenterologist needs to know about common anorectal disorders. World J Gastroenterol 2009;15: 3201–9.
33. Jensen SL. Treatment of first episodes of acute anal fissure: prospective randomised study of lignocaine ointment versus hydrocortisone ointment or warm sitz baths plus bran. Br Med J (Clin Res Ed) 1986;292:1167–9.
34. Sands LR. 0.4% nitroglycerin ointment in the treatment of chronic anal fissure pain: a viewpoint by Laurence R. Sands. Drugs 2006;66:350–2.
35. Lund JN. Nitric oxide deficiency in the internal anal sphincter of patients with chronic anal fissure. Int J Colorectal Dis 2006;21:673–5.
36. Loder PB, Kamm MA, Nicholls RJ, et al. 'Reversible chemical sphincterotomy' by local application of glyceryl trinitrate. Br J Surg 1994;81:1386–9.
37. Kua KB, Kocher HM, Kelkar A, et al. Effect of topical glyceryl trinitrate on anodermal blood flow in patients with chronic anal fissures. ANZ J Surg 2001;71: 548–50.
38. Gorfine SR. Treatment of benign anal disease with topical nitroglycerin. Dis Colon Rectum 1995;38:453–6 [discussion: 456–7].

39. Lund J, Armitage N, Scholefield J. Use of glyceryl trinitrate ointment in the treatment of anal fissure. Br J Surg 1996;83:776–7.
40. Lund J, Scholefield J. A randomized, prospective, double blinded, placebo-controlled trial of glyceryl trinitrate ointment in treatment of anal fissure. Lancet 1997;349:689–93.
41. Bacher H, Mischinger HJ, Werkgartner G, et al. Local nitroglycerin for treatment of anal fissures: an alternative to lateral sphincterotomy? Dis Colon Rectum 1997;40:840–5.
42. Oettle GJ. Glyceryl trinitrate vs. sphincterotomy for treatment of chronic fissure-in-ano: a randomized, controlled trial. Dis Colon Rectum 1997;40:1318–20.
43. Lund JN, Scholefield JH. Glyceryl trinitrate is an effective treatment for anal fissure. Dis Colon Rectum 1997;40:468–70.
44. Kennedy ML, Sowter S, Nguyen H, et al. Glyceryl trinitrate ointment for the treatment of chronic anal fissure: results of a placebo-controlled trial and long-term follow-up. Dis Colon Rectum 1999;42:1000–6.
45. Carapeti EA, Kamm MA, McDonald PJ, et al. Randomised controlled trial shows that glyceryl trinitrate heals anal fissures, higher doses are not more effective, and there is a high recurrence rate. Gut 1999;44:727–30.
46. Altomare DF, Rinaldi M, Milito G, et al. Glyceryl trinitrate for chronic anal fissure–healing or headache? Results of a multicenter, randomized, placebo-controlled, double-blind trial. Dis Colon Rectum 2000;43:174–9 [discussion: 179–81].
47. Zuberi BF, Rajput MR, Abro H, et al. A randomized trial of glyceryl trinitrate ointment and nitroglycerin patch in healing of anal fissures. Int J Colorectal Dis 2000;15:243–5.
48. Pitt J, Williams S, Dawson PM. Reasons for failure of glyceryl trinitrate treatment of chronic fissure-in-ano: a multivariate analysis. Dis Colon Rectum 2001;44:864–7.
49. Skinner SA, Polglase AL, Le CT, et al. Treatment of anal fissure with glyceryl trinitrate in patients referred for surgical management. ANZ J Surg 2001;71:218–20.
50. Gagliardi G, Pascariello A, Altomare DF, et al. Optimal treatment duration of glyceryl trinitrate for chronic anal fissure: results of a prospective randomized multicenter trial. Tech Coloproctol 2010;14:241–8.
51. Perez-Legaz J, Arroyo A, Moya P, et al. Perianal versus endoanal application of glyceryl trinitrate 0.4% ointment in the treatment of chronic anal fissure: results of a randomized controlled trial. Is this the solution to the headaches? Dis Colon Rectum 2012;55:893–9.
52. Griffin N, Acheson AG, Tung P, et al. Quality of life in patients with chronic anal fissure. Colorectal Dis 2004;6:39–44.
53. Perez-Legaz J, Arroyo A, Ruiz-Tovar J, et al. Treatment of chronic anal fissure with topical nitroglycerin ointment 0.4%: a prospective clinical study. Tech Coloproctol 2011;15:475–6.
54. Palazzo FF, Kapur S, Steward M, et al. Glyceryl trinitrate treatment of chronic fissure in ano: one year's experience with 0.5% GTN paste. J R Coll Surg Edinb 2000;45:168–70.
55. Dorfman G, Levitt M, Platell C. Treatment of chronic anal fissure with topical glyceryl trinitrate. Dis Colon Rectum 1999;42:1007–10.
56. Graziano A, Svidler Lopez L, Lencinas S, et al. Long-term results of topical nitroglycerin in the treatment of chronic anal fissures are disappointing. Tech Coloproctol 2001;5:143–7.

57. Carapeti EA, Kamm MA, Phillips RK. Topical diltiazem and bethanechol decrease anal sphincter pressure and heal anal fissures without side effects. Dis Colon Rectum 2000;43:1359–62.
58. Jonas M, Neal KR, Abercrombie JF, et al. A randomized trial of oral vs. topical diltiazem for chronic anal fissures. Dis Colon Rectum 2001;44:1074–8.
59. DasGupta R, Franklin I, Pitt J, et al. Successful treatment of chronic anal fissure with diltiazem gel. Colorectal Dis 2002;4:20–2.
60. Kocher HM, Steward M, Leather AJ, et al. Randomized clinical trial assessing the side-effects of glyceryl trinitrate and diltiazem hydrochloride in the treatment of chronic anal fissure. Br J Surg 2002;89:413–7.
61. Griffin N, Acheson AG, Jonas M, et al. The role of topical diltiazem in the treatment of chronic anal fissures that have failed glyceryl trinitrate therapy. Colorectal Dis 2002;4:430–5.
62. Jonas M, Speake W, Scholefield JH. Diltiazem heals glyceryl trinitrate-resistant chronic anal fissures: a prospective study. Dis Colon Rectum 2002;45:1091–5.
63. Bielecki K, Kolodziejczak M. A prospective randomized trial of diltiazem and glyceryl trinitrate ointment in the treatment of chronic anal fissure. Colorectal Dis 2003;5:256–7.
64. Shrivastava UK, Jain BK, Kumar P, et al. A comparison of the effects of diltiazem and glyceryl trinitrate ointment in the treatment of chronic anal fissure: a randomized clinical trial. Surg Today 2007;37:482–5.
65. Sanei B, Mahmoodieh M, Masoudpour H. Comparison of topical glyceryl trinitrate with diltiazem ointment for treatment of chronic anal fissure. A randomized clinical trial. Ann Ital Chir 2009;80:379–83.
66. Jawaid M, Masood Z, Salim M. Topical diltiazem hydrochloride and glyceryl trinitrate in the treatment of chronic anal fissure. J Coll Physicians Surg Pak 2009; 19:614–7.
67. Ala S, Saeedi M, Hadianamrei R, et al. Topical diltiazem vs. topical glyceryl trinitrate in the treatment of chronic anal fissure: a prospective, randomized, double-blind trial. Acta Gastroenterol Belg 2012;75:438–42.
68. Cook TA, Humphreys MM, McC Mortensen NJ. Oral nifedipine reduces resting anal pressure and heals chronic anal fissure. Br J Surg 1999;86:1269–73.
69. Perrotti P, Bove A, Antropoli C, et al. Topical nifedipine with lidocaine ointment vs. active control for treatment of chronic anal fissure: results of a prospective, randomized, double-blind study. Dis Colon Rectum 2002;45:1468–75.
70. Ansaloni L, Bernabe A, Ghetti R, et al. Oral lacidipine in the treatment of anal fissure. Tech Coloproctol 2002;6:79–82.
71. Ezri T, Susmallian S. Topical nifedipine vs. topical glyceryl trinitrate for treatment of chronic anal fissure. Dis Colon Rectum 2003;46:805–8.
72. Agaoglu N, Cengiz S, Arslan MK, et al. Oral nifedipine in the treatment of chronic anal fissure. Dig Surg 2003;20:452–6.
73. Golfam F, Golfam P, Khalaj A, et al. The effect of topical nifedipine in treatment of chronic anal fissure. Acta Med Iran 2010;48:295–9.
74. Sajid MS, Whitehouse PA, Sains P, et al. Systematic review of the use of topical diltiazem compared with glyceryl trinitrate for the nonoperative management of chronic anal fissure. Colorectal Dis 2013;15:19–26.
75. Sajid MS, Rimple J, Cheek E, et al. The efficacy of diltiazem and glyceryl trinitrate for the medical management of chronic anal fissure: a meta-analysis. Int J Colorectal Dis 2008;23:1–6.
76. Chrysos E, Xynos E, Tzovaras G, et al. Effect of nifedipine on rectoanal motility. Dis Colon Rectum 1996;39:212–6.

77. Mustafa NA, Cengiz S, Turkyilmaz S, et al. Comparison of topical glyceryl trinitrate ointment and oral nifedipine in the treatment of chronic anal fissure. Acta Chir Belg 2006;106:55–8.

78. Antropoli C, Perrotti P, Rubino M, et al. Nifedipine for local use in conservative treatment of anal fissures: preliminary results of a multicenter study. Dis Colon Rectum 1999;42:1011–5.

79. Katsinelos P, Kountouras J, Paroutoglou G, et al. Aggressive treatment of acute anal fissure with 0.5% nifedipine ointment prevents its evolution to chronicity. World J Gastroenterol 2006;12:6203–6.

80. Brisinda G, Cadeddu F, Brandara F, et al. Treating chronic anal fissure with botulinum neurotoxin. Nat Clin Pract Gastroenterol Hepatol 2004;1:82–9.

81. Jost WH, Schimrigk K. Therapy of anal fissure using botulin toxin. Dis Colon Rectum 1994;37:1340.

82. Gui D, Cassetta E, Anastasio G, et al. Botulinum toxin for chronic anal fissure. Lancet 1994;344:1127–8.

83. Maria G, Cassetta E, Gui D, et al. A comparison of botulinum toxin and saline for the treatment of chronic anal fissure. N Engl J Med 1998;338:217–20.

84. Mentes BB, Irkorucu O, Akin M, et al. Comparison of botulinum toxin injection and lateral internal sphincterotomy for the treatment of chronic anal fissure. Dis Colon Rectum 2003;46:232–7.

85. Giral A, Memisoglu K, Gultekin Y, et al. Botulinum toxin injection versus lateral internal sphincterotomy in the treatment of chronic anal fissure: a nonrandomized controlled trial. BMC Gastroenterol 2004;4:7.

86. Arroyo A, Perez F, Serrano P, et al. Surgical versus chemical (botulinum toxin) sphincterotomy for chronic anal fissure: long-term results of a prospective randomized clinical and manometric study. Am J Surg 2005;189:429–34.

87. Massoud BW, Mehrdad V, Baharak T, et al. Botulinum toxin injection versus internal anal sphincterotomy for the treatment of chronic anal fissure. Ann Saudi Med 2005;25:140–2.

88. Iswariah H, Stephens J, Rieger N, et al. Randomized prospective controlled trial of lateral internal sphincterotomy versus injection of botulinum toxin for the treatment of idiopathic fissure in ano. ANZ J Surg 2005;75:553–5.

89. Nasr M, Ezzat H, Elsebae M. Botulinum toxin injection versus lateral internal sphincterotomy in the treatment of chronic anal fissure: a randomized controlled trial. World J Surg 2010;34:2730–4.

90. Brisinda G, Maria G, Bentivoglio AR, et al. A comparison of injections of botulinum toxin and topical nitroglycerin ointment for the treatment of chronic anal fissure. N Engl J Med 1999;341:65–9.

91. De Nardi P, Ortolano E, Radaelli G, et al. Comparison of glycerine trinitrate and botulinum toxin-a for the treatment of chronic anal fissure: long-term results. Dis Colon Rectum 2006;49:427–32.

92. Fruehauf H, Fried M, Wegmueller B, et al. Efficacy and safety of botulinum toxin A injection compared with topical nitroglycerin ointment for the treatment of chronic anal fissure: a prospective randomized study. Am J Gastroenterol 2006;101:2107–12.

93. Brisinda G, Cadeddu F, Brandara F, et al. Randomized clinical trial comparing botulinum toxin injections with 0.2 per cent nitroglycerin ointment for chronic anal fissure. Br J Surg 2007;94:162–7.

94. Festen S, Gisbertz SS, van Schaagen F, et al. Blinded randomized clinical trial of botulinum toxin versus isosorbide dinitrate ointment for treatment of anal fissure. Br J Surg 2009;96:1393–9.

95. Samim M, Twigt B, Stoker L, et al. Topical diltiazem cream versus botulinum toxin a for the treatment of chronic anal fissure: a double-blind randomized clinical trial. Ann Surg 2012;255:18–22.

96. Yiannakopoulou E. Botulinum toxin and anal fissure: efficacy and safety systematic review. Int J Colorectal Dis 2012;27:1–9.

97. Minguez M, Herreros B, Espi A, et al. Long-term follow-up (42 months) of chronic anal fissure after healing with botulinum toxin. Gastroenterology 2002; 123:112–7.

98. Lindsey I, Cunningham C, Jones OM, et al. Fissurectomy-botulinum toxin: a novel sphincter-sparing procedure for medically resistant chronic anal fissure. Dis Colon Rectum 2004;47:1947–52.

99. Baraza W, Boereboom C, Shorthouse A, et al. The long-term efficacy of fissurectomy and botulinum toxin injection for chronic anal fissure in females. Dis Colon Rectum 2008;51:239–43.

100. Jones OM, Ramalingam T, Merrie A, et al. Randomized clinical trial of botulinum toxin plus glyceryl trinitrate vs. botulinum toxin alone for medically resistant chronic anal fissure: overall poor healing rates. Dis Colon Rectum 2006;49: 1574–80.

101. Lysy J, Israelit-Yatzkan Y, Sestiery-Ittah M, et al. Topical nitrates potentiate the effect of botulinum toxin in the treatment of patients with refractory anal fissure. Gut 2001;48:221–4.

102. Maria G, Brisinda G, Bentivoglio AR, et al. Botulinum toxin injections in the internal anal sphincter for the treatment of chronic anal fissure: long-term results after two different dosage regimens. Ann Surg 1998;228:664–9.

103. Brisinda G, Cadeddu F, Brandara F, et al. Botulinum toxin for recurrent anal fissure following lateral internal sphincterotomy. Br J Surg 2008;95:774–8.

104. Lestar B, Penninckx F, Kerremans R. Anal dilatation. Int J Colorectal Dis 1987;2: 167–8.

105. Sohn N, Eisenberg MM, Weinstein MA, et al. Precise anorectal sphincter dilatation—its role in the therapy of anal fissures. Dis Colon Rectum 1992;35: 322–7.

106. Watts JM, Bennett RC, Goligher JC. Stretching of anal sphincters in treatment of fissure-in-ano. Br Med J 1964;2:342–3.

107. Weaver RM, Ambrose NS, Alexander-Williams J, et al. Manual dilatation of the anus vs. lateral subcutaneous sphincterotomy in the treatment of chronic fissure-in-ano. Results of a prospective, randomized, clinical trial. Dis Colon Rectum 1987;30:420–3.

108. Gordon PH, Vasilevsky CA. Symposium on outpatient anorectal procedures. Lateral internal sphincterotomy: rationale, technique and anesthesia. Can J Surg 1985;28:228–30.

109. Lewis TH, Corman ML, Prager ED, et al. Long-term results of open and closed sphincterotomy for anal fissure. Dis Colon Rectum 1988;31:368–71.

110. Khubchandani IT, Reed JF. Sequelae of internal sphincterotomy for chronic fissure in ano. Br J Surg 1989;76:431–4.

111. Melange M, Colin JF, Van Wymersch T, et al. Anal fissure: correlation between symptoms and manometry before and after surgery. Int J Colorectal Dis 1992; 7:108–11.

112. Pernikoff BJ, Eisenstat TE, Rubin RJ, et al. Reappraisal of partial lateral internal sphincterotomy. Dis Colon Rectum 1994;37:1291–5.

113. Garcia-Aguilar J, Belmonte C, Wong WD, et al. Open vs. closed sphincterotomy for chronic anal fissure: long-term results. Dis Colon Rectum 1996;39:440–3.

114. Littlejohn DR, Newstead GL. Tailored lateral sphincterotomy for anal fissure. Dis Colon Rectum 1997;40:1439–42.
115. Hananel N, Gordon PH. Lateral internal sphincterotomy for fissure-in-ano—revisited. Dis Colon Rectum 1997;40:597–602.
116. Nyam DC, Pemberton JH. Long-term results of lateral internal sphincterotomy for chronic anal fissure with particular reference to incidence of fecal incontinence. Dis Colon Rectum 1999;42:1306–10.
117. Argov S, Levandovsky O. Open lateral sphincterotomy is still the best treatment for chronic anal fissure. Am J Surg 2000;179:201–2.
118. Wiley M, Day P, Rieger N, et al. Open vs. closed lateral internal sphincterotomy for idiopathic fissure-in-ano: a prospective, randomized, controlled trial. Dis Colon Rectum 2004;47:847–52.
119. Garg P, Garg M, Menon GR. Long-term continence disturbance after lateral internal sphincterotomy for chronic anal fissure: a systematic review and meta-analysis. Colorectal Dis 2013;15:e104–17.
120. Nelson R. A systematic review of medical therapy for anal fissure. Dis Colon Rectum 2004;47:422–31.
121. Patti R, Guercio G, Territo V, et al. Advancement flap in the management of chronic anal fissure: a prospective study. Updates Surg 2012;64:101–6.
122. Hancke E, Rikas E, Suchan K, et al. Dermal flap coverage for chronic anal fissure: lower incidence of anal incontinence compared to lateral internal sphincterotomy after long-term follow-up. Dis Colon Rectum 2010;53:1563–8.
123. Patel SD, Oxenham T, Praveen BV. Medium-term results of anal advancement flap compared with lateral sphincterotomy for the treatment of anal fissure. Int J Colorectal Dis 2011;26:1211–4.
124. Katdare MV, Ricciardi R. Anal stenosis. Surg Clin North Am 2010;90:137–45 [table of contents].
125. Bonello JC. Who's afraid of the dentate line? The Whitehead hemorrhoidectomy. Am J Surg 1988;156:182–6.
126. Brisinda G, Vanella S, Cadeddu F, et al. Surgical treatment of anal stenosis. World J Gastroenterol 2009;15:1921–8.
127. Milsom JW, Mazier WP. Classification and management of postsurgical anal stenosis. Surg Gynecol Obstet 1986;163:60–4.
128. Khubchandani IT. Anal stenosis. Surg Clin North Am 1994;74:1353–60.
129. Liberman H, Thorson AG. How I do it. Anal stenosis. Am J Surg 2000;179:325–9.
130. Shawki S, Belizon A, Person B, et al. What are the outcomes of reoperative restorative proctocolectomy and ileal pouch-anal anastomosis surgery? Dis Colon Rectum 2009;52:884–90.
131. Sentovich SM. Management of anorectal stricture. In: Cameron JL, Cameron A, editors. Current surgical therapy. 10th edition. Philadelphia: Elsevier; 2011. p. 241–2.
132. Duieb Z, Appu S, Hung K, et al. Anal stenosis: use of an algorithm to provide a tension-free anoplasty. ANZ J Surg 2010;80:337–40.

Modern Management of Hemorrhoidal Disease

Jason F. Hall, MD, MPH[a,b,*]

KEYWORDS

- Hemorrhoids • Nonoperative management • Hemorrhoidectomy
- Internal hemorrhoids • External hemorrhoids • Prolapsing hemorrhoids
- Thrombosed hemorrhoids

KEY POINTS

- Most hemorrhoidal complaints can be managed nonoperatively.
- Symptomatic internal hemorrhoids typically cause rectal bleeding.
- Symptomatic external hemorrhoids typically cause thrombosis and pain.
- Providers should be familiar with several different techniques to address hemorrhoidal complaints.
- Rubber band ligation is generally helpful in addressing hemorrhoidal bleeding that has not improved with nonoperative treatment.
- Excisional hemorrhoidectomy is effective in managing prolapsing or recurrent hemorrhoidal disease.

INTRODUCTION

Complaints secondary to hemorrhoidal disease have been treated by health care providers for at least 4000 years (**Table 1**).[1] John of Ardene (1307–1390), a surgeon in the English Middle Ages, reportedly stated: "The common people call them piles, the aristocracy call them hemorrhoids, the French call them figs—what does it matter so long as you can cure them?"[2] Most hemorrhoidal presentations can be managed nonoperatively. When hemorrhoidal symptoms do not respond to medical therapy, procedural intervention is recommended. A firm grasp of anorectal anatomy is essential for choosing the appropriate method of treatment. This article reviews the anatomy and pathophysiology of hemorrhoidal disease and the most commonly used techniques for the nonoperative and operative palliation of hemorrhoidal complaints.

Disclosures: The author has no relevant disclosures.
[a] Department of Colon and Rectal Surgery, Lahey Clinic, 41 Mall Road, Burlington, MA 01805, USA; [b] Department of Surgery, Tufts University School of Medicine, 145 Harrison Avenue, Boston, MA 02111, USA
* Department of Colon and Rectal Surgery, Lahey Clinic, 41 Mall Road, Burlington, MA 01805.
E-mail address: jason.f.hall@lahey.org

Gastroenterol Clin N Am 42 (2013) 759–772
http://dx.doi.org/10.1016/j.gtc.2013.09.001   **gastro.theclinics.com**
0889-8553/13/$ – see front matter © 2013 Elsevier Inc. All rights reserved.

Table 1
Clinical classification of hemorrhoidal pathology

	Location/Size	Symptoms
First degree	Bulge into anal canal	Painless bleeding
Second degree	Exit the anal canal with defecation Reduce spontaneously	Painless bleeding Pruritus
Third degree	Prolapse from anal canal with defecation Require manual reduction	Painless bleeding Pruritus Mucous/fecal leakage
Fourth degree	Permanent prolapse from anal canal Not reducible	Pain Bleeding Mucous/fecal leakage

ANATOMY AND PATHOPHYSIOLOGY

Hemorrhoids are specialized, vascular cushions located in the anal canal. Hemorrhoids are typically clustered into three anatomically distinct cushions located in the left lateral, right anterolateral, and right posterolateral anal canal (**Fig. 1**). They are found in the submucosal layer and are considered sinusoids because they do not typically have a muscular wall.[3] Hemorrhoids are held in the anal canal by Treitz muscle, a submucosal extension of the conjoined longitudinal ligament. The fibers seem to act as a support lattice not only for hemorrhoids but for other important structures in the anal canal. Some authors have reported a loss of these support structures with aging, perhaps explaining the increased incidence of hemorrhoidal complaints with age.[4]

Hemorrhoidal structures are typically described as internal hemorrhoids or external hemorrhoids. Internal hemorrhoids are proximal to the dentate line and have visceral innervation. For this reason, internal hemorrhoids generally do not present with pain as

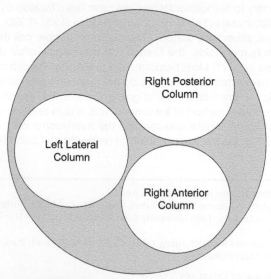

Fig. 1. Classic anatomic relationship of hemorrhoidal columns with patient in prone position.

an initial complaint. More often, patients with internal hemorrhoids complain of painless bleeding. Internal hemorrhoids generally are spanned by the anal transitional zone, and therefore can be covered by columnar, squamous, or basaloid cells. External hemorrhoids are located below the dentate line in the distal third of the anal canal. External hemorrhoids are covered by anoderm (squamous epithelium). Because of their somatic innervation, external hemorrhoids are more likely to present with pain.

Hemorrhoids are thought to enhance anal continence and may contribute 15% to 20% of resting anal canal pressure.[5] They also complete closure of the anus and may enhance control of defecation. Because hemorrhoids have sensory innervation, they also relay important data regarding the quality and composition (gas, liquid, stool) of intrarectal contents.

Because hemorrhoids represent collections of sinusoids, intra-abdominal pressure phenomena are easily manifested. Development of hemorrhoidal disease is likely associated with activities that increase in intra-abdominal pressure. This increase may be secondary to straining, excessive time spent on the toilet, or constipation. Other etiologic factors that can cause hemorrhoidal irritation include diarrhea and dehydration. Women in the third trimester of pregnancy commonly report hemorrhoidal swelling caused by increased intravascular volume and the estrogen sensitivity of hemorrhoidal tissues.

PHYSICAL EXAMINATION

Patients with anorectal complaints should be examined in a comprehensive and systematic fashion. The examination begins with inspection of the perianal skin. Often this is the only examination necessary because the pathology may be evident on the perianal skin. Often thrombosed external hemorrhoids are evident externally and can be identified because they are covered with anoderm. They commonly have a hint of visible clot underneath the surface of the anoderm (**Fig. 2**). These can be differentiated from prolapsed internal hemorrhoids, which are not covered with squamous epithelium, but rather columnar mucosa (**Fig. 3**).

Digital rectal examination can exclude the presence of palpable masses within the anal canal. Valuable information about the tone, contractile strength, and bulk of the anal sphincter mechanism can also be gained through digital examination.

Anoscopy is usually performed to inspect the anal canal mucosa and can often identify thrombosed internal hemorrhoids, fissures, condyloma, and the internal openings of fistula tracts, among other anorectal pathology. Rigid or flexible proctoscopy can evaluate the rectum for more proximal causes of bleeding, such as proctitis or rectal neoplasms.

HEMORRHOIDAL CLASSIFICATION

Hemorrhoids are normal structures and therefore they are only treated if they become symptomatic. They are commonly classified as first-, second-, third-, or fourth-degree hemorrhoids. First degree hemorrhoids simply represent hemorrhoids bulging into the anal canal but not out of the anal canal. Patients with this level of hemorrhoidal disease typically present with painless bleeding. Often this can be recurrent and ephemeral, occurring on a few selected days over the course of months.

Second-degree hemorrhoids are hemorrhoids that prolapse out of the anal canal with defecation but spontaneously reduce. Patients with second-degree hemorrhoids often complain of painless bleeding and perianal itching caused by chronic moisture secreted by the anal canal mucosa.

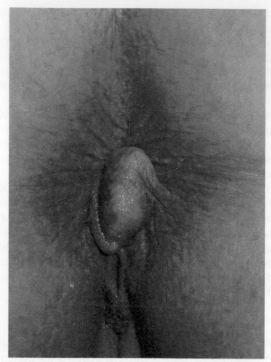

Fig. 2. Classic appearance of a thrombosed external hemorrhoid.

Third-degree hemorrhoids represent hemorrhoids that have prolapsed out of the anal canal and that require manual reduction. Often patients need to reduce the hemorrhoids several times per day or after every bowel movement. Patients with third degree hemorrhoids may report a history of bleeding with defecation; pain (likely caused by local ischemia); and mucus drainage.

Fourth-degree hemorrhoids are commonly referred to as incarcerated hemorrhoids (**Fig. 4**A). In this situation, hemorrhoids are permanently prolapsed outside of the anal canal and cannot be reduced manually. These patients typically present with bleeding

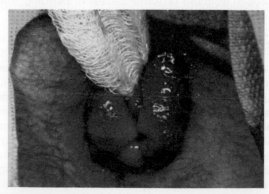

Fig. 3. Classic appearance of prolapsed internal hemorrhoids.

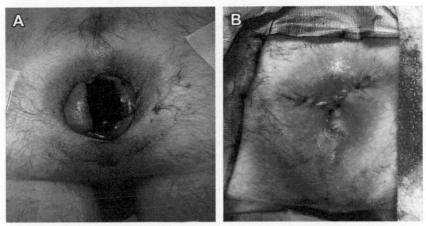

Fig. 4. (A) Grade 4 hemorrhoids. (B) Appearance of the anus after excisional hemorrhoidectomy.

and severe pain or discomfort. Many patients in this category require urgent surgical intervention (**Fig. 4**B).

NONOPERATIVE TREATMENT
Diet and Lifestyle Modifications

First- and second-degree hemorrhoidal disease can generally be treated with nonoperative measures. The primary goal of nonoperative treatment is to reverse the pathophysiologic trigger of hemorrhoidal disease and to reduce symptoms. In most patients, this therapy involves reduction of the intra-abdominal pressure transmitted to the hemorrhoidal vessels during bowel movements. Some patients require adjuncts to investigate unexplained constipation or diarrhea, which may have stimulated hemorrhoidal disease.

The mainstay of nonoperative hemorrhoidal treatment is to increase fiber and water consumption. Several studies document that fiber supplementation can reduce symptoms and bleeding, although this effect may take several weeks to manifest.[6,7] Patients should also be counseled on other lifestyle modifications, including the avoidance of prolonged sitting or straining on the toilet, perianal hygiene, and avoiding triggers of constipation or diarrhea.

Topical and Oral Agents

There are several over-the-counter medications that purport to reduce hemorrhoidal symptoms. Most of these treatment are aimed at providing symptomatic relief rather than truly altering the underlying pathophysiology of the disease. The various preparations include several medications including local anesthetics, vasoactive agents, corticosteroids, antibiotics, and lubricants. Although these treatments are plentiful, data regarding their efficacy are sparse.

Vasoconstrictive medications can be applied to the anal canal to alter the vascular channels supplying the hemorrhoidal tissues. Vasocontriction would theoretically reduce the size and perhaps secretions from hemorrhoidal tissues. One widely available commercial example is Preparation-H (Pfizer). This medication consists of petroleum, mineral oil, and 0.25% phenylephrine.[8]

Other authors have described effective use of nitrates for patients with hemorrhoids and elevated anal canal pressures. Although effective, treatment with topical nitrates was associated with a high incidence of nitrate-associated headaches.[9] Patients with acutely thrombosed internal or external hemorrhoids can sometimes be treated with topical calcium channel blockers, such as nifedipine.[10] These agents likely reduce spasm in the internal sphincter leading to manual or autoreduction of hemorrhoidal tissues.

Calcium dobesilate is a vaosactive drug used in the management of diabetic retinopathy and venous insufficiency. Calcium dobesilate's mechanism of action is thought to be related to decreasing tissue edema by altering vascular permeability and platelet aggregation. Menteş and colleagues[11] randomized 29 patients with symptomatic hemorrhoids to calcium dobesilate and a high-fiber diet or to a high-fiber diet alone. Eighty-six percent of patients treated with calcium dobesilate described cessation of bleeding and improvement in perianal irritation.

Oral flavinoids are also used in the management of hemorrhoidal disease. Flavinoids are a class of venotonic agents that also can alter vascular permeability and reduce tissue edema. Their mechanism of action is unclear but they are used in Europe and Asia for the treatment of hemorrhoidal disease.[11] A recent Cochrane review examined the use of oral phlebotonics including flavinoids and calcium dobesilate in the management of hemorrhoidal disease. Phelobotonics exhibited a remarkable treatment effect in favor of their use when the outcomes of pruritus, bleeding, discharge or leakage, and overall symptom improvement were compared with a control group.[12] These compounds have not gained wide acceptance in the United States.

Office Procedures

Several office procedures are available for the management of symptomatic hemorrhoids. These include infrared coagulation, sclerotherapy, cryotherapy, and rubber band ligation. All of the available techniques rely on tissue destruction and resultant tissue fixation caused by fibrosis.

Rubber band ligation

Rubber band ligation is most often used to treat first- and second-degree hemorrhoids. Certain third-degree hemorrhoids also can be treated with rubber band ligation. A rubber band is placed around the hemorrhoid above the dentate line (**Fig. 5**), causing localized ischemia in the intervening tissue. A portion of the hemorrhoid and the rubber band are passed in several days during defecation. The resultant fibrosis causes fixation of the remaining hemorrhoidal tissues. This prevents further prolapse and bleeding.

Several instruments are commercially available for application of the rubber bands. Suction ligators allow the surgeon to draw in the hemorrhoidal tissue using wall suction. The rubber band is applied with the same device; this approach is advantageous because it allows the surgeon to position an anoscope with the nondominant hand and apply the rubber band with the other hand. Other devices require the operator to grasp the hemorrhoidal pile with forceps and apply the rubber band with the other hand (**Fig. 6**). These types of devices require an assistant to hold the anoscope while the surgeon is applying the rubber band. This technical disadvantage is balanced by the fact that one can usually band more tissue with the latter device.

Hemorrhoidal banding is effective in controlling bleeding in greater than 90% of cases.[13] There are several rare complications of banding. These complications include bleeding, vasovagal response, pain, urinary retention, and rarely pelvic sepsis.

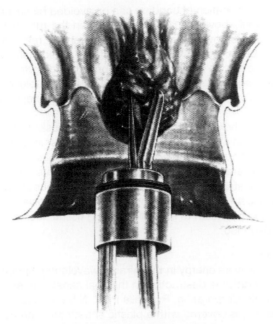

Fig. 5. The internal hemorrhoid is grasped above the dentate line in preparation for placement of a rubber band at that level. (*From* Corman M, Nicholls RJ, Fazio VW, et al. Corman's colon and rectal surgery. 5th edition. Philadelphia: Lippincott Williams & Wilkins; 2004; with permission.)

Rubber bands are commonly placed for intermittent bleeding. Increased bleeding after placement of a rubber band ligature is a frequent complaint and usually self-limited. A few patients may experience delayed bleeding after the rubber band cuts through the hemorrhoidal tissue (7–10 days). This is usually a one-time event; however, rarely the bleeding can be massive and require examination under anesthesia and ligation of the offending hemorrhoidal pile.

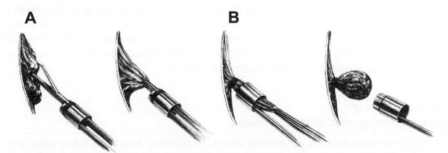

Fig. 6. (*A*) Care must be taken to elevate the hemorrhoidal tissues off of the underlying internal sphincter. (*B*) The rubber band is placed at the base of the hemorrhoidal tissues using the applicator. This ultimately results in ischemic necrosis of the hemorrhoid. Ultimately, this process leads to scarring and fixation of the remaining hemorrhoidal tissues. (*From* Corman M, Nicholls RJ, Fazio VW, et al. Corman's colon and rectal surgery. 5th edition. Philadelphia: Lippincott Williams & Wilkins; 2004; with permission.)

Severe pain as a complication of banding can be avoided by ensuring that the rubber band is placed well above the dentate line. When the rubber band is correctly placed, need for early removal because of pain is rare. If removal of the band is necessary, this can be accomplished with a knife or hook. Removing the band in an office setting can often be accompanied by brisk bleeding from the traumatized hemorrhoidal tissues, and one should be prepared for this troublesome complication. Having a good bedside assistant, suction, and dilute epinephrine available are essential.

A rare complication of hemorrhoidal banding is pelvic sepsis. Pelvic sepsis typically results from incorporation of the underlying internal sphincter into the band, leading to more extensive tissue necrosis and infection. Symptoms of pain, urinary retention, and fever following banding are hallmarks of pelvic sepsis. Patients in whom the diagnosis is suspected should be started on broad-spectrum intravenous antibiotics and urgent examination under anesthesia should be performed. This involves a complete examination of the anus and perineum to exclude evolving tissue necrosis, and all necrotic tissues should be debrided.

Infrared coagulation

Infrared coagulation delivers energy in the infrared wavelength spectrum. This energy causes thrombosis and tissue destruction in the anal canal. The energy delivery system (IRC2100; Redfield Corporation, Rochelle Park, NJ) consists of a light generator and a probe. The probe is covered with a plastic sheath and can be applied through an anoscope. A 1- to 1.5-second pulse delivers the appropriate amount of energy.[14] The operator aims to apply the infrared energy above the dentate line because this area is insensate. When patients are randomized to infrared coagulation versus rubber band ligation, several studies suggest that rubber band ligation is associated with more postprocedural pain.[15,16]

Cryotherapy

Cyrotherapy involves treating the offending hemorrhoidal tissues with a liquid nitrogen probe. This procedure leads to swelling and subsequent necrosis of the surrounding tissues. This technique is time consuming and requires special equipment, and has therefore not gained wide acceptance.[2]

Sclerotherapy

Sclerotherapy typically involves injecting a sclerosing agent into the submucosa. This then causes fibrosis of the surrounding tissues. This technique was first described in the nineteenth century,[17] although now it is typically performed with a phenol-based solution. Sclerotherapy can be effective in the short term, although its effects do not tend to be long lasting.[14] Complications of sclerotherapy include bacteremia, pelvic sepsis, prostatic abscess, and necrotizing fasciitis.[18,19]

OPERATIVE THERAPY
Operative Management of Hemorrhoids

Surgical hemorrhoidectomy is typically offered to patients who have failed office procedures, who have large external hemorrhoids, or who have combined internal/external hemorrhoids that are symptomatic (grades III–IV).[20] Coagulopathic patients requiring definitive control of bleeding are also candidates for operative therapy.[21] Operative approaches to hemorrhoids generally can be grouped into three categories: (1) excisional hemorrhoidectomy, (2) stapled hemorrhoidopexy, and (3) Doppler-guided transanal devascularization.

Preparation for Surgery

We generally use a similar preoperative approach for all of anorectal surgery. Patients self-administer an enema on the morning of surgery. Mechanical bowel preparation is seldom necessary unless we are planning concomitant colonoscopy.

Although there are several anesthetic options including general and spinal anesthesia, we generally use local anesthesia or sedation. Patients are usually sedated with propofol and/or midazolam. We find this approach facilitates faster recovery and discharge.[22]

Proper positioning of the patient is essential in anorectal surgery. We most commonly use the prone-jackknife position. The buttocks are retracted laterally with tape for better exposure. The lithotomy or lateral decubitus positions are also viable options based on surgeon experience and comfort level.

Excisional Hemorrhoidectomy

Excisional hemorrhoidectomy can be broadly classified into closed (or Ferguson) type, open (or Milligan-Morgan) type, circumferential, or Whitehead type. The Ferguson and Milligan-Morgan techniques of hemorrhoidectomy are essentially the same and only differ on whether the anal mucosa and anoderm are reapproximated after ligation of the hemorrhoidal pedicle.

Division of tissues during excisional hemorrhoidectomy can be accomplished by a variety of means, including a scalpel, scissors, monopolar cauterization, bipolar energy, and ultrasonic devices.[23–25] The available literature does not bear out any advantage of any particular approach.[26,27] Surgeons should be familiar with several different techniques and approaches.

Ferguson

Ferguson or closed hemorrhoidectomy is the most common form of hemorrhoidectomy performed in the United States.[20,28] This type of hemorrhoidectomy is performed by using a hemostat or Kelly clamp to tent up the external hemorrhoid at the anal verge (**Fig. 7**A). A curvilinear incision is made from the distal end (close to the anoderm) to the proximal portion of the hemorrhoid. It is important to have a long smooth incision for proper closure and to avoid "dog ears." The hemorrhoidal tissue is then dissected free from the underlying sphincter muscles (see **Fig. 7**B). During this portion of the case it is essential to stay in the submucosal plane. Dissecting outside of this plane either leads to excessive bleeding if one is too close to the hemorrhoidal column, or injury to

A   **B**

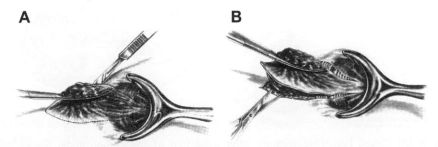

Fig. 7. (*A*) Closed hemorrhoidectomy: a hemostat or Kelly clamp to tent up the external hemorrhoid at the anal verge. (*B*) Closed hemorrhoidectomy: the hemorrhoidal tissue is then dissected free from the underlying sphincter muscles. (*From* Corman M, Nicholls RJ, Fazio VW, et al. Corman's colon and rectal surgery. 5th edition. Philadelphia: Lippincott Williams & Wilkins; 2004; with permission.)

internal sphincter if one is too close to the internal sphincter. Generally, if the dissection is performed correctly a healthy sphincter muscle can be identified at the base of the dissection (**Fig. 8**A). After the base of the hemorrhoid is reached, the pedicle of the hemorrhoid is ligated and the hemorrhoidal tissue is amputated. One of the stitches used to ligate the pedicle should be left long because this suture can be used to close the wound in a running fashion (see **Fig. 8**B). As the stitch is run toward the anoderm small bites of the underlying muscle are taken to obliterate the dead space. This stitch is also locked to ensure hemostasis. Once the anoderm is reached, a simple running stitch is used.

Milligan-Morgan or open hemorrhoidectomy

This technique was described by Milligan and Morgan, and is more commonly performed in the United Kingdom.[20,29] The steps are essentially the same as a Ferguson hemorrhoidectomy with the exception that the hemorhhoidectomy wound is not closed. Several studies have examined the outcomes of open and closed approaches to hemorrhoidectomy in patients with grade 3 and 4 disease. A closed technique was associated with less pain and better wound healing.[30,31]

Whitehead procedure

The general concept behind a Whitehead hemorrhoidectomy is the circumferential excision of hemorrhoidal tissues followed by advancement of the anal canal mucosa to close the defect. Rectangular or trapezoidal flaps are developed in the distal anal canal. A similar flap is developed more cephalad that contains the hemorrhoidal tissue. The hemorrhoidal tissue is excised, and more distal flap is advanced up into the anal canal. This flap is often pexied to the internal sphincter for added security. Finally, the flap is anastomosed to the mucosa above.[32] The procedure is not commonly performed because of its relative complexity compared with excisional hemorrhoidectomy, but also because of the potential long-term complications, especially anal ectropion. There have been several modifications of the procedure to improve operative results.[33–35]

Outcomes of excisional hemorrhoidectomy

A recent meta-analysis found that the long-term outcomes of excisional hemorrhoidectomy were superior to those of office procedures. Other authors have demonstrated that when compared with rubber band ligation excisional hemorrhoidectomy is more effective at achieving complete remission of hemorrhoidal symptoms.[36]

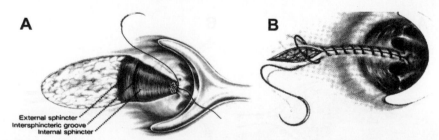

Fig. 8. (*A*) Closed hemorrhoidectomy: after dissection of the hemorrhoidal tissues, the sphincter muscles can be visualized. In the open or Milligan-Morgan technique the incision is left open to granulate through secondary intention. (*B*) Closed hemorrhoidectomy: the wound is closed in a running fashion. (*From* Corman M, Nicholls RJ, Fazio VW, et al. Corman's colon and rectal surgery. 5th edition. Philadelphia: Lippincott Williams & Wilkins; 2004; with permission.)

Patients undergoing excisional hemorrhoidectomy are less likely to require multiple treatments. Excisional hemorrhoidectomy had higher associations with certain complications, such as anal stenosis and postoperative hemorrhage. Excisional hemorrhoidectomy was also associated with an increased incidence of incontinence to flatus, although this result did not reach statistical significance.[36]

Stapled Hemorrhoidopexy

Stapled hemorrhoidopexy was first described as a treatment of mucosal prolapse. Subsequently its use was expanded to the treatment of hemorrhoids.[37,38] The procedure is most useful for the treatment of bleeding and/or prolapsing internal hemorrhoids in patients with relatively confluent/circumferential disease. It has no effect on external hemorrhoids and therefore its use is somewhat limited.

A circular anal dilator is sutured to the perianal skin to secure it in place. During this process the internal hemorrhoidal component is maximally reduced. A purse-string suture is placed 2 to 4 cm above the dentate line, at the base of the hemorrhoidal columns. Correct placement of this suture is critical to prevent placement of the staple line too close to the dentate line, which can result in chronic pain (**Fig. 9**). It is also essential that the purse-string be placed in the submucosal layer. If stitches are placed too deep, one can cause injury to the internal sphincter resulting in increased rates of fecal incontinence.[39,40]

The stapler head is inserted through the purse-string and secured. The stapler is closed while maintaining moderate tension on the purse-string. The stapler is then fired and opened revealing a staple line above the hemorrhoidal tissue. Although some hemorrhoid tissue may be included in the segment of mucosa that is excised, stapled hemorrhoidectomy functions to prevent prolapse of the hemorrhoids by pexying them in the anal canal.

Outcomes of stapled hemorrhoidopexy

Two recent meta-analyses demonstrated no significant differences between stapled hemorrhoidopexy and conventional hemorrhoidectomy when the outcomes of

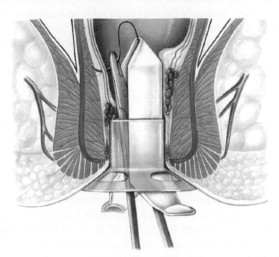

Fig. 9. Stapled hemorrhoidopexy: a pursestring is placed 2 to 4 cm above the dentate line. A specialized stapler is used to then remove redundant hemorrhoidal tissues and pexy the remaining hemorrhoids. (*From* Sardinha TC, Corman ML. Hemorrhoids. Surg Clin North Am 2002;82(6):1153–67; with permission.)

urgency, pruritus, and pain were examined. The stapled technique was also associated with a higher chance of long-term recurrence.[41,42] Although stapled hemorrhoidopexy is associated with several unique complications (ie, rectovaginal fistula, staple line bleeding, chronic pain), overall complication rates are similar to those of excisional hemorrhoidectomy. A meta-analysis of almost 2000 patients found the complication rates to be 20.2% for stapled hemorrhoidopexy versus 25.2% for conventional hemorrhoidectomy ($P = .06$).[42]

Doppler-Guided Transanal Hemorrhoid Devascularization

This technique involves suture ligation of each hemorrhoidal column without resection. The feeding vessels of each hemorrhoidal column are identified using a Doppler probe. This technique has been marketed as a less painful alternative to excisional hemorrhoidectomy.

The transanal hemorrhoid devascularization kit includes a patented anoscope. The anoscope is assembled and inserted into the anal canal. The anoscope is used to identify the signal of artery supplying each hemorrhoidal column, usually at the top of the hemorrhoidal column. Once the artery is identified, it is then ligated using a 0 Vicryl suture. The anoscope and Doppler are then used to confirm the disappearance of the arterial signal. The same stitch is then used to oversew the hemorrhoidal column.[43]

Outcomes of Doppler-guided transanal hemorrhoid devascularization
Doppler-guided or -assisted hemorrhoidal ligation has been reported to be effective in 90% of patients, with recurrence rates ranging from 10% to 15%.[44-46] Other authors found that recurrences are more common when this technique is applied to grade IV hemorrhoids.[47]

SUMMARY

Symptomatic hemorrhoids are a commonly occurring problem. There are a variety of surgical and nonoperative options for management of hemorrhoidal disease. Grade 1 and 2 hemorrhoids can generally be managed with nonoperative measures. Grade 3 and 4 hemorrhoids are generally managed with procedure interventions. The experienced anorectal surgeon should have a variety of techniques at her or his disposal.

REFERENCES

1. Parks AG. De haemorrhois. A study in surgical history. Guys Hosp Rep 1955;104: 135–56.
2. Hulme-Moir M, Bartolo DC. Disorders of the anorectum. Gastroenterol Clin North Am 2001;30:183–97.
3. Thomson WH. The nature of haemorrhoids. Br J Surg 1975;62:542–52.
4. Haas PA, Fox TA Jr. Age-related changes and scar formations of perianal connective tissue. Dis Colon Rectum 1980;23:160–9.
5. Lestar B, Pennickx F, Kerremans R. The composition of anal basal pressure. An in vivo and in vitro study in man. Int J Colorectal Dis 1989;4:118–22.
6. Alonso-Coello P, Mills E, Heels-Ansdell D, et al. Fiber for the treatment of hemorrhoids complications: a systematic review and metaanalysis. Am J Gastroenterol 2006;101:181–8.
7. Moesgaard F, Nielsen ML, Hansen JB, et al. High fiber diet reduces bleeding and pain in patients with hemorrhoids: a double-blind trial of Vi-Siblin. Dis Colon Rectum 1982;25:454–6.

8. Lohsiriwat V. Hemorrhoids: from basic pathophysiology to clinical management. World J Gastroenterol 2012;18(17):2009–17.
9. Tjandra JJ, Tan JJ, Lim JF, et al. Rectogesic (glyceryl trinitrate 0.2%) ointment relieves symptoms of haemorrhoids associated with high resting anal canal pressures. Colorectal Dis 2007;9:457–63.
10. Perrotti P, Antropoli C, Molino D, et al. Conservative treatment of acute thrombosed external hemorrhoids with topical nifedipine. Dis Colon Rectum 2001;44: 405–9.
11. Menteş BB, Görgül A, Tatlicioğlu E, et al. Efficacy of calcium dobesilate in treating acute attacks of hemorrhoidal disease. Dis Colon Rectum 2001;44:1489–95.
12. Perera N, Liolitsa D, Iype S, et al. Phlebotonics for haemorrhoids. Cochrane Database Syst Rev 2012;(8):CD004322.
13. Su MY, Chiu CT, Wu CS, et al. Endoscopic hemorrhoidal ligation of symptomatic internal hemorrhoids. Gastrointest Endosc 2003;58:871–4.
14. Halverson A. Hemorrhoids. Clin Colon Rectal Surg 2007;20(2):77–85.
15. Poen AC, Felt-Bersma RJ, Cuesta MA, et al. A randomized controlled trial of rubber band ligation versus infra-red coagulation in the treatment of internal haemorrhoids. Eur J Gastroenterol Hepatol 2000;12(5):535–9.
16. Marques CF, Nahas SC, Nahas CS, et al. Early results of the treatment of internal hemorrhoid disease by infrared coagulation and elastic banding: a prospective randomized cross-over trial. Tech Coloproctol 2006;10(4):312–7.
17. Goligher JC. Surgery of the anus, rectum and colon. 4th edition. London: Bailliere Tindall; 1980. p. 93–135.
18. Guy RJ, Seow-Choen F. Septic complications after treatment of haemorrhoids. Br J Surg 2003;90:147–56.
19. Adami B, Eckardt VF, Suermann RB, et al. Bacteremia after proctoscopy and hemorrhoidal injection sclerotherapy. Dis Colon Rectum 1981;24:373 4.
20. Rivadeneira DE, Steele SR, Ternent C, et al, on behalf of the Standards Practice Task Force of The American Society of Colon and Rectal Surgeons. Practice parameters for the management of hemorrhoids (revised 2010). Dis Colon Rectum 2011;54(9):1059–64.
21. Singer M. Hemorrhoids. In: Beck DE, Roberts PL, Saclarides TJ, et al, editors. The ASCRS textbook of colon and rectal surgery. 2nd edition. New York: Springer; 2011. p. 175–202.
22. Read TE, Henry SE, Hovis RM, et al. Prospective evaluation of anesthetic technique for anorectal surgery. Dis Colon rectum 2002;45(11):1553–8.
23. Gencosmanoglu R, Sad O, Koc D, et al. Hemorrhoidectomy: open or closed technique? A prospective, randomized clinical trial. Dis Colon Rectum 2002;45:70–5.
24. Arbman G, Krook H, Haapaniemi S. Closed vs. open hemorrhoidectomy—is there any difference? Dis Colon Rectum 2000;43:31–4.
25. Abo-hashem AA, Sarhan A, Aly AM. Harmonic scalpel compared with bipolar electro-cautery hemorrhoidectomy: a randomized controlled trial. Int J Surg 2010;8:243–7.
26. Chung CC, Ha JP, Tai YP, et al. Double-blind, randomized trial comparing Harmonic scalpel hemorrhoidectomy, bipolar scissors hemorrhoidectomy, and scissors excision: ligation technique. Dis Colon Rectum 2002;45:789–94.
27. Nienhuijs S, de Hingh I. Conventional versus LigaSure hemorrhoidectomy for patients with symptomatic hemorrhoids. Cochrane Database Syst Rev 2009;(1):CD006761.
28. Ferguson JA, Mazier WP, Ganchrow MI, et al. The closed technique of hemorrhoidecomy. Surgery 1971;70(3):480–4.

29. Milligan ET, Morgan CN, Jones LE. Surgical anatomy of the anal canal and the operative treatment of hemorrhoids. Lancet 1937;2:119–24.
30. You SY, Kim SH, Chung CS, et al. Open vs. closed hemorrhoidectomy. Dis Colon Rectum 2005;48(1):108–13.
31. Sanchez C, Chinn BT. Hemorrhoids. Clin Colon Rectal Surg 2011;24(1):5–13, 23.
32. Whitehead W. The surgical treatment of haemorrhoids. Br Med J 1882;1(1101): 148–50.
33. Burchell MC, Thow GB, Manson RR. A "modified Whitehead" hemorrhoidectomy. Dis Colon Rectum 1976;19:225–32.
34. Barrios G, Khubchandani M. Whitehead operation revisited. Dis Colon Rectum 1979;22:330–2.
35. Khubchandani M. Results of Whitehead operation. Dis Colon Rectum 1984;27: 730–2.
36. Shanmugam V, Thaha MA, Rabindranath KS, et al. Systematic review of randomized trials comparing rubber band ligation with excisional haemorrhoidectomy. Br J Surg 2005;92(12):1481–7.
37. Pescatori M, Favetta U, Dedola S, et al. Transanal stapled excision for rectal mucosal prolapse. Tech coloproctol 1997;1:96–8.
38. Longo A. Treatment of hemorrhoid disease by reduction of mucosa and hemorrhoid prolapse with a circular-suturing device: a new procedure. In: Proceedings of the 6th World Congress of Endoscopic Surgery. Rome (Italy): 1998. p. 777–84.
39. Ng KH, Chew MH, Eu WK. Modified stapled haemorrhoidectomy: a suggested improved technique. ANZ J Surg 2008;78:394–7.
40. Pigot F, Dao-Quang M, Castinel A, et al. Low haemorrhoidopexy staple line does not improve results and increases risk for incontinence. Tech Coloproctol 2006; 10:329–33.
41. Nisar PJ, Acheson AG, Neal KR, et al. Stapled hemorrhoidopexy compared with conventional hemorrhoidectomy: systematic review of randomized controlled trials. Dis Colon Rectum 2004;47:1837–45.
42. Tjandra JJ, Chan MK. Systematic review on the procedure for prolapse and hemorrhoids (stapled hemorrhoidopexy). Dis Colon Rectum 2007;50:878–92.
43. Morinaga K, Hasuda K, Ikeda T. Novel therapy for internal hemorrhoids: ligation of the hemorrhoidal artery with a newly devised instrument (Moricorn) in conjunction with a Doppler Flowmeter. Am J Gastroenterol 1995;90(4):610–3.
44. Ratto C, Donisi L, Parello A, et al. Evaluation of transanal hemorrhoidal dearterialization as a minimally invasive therapeutic approach to hemorrhoids. Dis Colon Rectum 2010;53:803–11.
45. Felice C, Privitera A, Ellul E, et al. Doppler-guided hemorrhoidal artery ligation: an alternative to hemorrhoidectomy. Dis Colon Rectum 2005;48:2090–3.
46. Faucheron JL, Gangner Y. Doppler-guided hemorrhoidal artery ligation for the treatment of symptomatic hemorrhoids: early and three-year follow-up results in 100 consecutive patients. Dis Colon Rectum 2008;51:945–9.
47. Giordano P, Overton J, Madeddu F, et al. Transanal hemorrhoidal dearterialization: a systematic review. Dis Colon Rectum 2009;52:1665–71.

Anal Abscess and Fistula

Erica B. Sneider, MD[a], Justin A. Maykel, MD[b],*

KEYWORDS

- Anal abscess • Anal fistula • Fistulizing Crohn disease • Fistulotomy
- LIFT procedure • Endorectal advancement flap

KEY POINTS

- Anal abscess is a relatively common condition that results from an infection in the perianal crypts and glands.
- Anal fistulas can develop following abscess formation and can involve variable amounts of the internal and external anal sphincters.
- Most abscesses and fistulas can be diagnosed by history and physical examination, but complex and recurrent infections may require imaging, such as ultrasound, computed tomography scan, or magnetic resonance imaging.
- Successful treatment of anal fistulas mandates a balance between wound healing and maintenance of continence.
- The most common surgical procedures used to treat simple and complex fistulas include fistulotomy, fistulectomy, fibrin glue, plug placement, LIFT procedure, and endorectal advancement flap.

INTRODUCTION

Benign anorectal diseases, such as anal abscesses and fistula, are commonly seen by primary care physicians, gastroenterologists, emergency physicians, general surgeons, and colorectal surgeons. A thorough understanding of the pathophysiology of each of these conditions is necessary to help guide appropriate treatment. The goals of this article are to review the pathophysiology, presentation, diagnosis, and treatment of both anal abscesses and fistulas in the context of the current literature.

ANAL ANATOMY

A comprehensive appreciation of anal anatomy establishes a framework for understanding the pathophysiology of anal abscess and fistula. The surgical anal canal is

Disclosures: The authors have no disclosures.
[a] Department of Surgery, University of Massachusetts Medical School, 55 Lake Avenue North, Worcester, MA 01655, USA; [b] Division of Colon and Rectal Surgery, Department of Surgery, University of Massachusetts Medical School, 67 Belmont Street, Worcester, MA 01605, USA
* Corresponding author.
E-mail address: maykelj@ummhc.org

Gastroenterol Clin N Am 42 (2013) 773–784
http://dx.doi.org/10.1016/j.gtc.2013.08.003
0889-8553/13/$ – see front matter © 2013 Elsevier Inc. All rights reserved.

gastro.theclinics.com

2 to 4 cm in length, beginning at the anorectal junction and ending at the anal verge (**Fig. 1**). The upper portion of the anal canal is composed of columnar endothelium and the lower portion of the anal canal is composed of squamous epithelium. The transition between these 2 distinct areas of the anal canal occurs at the dentate or pectinate line. The dentate line is surrounded by longitudinal mucosal folds, called columns of Morgagni. Each fold contains anal crypts and each crypt contains between 3 and 12 anal glands.[1,2] The distribution of the glands is not uniform; most of the glands lie in the anterior position of the anal canal, with only a few in the posterior midline.

ANAL ABSCESS

Anal abscesses commonly occur in healthy individuals, but they also occur in patients with inflammatory conditions, such as Crohn disease.[3] The incidence of anorectal abscess in the United States is estimated to be approximately 68,000 to 96,000 cases per year.[4] Anal abscesses are seen 2 times more frequently in men than in women.[4,5]

There have been multiple theories addressing the causes of anorectal abscesses, while most focus on infection within the anal glands.[4] This "cryptoglandular theory" was introduced by Eisenhammer in 1956 and is now widely accepted.[5–8] The theory was developed on the principle of obstruction, in which an individual gland becomes impacted with debris and infection and abscess formation occurs.[3] Because the crypt glands penetrate the anal sphincter complex to varying degrees, the infection and abscess follows the path of least resistance, and the abscess accumulates wherever the gland terminates.[3]

Anorectal abscesses are classified based on their location in relation to the anal sphincters (**Fig. 2**). *Perianal abscesses* are the most common and are superficial infections that extend between the internal and external sphincter and reach the anal verge. If the abscess penetrates the external anal sphincter, it becomes an *ischiorectal*

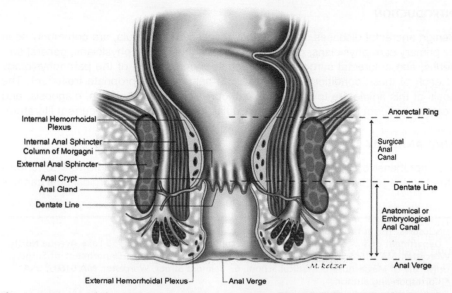

Fig. 1. Anatomy of the anal canal. (*From* Jorge JMN, Habr-Gama A. Anatomy and embryology. In: Beck DE, Roberts PL, Saclarides TJ, et al, editors. The ASCRS Textbook of Colon and Rectal Surgery. New York: Springer; 2011; with kind permission from Springer Science and Business Media.)

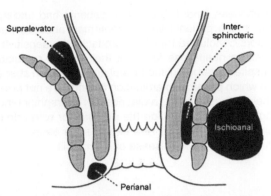

Fig. 2. Classification of anorectal abscesses. (*From* Vasilevsky CA. Fistula-in-ano and abcess. In: Beck DE, Wexner SD, editors. Fundamentals of anorectal surgery. London: WB Saunders; 1998; with permission.)

abscess. Intersphincteric abscesses are infections in the potential space between the internal and external sphincters. When the abscess extends cephalad along the rectal wall above the levators, it is a *supralevator abscess.* A deep postanal abscess extending into either or both ischiorectal fossa is termed a *horseshoe abscess.*[3,4]

SYMPTOMS

Most patients with an anal abscess present with pain. If the abscess is low (such as perianal or ischiorectal abscess) then the pain is often associated with other complaints, including swelling and redness. High abscesses (such as supralevator abscess) do not extend to the sensate perianal tissues and are less likely to present with swelling or redness. These abscesses are more likely to be associated with systemic symptoms, such as fever and malaise.[4]

DIAGNOSIS

Most patients with an anal abscess can be diagnosed clinically on physical examination evidenced by erythema, warmth, tenderness on palpation, induration, and fluctuance, which are the most common physical findings.[9] Patients with these findings often will not tolerate a rectal examination and a digital rectal examination should be deferred in the acute setting because of the low likelihood of providing additional information. Conversely, if there are no signs of infection (such as erythema, edema, tenderness to palpation, or fluctuance) that suggest a perianal or ischiorectal abscess, a supralevator or intersphincteric abscess should be considered. Severe pain and local induration found on digital rectal examination may help make the diagnosis. The differential diagnosis for anal abscesses includes anal fissure, thrombosed external hemorrhoids, malignancy, sexually transmitted diseases, proctitis, cellulitis, and levator muscle spasm.[4] When digital examination is impossible or the infection is extensive, examination under anesthesia (EUA) is necessary to identify the site of infection and drainage can be performed in the same setting.

Radiographic imaging, such as ultrasound, computed tomography (CT) or magnetic resonance imaging (MRI), is rarely necessary to make the diagnosis of anal abscess, and should be reserved for complex cases, as seen with Crohn disease or recurrent infections.[5,9] Caliste and colleagues[9] studied 1000 patients who were diagnosed with anal or rectal abscess, and 113 of these patients had undergone a CT scan. Twenty-six (23%) of these patients with a confirmed abscess had a negative CT scan. The investigators concluded that CT scan lacks the sensitivity in identification of perirectal abscess, as nearly one-fourth of their patient population had negative CT scan imaging despite undergoing successful drainage of an abscess by a surgeon. In complex cases in which physical examination findings are not present or equivocal, a CT scan can be helpful in confirming a diagnosis of intersphincteric or suprasphincteric abscess. Imaging may also provide the practitioner with additional information used to guide management for these rare cases, such as intra-abdominal findings consistent with inflammatory bowel disease or diverticulitis.

TREATMENT

Treatment of anal abscesses requires incision and drainage.[5,10] A potential consequence of draining an anal abscess (either by incision and drainage or spontaneous) is the risk of fistula formation in the future, which ranges from 5% to 83%.[11] One hypothesis for the development of a fistula following incision and drainage of an anal abscess involves insufficient drainage of the abscess resulting in persistent chronic infection and the formation of a nonhealing tract that matures as a fistula.[11]

Most patients with perianal or ischiorectal abscesses can be treated in the outpatient setting, whereas patients with more complex (loculated or large ischiorectal, intersphincteric, supralevator, or horseshoe) abscesses may benefit from EUA and drainage in an operating room under anesthesia. Certain patients with anxiety or severe pain may not be suitable candidates for bedside procedures. Following adequate incision and drainage where there are no signs of cellulitis, antibiotics are not necessary unless the patient has other medical comorbidities, such as diabetes mellitus or immunosuppression.[11,12] Sozener and colleagues[11] performed a multicenter, double-blinded, placebo-controlled randomized trial evaluating 151 patients with anorectal abscesses to determine if antibiotic use after adequate incision and drainage helped prevent future fistula formation. At 1-year follow-up, 45 (30%) patients developed an anal fistula. The rate of fistula formation was significantly higher in the group treated with antibiotics and drainage than the placebo, leading to the conclusion that antibiotic usage did not decrease the rate of fistula formation. Multiple logistic regression demonstrated that the risk of fistula formation increased eightfold in patients with ischiorectal abscesses and threefold in patients with intersphincteric abscesses compared with perianal abscesses.

Previous studies have shown that risk factors for recurrence of anal abscesses include Crohn disease, diabetes mellitus, and ischiorectal location.[13,14] A more recent study in 2010 by Yano and colleagues[15] found that patients with diabetes mellitus and ischiorectal abscesses were not at increased risk for recurrence of anal abscess. Interestingly, the investigators also studied body mass index (BMI) and found that patients with morbid obesity are not at increased risk for recurrence of anal abscess either.

The decision of whether or not to perform a fistulotomy during the original incision and drainage of the anal abscess has been debated in the literature.[10] In a randomized clinical trial, Oliver and colleagues[10] compared simple drainage of anorectal abscesses with and without fistula track treatment to evaluate the effectiveness and morbidity of both operations in the management of acute anal sepsis. Two hundred patients were included in the study: 100 randomized to the group that underwent drainage and treatment of the fistula, whereas the other 100 patients had only abscess drainage performed. At 1-year follow-up, the investigators found that drainage of anal abscess with fistulotomy if a fistula track was present can be safely performed in cases of subcutaneous, intersphincteric, or low transsphincteric fistula with a minimal recurrence rate (5%), compared with 29% recurrence rate in patients treated with drainage alone.

Onaca and colleagues[16] studied 500 consecutive patients with perirectal abscess requiring incisional drainage. Forty-eight (9.6%) patients required early reoperation and 4 patients required a second operation within 2 to 8 days; the reoperation rate was 7.6%. The most common pattern of operative failure leading to reoperation was inadequate drainage either due to inadequate incision and drainage at the initial operation or premature closure of the skin edges over the abscess cavity. Half of all horseshoe ischiorectal abscesses were associated with a failed drainage procedure due to unrecognized additional loculations.[16] This finding highlights the importance of a thorough examination that can sometimes only be accomplished under anesthesia with deliberate probing and drainage of any existing loculations followed by fastidious local wound care.

Drainage of anal abscesses can be performed in the emergency room, outpatient setting, or in the operating room.[12] For superficial abscesses, such as perianal abscesses, drainage in the office or emergency room is entirely feasible. Local anesthesia, such as 1% lidocaine with epinephrine (and bupivacaine for extended analgesia), can be injected subcutaneously into the area affected by the abscess to provide local anesthesia for the skin.[17] Care is taken to adequately anesthetize the area surrounding the abscess without injecting directly into the abscess cavity. A scalpel is used to make an incision, either cruciate or elliptical, over the area of fluctuance. Once in the abscess cavity, any loculations can be broken up using a Hemostat or even a finger. To maintain hemostasis and prevent the skin from closing prematurely, the wound can be packed with either the end of a gauze sponge or a wick. The packing can be removed in 24 hours. We recommend sitz baths following incision and drainage for local cleansing and patient comfort.

If the abscess is more complicated, drainage should be performed in the operating room under general anesthesia or conscious sedation and local anesthesia.[12] Position of the patient is dependent on the location of the abscess and surgeon preference. Examination under anesthesia can be performed to identify the site of infection. The area of fluctuance or induration can be palpated directly or an internal or external opening is visualized with purulent drainage. Needle aspiration can be used to localize the abscess cavity if more deep and difficult to palpate and an incision can be made following the trajectory of the needle.

COMPLICATIONS

Consequences of anal abscess include recurrence, sepsis, and fistula formation. Recurrence is thought to be secondary to insufficient drainage and may be more common when drainage is delayed. Complications related to the abscess drainage procedure are similar to those described for other anorectal procedures, most commonly postoperative bleeding and urinary retention.[5]

FISTULA

Anal fistulas occur with an incidence of 5.5 per 100,000 women and 12.1 per 100,000 men.[18] Fistulas can occur at any age but the average age is 39 years.[18] Perianal fistulizing disease affects up to 30% of patients with Crohn disease.[19] A fistula is defined as an abnormal communication between 2 epithelialized surfaces; anal fistula represents a communication between the anorectal canal and the perianal skin.[20] Similar to the development of anal abscesses, the cryptoglandular theory is also thought to play a role in the formation of anal fistula. It is thought that all fistulas develop as the result of an anal abscess but not all anal abscesses lead to fistula formation.[18,20]

Fistulas are classified based on their relationship to the anal sphincter complex (**Fig. 3**). The Parks classification system for fistulas divides them into 5 types: submucosal, intersphincteric, transsphincteric (high and low), suprasphincteric, and extrasphincteric.[7] Submucosal fistulas originate at an infected crypt at the level of the dentate line. Because these fistulas do not involve the sphincter muscles, they are the most simple to treat, as fistulotomy does not require sphincter division. Intersphincteric fistulas cross through the internal sphincter and exit through the intersphincteric plane without involving the external sphincter muscle, making treatment by fistulotomy feasible without high rates of incontinence. The trajectory of transsphincteric fistulas that span the internal and external sphincter muscles predisposes patients to higher rates of incontinence following fistulotomy. Suprasphincteric fistulas originate at the dentate line and cross above the external sphincter and exit onto the perianal skin through the ischiorectal fossa. Extrasphincteric fistulas are extremely rare and do not involve the sphincter complex as they pass through the rectal wall and through the ischiorectal fossa to the perianal skin. Each of these fistula types can be associated with a high blind tract and can be associated with malignancy, rare infections, and inflammatory disorders.[3]

Goodsall's rule states that an external opening located posterior to an imaginary horizontal line across the anus should have a track that follows a curvilinear course to the posterior midline of the anus. This relates to the fact that posterior glands tend to lie in the posterior midline. External openings anterior to the line should course

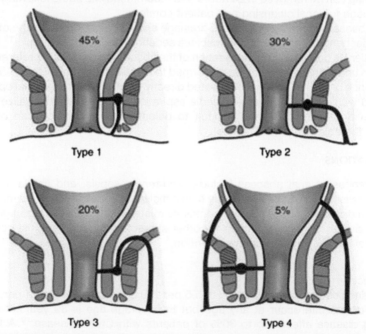

Fig. 3. Fistula classification: type 1, intersphincteric; type 2, transsphincteric; type 3, suprasphincteric; type 4, extrasphincteric. (*From* Parks AG, Gordon PH, Hardcastle JD. A classification of fistula in ano. Br J Surg 1976;63:1–2; with permission.)

in a radial pattern directly toward the anal canal.[17,20] Although often taught to medical students and residents, the predictive accuracy of this "rule" remains uncertain.[21]

OTHER CLASSIFICATION SCHEMES

Low transsphincteric fistulas involve only the outer or distal one-third of the internal and external sphincter muscles. High transsphincteric fistulas involve a greater portion of the external sphincter and are more complicated to treat because of the amount of sphincter muscle involved and the possible complications of incontinence following fistulotomy.[20]

Another option is to define a fistula as simple or complex. "Simple fistulas" are low fistulas that involve the internal sphincter only or the lowest portion of the internal and external sphincters. All other fistulas can be considered "complex." These include any fistula involving more than 30% of the sphincter complex, anterior fistulas in women, any fistula with secondary tracts or residual abscess cavities (ie, horseshoe extensions), fistulas associated with other conditions, such as perianal Crohn disease or radiation therapy, if they involve other organs such as the vagina or urethra, and if they are recurrent.[18,20,22]

SYMPTOMS

A patient who presents with a fistula-in-ano often has a history of an abscess that has either been drained surgically or spontaneously. Symptoms that are common include drainage, pain with defecation, and perianal itching and bleeding due to the presence of granulation tissue at the internal or external opening.[17]

DIAGNOSIS

Physical examination may reveal an external opening with drainage.[17] Using Goodsall's rule as a guide can help locate the fistula tract. Perianal palpation may reveal a cordlike structure from the induration associated with the fistula tract. After inspection and palpation, there are multiple techniques that can be used to help identify and locate the often elusive fistula tract and internal opening. Anoscopy should be performed to see if an internal opening can be identified. Preoperative imaging, such as endoanal ultrasound, MRI, CT scan, or fistulography, can be helpful to determine the relationship of the fistula tract to the anal sphincters.[17,23] Operative maneuvers used to identify the internal opening include injection of the external opening with dilute hydrogen peroxide or methylene blue.

TREATMENT

Fistulizing disease and its treatment, including both the use of fistulotomy and setons, can be traced all the way back to Hippocrates in 400 BC.[24] Even in 2013, the successful treatment of anal fistula often remains complicated, frustrating, and challenging. The goals of treatment include resolving the acute-on-chronic inflammatory process through complete wound healing, maintaining continence, and preventing future recurrence.[24]

Treatment of an anal fistula is dictated by the path that the fistula takes and the amount of sphincter complex involved by the fistula tract.[3,18] Although rarely recommended, medical management with observation alone can be a reasonable option when the patient is minimally symptomatic or has significant medical comorbidities making the patient a prohibitive operative risk.[3] Medical management can also be used for patients with inflammatory bowel disease, specifically Crohn disease, in which oral metronidazole has been shown to be useful in the treatment of perianal fistulas. A dose of 20 mg/kg/d divided into 3 or 4 dosages has been shown to eliminate drainage, erythema, and induration in 80% of patients within 8 weeks of treatment.[25] Long-standing fistulas must be monitored because of the rare but documented possibility of developing a malignancy along this chronically inflamed tract.[26]

Infliximab is an immunoglobulin G1 monoclonal antibody against tumor necrosis factor-α that has been shown to be effective in the treatment of active intestinal Crohn disease. The efficacy of infliximab in the treatment of perianal Crohn disease remains debated.[27,28] Gaertner and colleagues[29] performed a retrospective chart review of 226 consecutive patients with perianal Crohn disease: 147 patients underwent operative treatment alone and 79 underwent combined treatment with surgery and infliximab. Although there was no significant difference between the 2 groups in terms of fistula healing (60% in the operative group and 59% in the combined group), the group receiving infliximab healed significantly faster than the operative group. In addition, patients with seton drainage plus infliximab healed more frequently than those treated with seton drainage alone ($P = .001$), providing a potential alternative to surgery. The ability to accurately define "healing" and the long-term efficacy of this approach remain in question.[27,28]

Simple submucosal, intersphincteric, and low transspincteric fistulas can be effectively managed in the operating room via fistulotomy, with minimal risk of fecal incontinence.[3,18] Of course, the surgeon must be cautious with the decision to cut any sphincter muscle when patients admit to borderline control, as seen in the elderly or in women following vaginal delivery. The location of the fistula (anterior in a woman) or disease process (Crohn disease) may impact surgical options as well. The most common alternative surgical treatment options include fistulotomy, fistulectomy, cutting seton, fibrin glue, fistula plug, ligation of the intersphincteric fistula tract (LIFT), and advancement flaps.[18,24]

Fistulotomy

A fistulotomy is the division of the tissue (skin, subcutaneous tissue, scar, and muscle) overlying a fistula tract thereby exposing the entire track. This is the standard treatment for simple fistulas (intersphincteric and low transsphincteric) because recurrence rates are low (0%–2%).[20] Incontinence rates following fistulotomy depends on both the amount of muscle divided at the time of operation as well as any preexisting sphincter damage causing scarring of the anal canal. Incontinence rates have been reported to range from 18% to 52%.[17]

Fistulectomy

Fistulectomy involves excision of the chronic, epithelialized tract to allow healing by secondary intention. The fistula track is identified by placing a fistula probe within the track and then the tract itself can be cored out around the probe from the skin, through the perirectal fat and to the sphincter complex. The internal opening is closed with a suture and the wound is left open to heal by secondary intent. A downfall of this technique is the potential to leave large tissue defects, resulting in prolonged wound healing.[30] Long tracts can be difficult to follow, particularly in obese patients. In a systematic review, Malik and Nelson[31] cited 2 randomized controlled trials that compared fistulotomy to fistulectomy. The internal and external anal sphincter defects seen on endoanal ultrasound in the 40 patients randomized to the fistulectomy group was larger than in the fistulotomy group. In addition, fistulotomy had significantly shorter healing times when compared with fistulectomy.[31]

Setons

A seton is a suture or vessel loop that is passed through the fistula tract and tied to form a continuous ring between the internal and external opening. A seton is typically placed in conjunction with wound debridement, at which time granulation tissue and fecal material can be removed and any side tract identified, defined, and drained. The purpose of a marking seton is to keep the fistula tract open, allowing drainage and wound contraction while preventing the development of perianal sepsis.[20] Occasionally, on reevaluation several months later, the marking seton will be positioned in a more superficial location (extruded by body) and a staged fistulotomy can be safely performed.

A cutting seton is one that is progressively tightened and can be used in the treatment of transsphincteric fistulas. Cutting setons lead to gradual cutting of the sphincter muscles and production of inflammation and fibrosis, thereby preventing the development of a retracted defect in the sphincter muscle, which may lead to fecal incontinence.[20,24,31] Again, studies suffer from small sample size and lack of randomization, but evidence suggests promising fistula healing rates balanced by the risk of postoperative fecal incontinence.[32]

Fibrin Glue

Fibrin glue is made of a combination of fibrinogen, thrombin, and calcium. This glue first made an appearance during World War I when it was found to be useful in hemostasis and then later in the 1940s as a sealant for skin-graft procedures.[3] In 1991, Hjortrub and colleagues published their results using fibrin glue as a sealant for anal fistulas.[33] The glue is thought to heal the fistula by inducing clot formation within the fistula track and then promoting the growth of collagen into the track and wound healing.[20] Many studies have been performed evaluating the success rates for fibrin glue injection, which have been shown to vary widely between 10% and 85%.[34] Most studies are limited by small patient numbers, heterogeneous fistula classification and inclusion, and limited follow-up. Cintron and colleagues[32] reported the results of fibrin glue in treatment of fistula-in-ano. A total of 79 patients were enrolled in the study. Three different types of sealants were used: autologous fibrin tissue adhesive, ViGuard-FS (V.I. Technologies Incorporated, New York, NY), and Tissell-VH (Baxter Healthcare Corporation, Glendale, CA). At mean follow-up of 12 months, the overall success rate was 61%. Transsphincteric fistulas had a success rate of 62%, intersphincteric fistulas had a success rate of 82%, and patients with Crohn disease or rectovaginal fistulas had an overall success rate of 36%. There was no difference in success rate among the 3 fibrin adhesives.[35]

Fistula Plugs

Fistula plugs are made of acellular porcine submucosal collagen designed to allow the growth of fibroblasts into its scaffolding and therefore promoting closure of the fistula.[4] The fistula plug is pulled through the fistula tract, secured at the internal opening, and trimmed at the external opening, which is left open for continued drainage.[20] Original success rates were shown to be approximately 80% to 85%, but more recent studies have not replicated these results with the success rates of 30% to 50%.[36]

LIFT Procedure

The LIFT procedure was described by Rojanasakul and colleagues[37] in 2007 and is a surgical alternative that avoids any division of the sphincter complex. Once the transsphincteric fistula tract is dissected and identified within the intersphincteric space, it can be divided and ligated in the space between the internal and external sphincters.[37] Reports in the literature demonstrate widely variable success rates ranging from 40% to 88%.[38] Potential benefits of this approach include sphincter preservation and the conversion of a transsphincteric fistula to an intersphincteric fistula that is amenable to simple fistulotomy.

Endorectal Advancement Flap

The advancement flap technique was designed as a sphincter-sparing procedure. Via a transanal approach, a healthy sleeve of rectal wall is raised and advanced over the debrided internal opening of the fistula. By positioning a flap of pliable tissue over the internal opening of the fistula, the fistula tract is protected from fecal contamination and allowed to heal by secondary intention.[30] One challenge associated with this procedure is that high internal openings are difficult to reach using this technique. In addition, if the flap becomes ischemic, a larger defect may occur. Studies in the literature demonstrate widely variable success rates ranging from 24% to 100%.[38] Review of the literature suggests improved outcomes when endorectal advancement flaps are performed with a fistulectomy, without a staging seton, without the addition of fibrin glue, and when a full-thickness flap is created.[39–42]

Ortiz and colleagues[43] performed the only prospective randomized clinical trial comparing the endorectal advancement flap with any other surgical approach, comparing the anal fistula plug with endorectal advancement flap for the treatment of high cryptoglandular fistula-in-ano. During 1 year follow-up, the anal fistula recurred in 12 of 15 patients treated with the anal fistula plug compared with 2 recurrences in the 16 patients treated with endorectal advancement flap.

SUMMARY

In conclusion, anal abscesses and fistulas are common conditions that remain related to one another. Once the acute infection has resolved, there is a relatively high probability of fistula formation. Treatment is tailored to the individual, taking into account baseline continence as well as degree of sphincter involvement. Options range from less to more invasive, and prudent surgeons prepare patients by discussing operative success rates and the potential need for several invasive procedures. The successful closure and healing of a complex fistula can be one of the most satisfying triumphs for a surgeon.

REFERENCES

1. Neves Jorge JM, Habr-Gama A. Chapter 1: anatomy and embryology. The ASCRS textbook of colon and rectal surgery. New York: Springer; 2011.
2. Bullard KM, Rothenberger DA. "Colon, rectum and anus." Chapter 28. Schwartz's principles of surgery. 8th edition. New York: McGraw-Hill; 2005.
3. Rizzo JA, Naig AL, Johnson EK. Anorectal abscess and fistula-in-ano: evidence-based management. Surg Clin North Am 2010;90:45–68.
4. Abcarian H. Anorectal infection: abscess-fistula. Clin Colon Rectal Surg 2011; 24(1):14–21.
5. Ommer A, Herold A, Berg E, et al. German S3 guidelines: anal abscess. Int J Colorectal Dis 2012;27:831–7.
6. Eisenhammer S. The internam anal sphincter and anorectal abscess. Surg Gynecol Obstet 1956;103:501–6.
7. Parks AG. Pathogenesis and treatment of fistula-in-ano. Br Med J 1961;1:463–9.
8. Rickard MJ. Anal abscesses and fistulas. ANZ J Surg 2005;75:64–72.

9. Caliste X, Nazier S, Goode T, et al. Sensitivity of computed tomography in detection of perirectal abscess. Am Surg 2011;77(2):166–8.

10. Oliver I, Lacueva FJ, Vicente FP, et al. Randomized clinical trial comparing simple drainage of anorectal abscess with and without fistula track treatment. Int J Colorectal Dis 2003;18:107–10.

11. Sozener U, Gedik E, Aslar AK, et al. Does adjuvant antibiotic treatment after drainage of anorectal abscess prevent development of anal fistulas? A randomized, placebo-controlled, double-blind, multicenter study. Dis Colon Rectum 2011;54(8):923–9.

12. Whiteford MH, Kilkenny J, Hyman N, et al. Practice parameters for the treatment of perianal abscess and fistula-in-ano (revised). Dis Colon Rectum 2005;48(7): 1337–42.

13. Vasilevsky CA, Gordon PH. The incidence of recurrent abscesses or fistula-in-ano following anorectal suppuration. Dis Colon Rectum 1984;27:126–30.

14. Cox SW, Senagore AJ, Luchtefeld MA, et al. Outcome after incision and drainage with fistulotomy for ischiorectal abscess. Am Surg 1997;63:686–9.

15. Yano T, Asano M, Matsude Y, et al. Prognostic factors for recurrence following the initial drainage of an anorectal abscess. Int J Colorectal Dis 2010;25:1495–8.

16. Onaca N, Hirshberg A, Adar R. Early reoperation for perirectal abscess: a preventable complication. Dis Colon Rectum 2001;44(10):1469–72.

17. Beck DE, Roberts PL, Saclarides TJ, et al. Chapter 13: anorectal abscess and fistula. The ASCRS textbook of colon and rectal surgery. New York: Springer; 2011.

18. Cirocchi R, Trastulli S, Morelli U, et al. The treatment of anal fistulas with biologically derived products: is innovation better than conventional surgical treatment? An update. Tech Coloproctol 2013;17(3):259–73.

19. Chung W, Ko D, Sun C, et al. Outcomes of anal fistula surgery in patients with inflammatory bowel disease. Am J Surg 2010;199:609–13.

20. Simpson JA, Banerjea A, Scholefield JH. Management of anal fistula. BMJ 2012; 345:1–9.

21. Leng Q, Jin HY. Anal fistula plug vs mucosa advancement flap in complex fistula-in-ano: a meta-analysis. World J Gastrointest Surg 2012;4(11):256–61.

22. Gaertner WB, Hagerman GF, Finne CO, et al. Fistula-associated anal adenocarcinoma: good results with aggressive therapy. Dis Colon Rectum 2008;51(7):1061–7.

23. Cheong DM, Nogueras JJ, Wexner SD, et al. Anal endosonography for recurrent anal fistulas: image enhancement with hydrogen peroxide. Dis Colon Rectum 1993;36(12):1158–60.

24. Dudukgian H, Abcarian H. Why do we have so much trouble treating anal fistula? World J Gastroenterol 2011;17(28):3292–6.

25. Jakobovits J, Schuster MM. Metronidazole therapy for Crohn's disease and associated fistulae. Am J Gastroenterol 1984;79:533–40.

26. Uchino M, Ikeuchi H, Bando T, et al. Long-term efficacy of infliximab maintenance therapy for perianal Crohn's disease. World J Gastroenterol 2011;17(9):1174–9.

27. Hyder SA, Travis SPL, Jewell DP, et al. Fistulating anal Crohn's disease: results of combined surgical and infliximab treatment. Dis Colon Rectum 2006;49(12): 1837–41.

28. Loungnarath R, Dietz DW, Mutch MG, et al. Fibrin glue treatment of complex anal fistulas has low success rate. Dis Colon Rectum 2004;47:432–6.

29. Gaertner WB, Decanini A, Mellgren A, et al. Does infliximab infusion impact results of operative treatment for Crohn's perianal fistulas? Dis Colon Rectum 2007;50(11):1754–60.

30. Bleier J, Moloo H. Current management of cryptoglandular fistula-in-ano. World J Gastroenterol 2011;17(28):3286–91.
31. Malik AI, Nelson RL. Surgical management of anal fistulae: a systemic review. Colorectal Dis 2008;10:420–30.
32. Cintron JR, Park JJ, Orsay CP, et al. Repair of fistulas-in-ano using fibrin adhesive. Dis Colon Rectum 2000;43:944–50.
33. Hjortrub A, Moesgaard F, Kjaergard J. Fibrin adhesive in the treatment of perineal fistulas. Dis Colon Rectum 1991;34:752–4.
34. Ellis CN, Rostas JW, Greiner FG. Long-term outcomes with the use of bioprosthetic plugs for the management of complex anal fistulas. Dis Colon Rectum 2010;53(5):798–802.
35. Cirocco WC, Reilly JC. Challenging the predictive accuracy of Goodsall's rule for anal fistulas. Dis Colon Rectum 1992;35(6):537–42.
36. Hammond TM, Knowles CH, Porrett T, et al. The Snug Seton: short and medium term results of slow fistulotomy for idiopathic anal fistulae. Colorectal Dis 2006; 8(4):328–37.
37. Rojanasakul A, Pattanaarun J, Sahakitrungruang C, et al. Total anal sphincter saving technique for fistula-in-ano: the ligation of the intersphincteric fistula tract. J Med Assoc Thai 2007;90:581–6.
38. Lewis R, Lunniss PJ, Hammond TM. Novel biological strategies in the management of anal fistula. Colorectal Dis 2012;14:1445–56.
39. Ellis CN, Clark S. Fibrin glue as an adjunct to flap repair of anal fistulas: a randomized controlled study. Dis Colon Rectum 2006;49:1736–40.
40. Ortiz H, Marzo J. Endorectal flap advancement repair and fistulectomy for high transsphincteric and suprasphincteric fistulas. Br J Surg 2000;87(12):1680–3.
41. Mitalas LE, van Wijk JJ, Gossenlink MP, et al. Seton drainage prior to transanal advancement flap repair: useful or not? Int J Colorectal Dis 2010;25(12): 1499–502.
42. Dubsky PC, Stift A, Friedl J, et al. Endorectal advancement flaps in the treatment of high anal fistula of cryptoglandular origin: full thickness vs. mucosal-rectum flaps. Dis Colon Rectum 2008;51(6):852–7.
43. Ortiz H, Marzo J, Ciga MA, et al. Randomized clinical trial of anal fistula plug versus endorectal advancement flap for the treatment of high cryptoglandular fistula in ano. Br J Surg 2009;96:608–12.

Chronic Pelvic Pain

Sharon L. Stein, MD

KEYWORDS

- Chronic pelvic pain • Myofascial pain • Pelvic pain syndrome • Levator syndrome
- Proctalgia fugax

KEY POINTS

- Chronic pelvic pain (CPP) is a difficult problem to treat that affects approximately 15% of women and unknown percentage of men.
- CPP may be difficult to diagnose and treat because causes, evaluation, and treatments may traverse multiple specialties.
- The most common causes for CPP include endometriosis, adhesions, musculoskeletal pain, and neurologic dysfunction.
- Patients with CPP are more likely to have other somatic pain syndromes, constipation, irritable bowel syndrome, or a history of sexual or physical abuse.
- Treatments of CPP are cause-specific. For patients who lack a clear cause, NSAIDs, tricyclic antidepressants, biofeedback, and neuroablative techniques are used.

INTRODUCTION

The evaluation and successful treatment of pelvic pain is a complex problem. Chronic pelvic pain (CPP) may encompass gastroenterologic, urologic, gynecologic, onco-logic, musculoskeletal, and psychosocial systems.[1] Subspecialists often lack interdisciplinary training and understanding of the diverse causes needed to evaluate and treat patients. This deficit makes comprehensive evaluation, diagnosis, and treatment difficult, and may frustrate patients who are sent from one specialist to another for further evaluation and diagnosis.

This article attempts to create a multidisciplinary overview for evaluation, testing and treatment options. It reviews the most common causes of CPP and discusses management options. Finally, some obstacles to treatment are reviewed and ways to improve efficiency of evaluation and treatment are suggested.

DEFINITION OF CPP

Pelvic pain is divided into acute and chronic pain. Acute pain is typically caused by a precise cause, such as anal fissure or thrombosed external hemorrhoid. Acute pain

Division of Colorectal Surgery, Department of Surgery, University Hospitals Case Medical Center, 11100 Euclid Avenue Lakeside 5047, Cleveland, OH 44106, USA
E-mail address: Sharon.stein@uhhospitals.org

Gastroenterol Clin N Am 42 (2013) 785–800
http://dx.doi.org/10.1016/j.gtc.2013.08.005
0889-8553/13/$ – see front matter © 2013 Elsevier Inc. All rights reserved.

gastro.theclinics.com

tends to diminish and it resolves with treatment and healing; it is not discussed in this article. In contrast, CPP is described as pain lasting a minimum of 6 months in duration, which may be sudden or gradual in onset and affects "the visceral or somatic system and structures supplied by the nervous system from the 10th thoracic spinal level and below."[2] Because of the broad definition of pelvic pain, the evaluation of pelvic pain extends across many subspecialties and organ systems.

EPIDEMIOLOGY OF CPP

CPP is a ubiquitous disease; in the United States it is estimated that 9 million women between ages 18 and 50 or 15% of the female population suffer from CPP.[3] A study from the United Kingdom demonstrated a CPP rate of 24%, with 33% of women reporting 5 years or greater duration.[4] A study in New Zealand found a prevalence of 25.4%.[5] A 1994 Gallup poll estimated the direct cost of CPP at $881.5 million dollars annually, with 15% of women with CPP noting lost work revenue and 45% reporting decreased work productivity.[3]

Ideally, a specific cause can be elucidated; however, in many cases, a distinct diagnosis is never discovered. Population studies demonstrate between 50% and 61% of all women with pelvic pain lack a clear diagnosis.[3,5] Even patients who undergo diagnostic laparoscopy still lack a diagnosis in 30% to 40% of cases.[6]

An epidemiologic study found that women with CPP are more likely to have a history of spontaneous abortion, military service, nongynecologic surgery, and nonpelvic somatic complaints than controls.[7] Additional studies have demonstrated a correlation with history of multiple sexual partners and psychosexual trauma or abuse.[7–9] CPP subjects are four times as likely to have a history of pelvic inflammatory disease.[10] Subjects with CPP also have a higher incidence of constipation, irritable bowel syndrome (IBS), depression, and anxiety than control groups.

Although CPP is better described and is more prevalent in women, it is not exclusive to the female gender. Chronic prostatitis/chronic pelvic pain (CP/CPP) is a well-described cause of pelvic pain in men. Musculoskeletal disorders may also be present with pelvic pain. As the diagnosis of CPP is better understood and known, it is likely that more men will present with similar complaints.

RELEVANT HISTORY FOR PATIENTS WITH CPP

History is a vital element in evaluation of CPP. Given the complexity of elements involved, a thorough history must include history of gastroenterologic, gynecologic, urologic, musculoskeletal, and pain symptoms. A full review of systems, including infectious diseases, endocrine disorders, and psychiatric disorders, is necessary. The International Pelvic Pain Society provides an extensive history intake form.[11]

A discussion of the character, intensity, radiation, and chronicity of pain should be obtained. Duration of pain, and exacerbating and alleviating factors, should be determined. Daily variation may give clues to the cause. Pelvic congestion syndrome typically increases in intensity as the day progresses, whereas proctalgia fugax tends to awaken the patient at night.

Determining the relationship of pain to each organ system is important. From a gynecologic perspective, correlation with sexual activity is also important. Pain associated with superficial stimulation is more consistent with vaginitis or vulvodynia; whereas deep dyspareunia is consistent with endometriosis or pelvic inflammatory disease. Abnormal vaginal bleeding may be symptomatic of uterine leiomyomas, adenomyosis, or malignancy, and should be evaluated with pelvic ultrasound.

A history of high-risk sexual behavior, multiple partners, and/or genital discharge can suggest pelvic inflammatory disease.

A history of pain or pressure with urination, difficulty emptying, or frequency suggests urologic causes. History of gastrointestinal disorders, including constipation and IBS, can be helpful. Manual evacuation and vaginal digitation are consistent with obstructed defecation. A history of recent trauma or pregnancy may help illuminate a musculoskeletal cause and surgical interventions 3 to 6 months ago may suggest adhesive disease.[12] Copies of colonoscopies, operative reports, or pathologic specimens are crucial. Previous perineal operations, mesh placement, and radiation may suggest iatrogenic causes.

Visceral and somatic pain may be sensed differently. Because visceral innervation of the pelvic structures share common neural pathways, distinguishing the cause of visceral pain may be difficult.[10] Visceral pain is associated with dull, crampy, or poorly localized pain, and may be associated with autonomic phenomena such as nausea, vomiting, and sweating.[13] Somatic pain, in contrast, originates from muscles, bones, and joints, and typically presents according to specific dermatomes. Somatic pain is associated with sharp or dull pain. Neuropathic pain may produce burning, paresthesia, or lancing pain. A history of pain syndromes, or drug or alcohol, abuse may also factor into evaluation and treatment. Janicki[14] has described a centralized sensitization of the pain receptors in patients with CPP and has suggested that understanding this may also be necessary for success.

An evaluation should also determine level of functional disability. The patient's ability to work, engage in daily activities, and emotional and sexual relationships is relevant. A full psychological evaluation should be considered for patients with history of sexual, physical abuse, depression, or anxiety. This does not alleviate the need for physical diagnosis; however, recognition and treatment may be important elements in symptom improvement.

PHYSICAL EXAMINATION

The physical examination encompasses multiple specialty examinations and may be time consuming for the practitioner and difficult for the patient with CPP. The entire examination and evaluation may require several visits to complete. All practitioners should have a chaperone during invasive examinations and at least one member of the medical team should be female.

Before commencing a formal examination, the practitioners should evaluate patient gait, movement, and sitting pose. Patients with pelvic girdle pain or spinal pain may have difficulty ambulating and sit off to one side; the practitioner should question the patient on this.

Specific areas of concern include the abdomen and abdominal wall. Patients should be examined for scars and previous surgeries or complications from surgeries should be reviewed. The abdomen should be palpated for tenderness, masses, or lesions. Distension and bloating may suggest history of constipation or bowel obstruction. The area of greatest abdominal pain should be localized. Performing a Valsalva maneuver or asking the patient to raise her head and legs separates the visceral organs from abdominal wall and may identify pressure points. Flexion of the head reduces abdominal pain and points to a visceral origin; conversely, increasing pain suggests abdominal wall or musculoskeletal origin.

The pelvic examination should commence with visual inspection noting areas of discoloration, dermatologic disorders, or sequelae of infection. A Q-tip examination using light touch is used to evaluate the sensory and neurologic systems of the perineum. Signs of incontinence at baseline or with straining should be noted. Pelvic organ prolapse quantification (Pop-Q) examination should be performed. Rectal prolapse can be noted during propulsive activity as well. Preferably, patients should be examined in both a reclining and standing position for greater sensitivity.

Anteriorly, the urethra and bladder trigone should be evaluated. A mass by the urethra suggests ureteral diverticulum, whereas tenderness and dysuria suggests urethritis, urethral syndrome, or interstitial cystitis (IC). A urinalysis can evaluate for infectious causes of urologic origin. Hematuria is associated with endometriosis. If urinary tract cause is suggested, a cystoscopy with evaluation for Hunner ulcers and a potassium chloride (KCl) sensitivity test to evaluate for IC are warranted. Urodynamics are indicated if urinary dysfunction exists.

In the vaginal compartment, an evaluation for vaginal discharge, Pap smear, and bimanual examination should be performed. Vaginal discharge and cervical motion tenderness are concerning for sexually transmitted diseases and can be further evaluated with cultures or histology. Tenderness may suggest vulvodynia or vaginitis.

A rectal examination should include digital examination and anoscopy to evaluate for lesions. For patients with bleeding, inflammation, or lesions noted on anoscopy, a colonoscopy may be warranted. Fissures, hemorrhoids, fistulas, or abscesses can cause chronic anal pain. Pain on rectal examination without fluctuance can be a sign of an intersphincteric abscess, which may have no external signs.

The musculoskeletal examination should evaluate the abdominal wall and pelvic floor muscles. During vaginal examination, the levator plate should be palpated on both sides of the vagina. A finger is curved over the levators during relaxation and contraction to evaluate for tenderness. The piriformis muscle is palpated through the vagina, cephalad to the ischial spine in a posterior lateral direction. The piriformis is lateral to the bulbospongiosus and transverse perineum that run parallel to the vagina. The internal and external sphincter muscles are evaluated transanally at rest and with contraction. Note should be made of weakness or deficiency. During normal contraction, a slight upward pull should be felt from the coccygeus, puborectalis, and pubovaginalis muscles. During propulsion, descent of the pelvic wall and motility of the rectum should be noted.

The coccyx should be evaluated for coccygodynia. Pain with palpation or mobility is a sign of coccygodynia; a normal coccyx should rotate 25° to 30° without discomfort. External rotation of the leg against resistance may exacerbate the pain. Flexion of the hip and knee against resistance may demonstrate psoas pain. Additional musculoskeletal evaluation includes evaluation of pelvic ring instability, which is particularly common after delivery. Straight leg raise, resisted hip abduction, adduction tests, and posterior provocative pain test may be helpful in evaluating the stability of the pelvic ring.

If the examination fails to elicit a clear cause for their pain, an MRI may be helpful. In a study of subjects with CPP and no specific clinical findings, MRI was able to elucidate a cause in 39% of cases.[15] For the remainder, 36% of subjects were ultimately diagnosed with levator ani syndrome and 25% with unspecified anorectal pain. Other testing includes pelvic ultrasound, cystoscopy, and colonoscopy. In the past, laparoscopy was performed for diagnostic purposes but is no longer indicated.[16]

COMMON CAUSES FOR CPP

The three most common documented findings on laparoscopy for CPP are endometriosis (33%), adhesions (24%), and absence of pathologic condition on laparoscopy (35%).[17] However, hundreds of different causes may cause pelvic pain (**Fig. 1**).

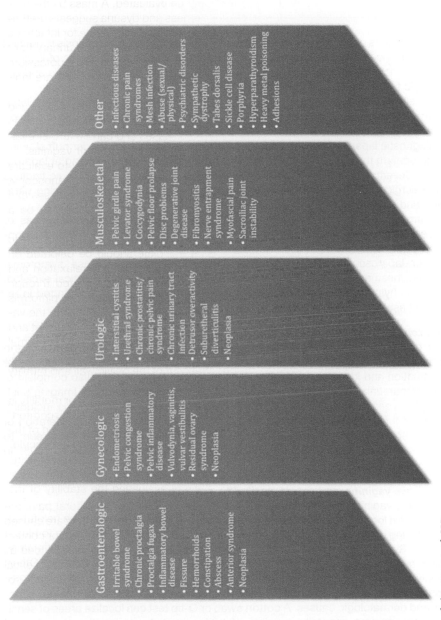

Fig. 1. Some of the causes of CPP.

Gastroenterologic
- Irritable bowel syndrome
- Chronic proctalgia
- Proctalgia fugax
- Inflammatory bowel disease
- Fissure
- Hemorrhoids
- Constipation
- Abscess
- Anterior syndrome
- Neoplasia

Gynecologic
- Endometriosis
- Pelvic congestion syndrome
- Pelvic inflammatory disease
- Vulvodynia, vaginitis, vulvar vestibulitis
- Residual ovary syndrome
- Neoplasia

Urologic
- Interstitial cystitis
- Urethral syndrome
- Chronic prostatitis/ chronic pelvic pain syndrome
- Chronic urinary tract infection
- Detrusor overactivity
- Suburethral diverticulitis
- Neoplasia

Musculoskeletal
- Pelvic girdle pain
- Levator syndrome
- Coccygodynia
- Pelvic floor prolapse
- Disc problems
- Degenerative joint disease
- Fibromyositis
- Nerve entrapment syndrome
- Myofascial pain
- Sacroiliac joint instability

Other
- Infectious diseases
- Chronic pain syndromes
- Mesh infection
- Abuse (sexual/ physical)
- Psychiatric disorders
- Sympathetic dystrophy
- Tabes dorsalis
- Sickle cell disease
- Porphyria
- Hyperparathyroidism
- Heavy metal poisoning
- Adhesions

Because normal pelvic function requires coordinated activity of the muscular, connective, visceral, and neural tissues of the pelvis, dysfunction in any area can create a complex situation that may ultimately manifest itself as pelvic pain.

Gynecologic

Endometriosis
Endometriosis is one of the leading causes of CPP in women. Endometriosis is defined as the presence of endometrial tissue outside of the uterine cavity. Areas of involvement may include proximal or distant sites and may affect gastroenterologic and gynecologic function secondary to local or metastatic invasion.

Typically, patients are nulliparous, in their 20s and 30s, with symptoms correlated with menstrual cycle, including dysmenorrhea and pain. Deep dyspareunia and involuntary infertility are also common. Patients are often diagnosed by symptoms alone, but diagnostic laparoscopy with findings of chocolate cysts and powder puff staining help to confirm the diagnosis. Up to 40% of patients may have no finding at laparoscopy.[16] Severity of pain is not generally correlated with gross or pathologic findings during surgical extirpation.[18] Noninvasive diagnosis is being evaluated using ultrasound and pelvic MRI.[19–23]

Treatment of endometriosis is often hormonal, including oral contraceptives or induced menopause, which may lead to the atrophy of implants and relief of symptoms. Acupuncture has been used with success in some cases.[24,25] Presacral neurectomy or laparoscopic uterine nerve ablation (LUNA) may decrease symptoms; however, these are not endorsed by a recent Cochrane review.[26] Surgical excision, abdominal hysterectomy, and salpingo-oophorectomy may be recommended in refractory cases.

Pelvic congestion
Pelvic congestion is most frequently seen in women between 20 and 30 years old, and is analogous to a scrotal varicocele in men. Symptoms generally worsen before menstruation and increase in severity during the day. Patients may also complain of deep dyspareunia or postcoital pain. Dilated vessels can be seen on imaging such as duplex venography, MRI, or during laparoscopy. Pathologic findings including fibrosis of tunica intima and media are noted with hypertrophy and proliferation of capillary endothelium.[27] Both ovarian suppression and embolic treatment seem to control symptoms, with embolic treatment success varying from 24% to 100% in studies.[28]

Vulvodynia, vaginitis, and vulvar vestibulitis syndromes
Vulvodynia, vaginitis, and vulvar vestibulitis syndromes, as well as clitoral pain, are forms of pain localized to the anterior compartment. It is hypothesized they are caused by stretching of the perivaginal and perivulvar muscles, hormonal changes, or contact irritation. Symptoms are typically intermittent in nature and may be experienced as itching, burning, stinging, rawness, or dyspareunia. Onset may occur after first sexual experience or tampon use, but may also occur after trauma such as delivery or vigorous sexual activity. Laboratory testing is generally performed to rule out infectious and dermatologic causes. A cotton swab or Q-tip test can localize areas of sensitivity. Management generally consists of biofeedback to desensitize the affected region, including application of manual therapy or electrotherapy. Topical agents such as lidocaine or lubricant may be helpful and, in some patients, botulinum toxin type A (Botox) injections are efficacious. Up to 50% of patients may respond to pain medications, such as tricyclic agents, or gabapentin.[29,30] Behavioral therapy

and interventional pain techniques may be helpful in patients who fail to respond to initial treatments.

Urologic

Chronic prostatitis/chronic pelvic pain (CP/CPP)

Although CPP is generally recognized as an entity affecting women, men can also have CPP. In addition to a multitude of musculoskeletal ailments, men can develop CP/CPP. This syndrome was recognized by the National Institute of Health in 1995. It is characterized by CPP and voiding symptoms in the absence of urinary tract infection, anatomic abnormality, or urologic malignancy.[31] Inflammatory and noninflammatory types, depending on the presence or absence of leukocytes in expressed prostatic secretions, have been described. A 2013 review of articles on CP/CPP suggested treatment options and advocated a multimodal therapeutic approach that may include use of alpha-blockers in patients with significant voiding symptoms, and physical therapy or antibiotics for newly diagnosed antimicrobial-naive patients.[32]

Interstitial cystitis (IC)

Symptoms of IC include bladder pain, urinary frequency, urgency, or nocturia. Pain is often present in the suprapubic area but it may occur in the lower back or buttock. Fifty-one percent of women complain of dyspareunia. Concomitant fibromyalgia, vulvodynia, anxiety, and depression are common.[33]

Urinalysis is generally performed to rule out urinary tract infection. On cystoscopy, Hunner ulcers may be seen in the bladder mucosa and a KCl sensitivity test is used to obtain a definitive diagnosis. The KCl sensitivity test evaluates the bladder for increased epithelial permeability that is believed to contribute to IC.[34] This test is positive in up to 75% of patients, although false positives may occur.[35]

First-line treatment of IC is generally nonsteroidal antiinflammatory medication (NSAID), although neither NSAIDs nor opioids have been noted to be effective. Pentosan polysulfate sodium (PPS) is the only treatment of IC approved by the Food and Drug Administration (FDA).[17] PPS is hypothesized to mimic the normal glycosaminoglycan layer that protects the bladder urothelium that is dysfunctional in IC. Treatment is effective in 28% to 32% of patients but may require up to 6 months of treatments.[36,37] Use of PPS in conjunction with tricyclic antidepressants may have better results.[17] Both dimethyl sulfoxide and heparin have been administered as intravesicular injection with limited success, and Botox in combination with hydrodistention has been used with some efficacy.[38,39] Sacral nerve stimulation has been used for patients who failed other therapies.[40]

Urethral syndrome

Urethral syndrome is associated with incomplete emptying and burning during urination, particularly after intercourse. The urethra may be tender on examination. It is believed that urethral syndrome is caused by noninfectious, stenotic, or fibrous changes in the urethra. Urethral syndrome is associated with grand multiparity, delivery without episiotomy, and general pelvic relaxation.[41] Treatment generally consists of diathermy and coagulation.[42]

Gastroenterologic

Irritable bowel syndrome (IBS)

IBS is defined as the chronic presence of abdominal pain or discomfort 3 days or more per month that correlates with stooling, change in frequency, or form of stool.[43] IBS is believed to be multifactorial in origin and related to the hypersensitivity of the viscera leading to disproportionate pain with intestinal distension, dysregulation of gastrointestinal motility, and endocrine effects of hypothalamic pituitary axis.[44]

IBS is a diagnosis of exclusion. Other causes that may cause bowel dysfunction, such as Crohn's disease, diverticulitis, sprue, lactose allergy, and chronic appendicitis, must be ruled out. There is a strong association between CPP and IBS; 65% to 79% of patients with IBS have CPP and 60% of patients have associated dysmenorrhea.[45]

Dietary modification may be helpful to decrease symptomatology. For patients with diarrhea, loperamide, cholestyramine, and alosetron (for women) are most commonly recommended. A trial of rifaximin has been shown to provide symptom relief but is not yet approved by the FDA for IBS.[46] Constipation is generally treated with dietary and supplementary fiber, stool softener, or cathartics such as lactulose and polyethylene glycol. A 2007 Cochrane database reviewed the use of tegaserod, a 5-hydroxytryptamine[4] partial agonist and found patients were more likely to have modest relief than with placebo.[47] Tricyclic antidepressants, smooth muscle relaxants, and serotonin reuptake inhibitors have also been used with some success.[43]

Chronic proctalgia

Chronic proctalgia is defined as chronic or recurrent anorectal pain lasting for 20 minutes or longer, in the absence of other anorectal causes of pain such as hemorrhoids, fissures, and coccygodynia. Patients often describe a burning sensation, which may worsen with defecation or sitting and improve when supine. Symptoms are generally more common in women and are often associated with other bowel dysfunction, such as obstructed defecation. Proctalgia has an incidence of 2% to 5%.[48] First-line therapy for patients with chronic proctalgia and obstructed defecation is generally biofeedback with success rates as high as 65%.[49] For patients without defecatory symptoms, Botox may be used as well. Tricyclic antidepressants, sacral nerve stimulation, and pain medication are reserved for refractory cases.

Proctalgia fugax

Proctalgia fugax is sudden nocturnal cramping that occurs and spontaneously resolves without objective findings and has an incidence of 8% to 18%.[50,51] Episodes are localized to the anus or lower rectum and last for seconds to minutes. Complete cessation of pain occurs between episodes.[52] There is some association with high resting and squeeze pressures that may improve with biofeedback.[53] If pain is unilateral, entrapment of the pudendal nerve at the Alcock's canal should be considered.[54] First-line treatment includes topical diltiazem or nitroglycerin, injection of Botox, or strip myomectomy in severe cases in which internal anal sphincter is thickened.[49,55,56] Injection of the pudendal nerve and sphincterotomy have both been used with some success.[57,58] Sacral nerve modulation has also been effective.[59]

Musculoskeletal

Pelvic girdle pain

Pelvic girdle pain presents as posterior sacral or buttock pain of variable intensity.[60] It is generally associated with recent pregnancy or pain that started during pregnancy.[61] One to sixteen percent of women have pain lasting longer than 12 months postpartum.[62] Evaluation consists of musculoskeletal testing, including straight leg raise, provocative testing, palpation of sacroiliac ligament, resisted hip abduction, and adduction tests.[63] Treatment is generally multidisciplinary and includes an exercise program focusing on restoring pelvic stability. Occasionally intra-articular injections with steroids are given for sacroiliac joint pain.[64] Pain medications are generally avoided, except for antiinflammatory medications. For severe cases, radiofrequency thermocoagulation, cryoneurolysis under fluoroscopic guidance, and pulsed radiofrequency have been used with lasting improvement.[65,66]

Levator syndrome
Levator syndrome is generally attributed to muscle spasm of the pelvic floor musculature and consists of wide range of complex musculoskeletal disorders, including piriformis and puborectalis syndromes. Symptoms are generally a vague dull pressure or ache that may worsen with sitting or lying down. It is often associated with incomplete evacuation. It is more common in women, with an incidence of approximately 6%.[67] Diagnosis is made with palpation of muscles and associated tenderness. Digital massage is associated with improvement in symptoms in up to 68% of patients.[68] Lidocaine, methylprednisolone, and triamcinolone have also been injected with varied results.[69,70] Case reports also demonstrate improvement after injection of Botox.[71] Biofeedback has been used with approximately 30% of patients noting Improvement.[72]

Coccygodynia
Coccygodynia is pain at or around the coccyx evoked by manipulation of the coccyx. It is typically associated with local trauma, prolonged sitting, or cycling. It may be exacerbated by sitting, bending, or arising, as well as during intercourse or defecation. Coccygodynia may be secondary to hypertonicity of the pelvic floor and decreased coccyx mobility. The cause may be unknown in up to 30% of cases. Diagnosis can be confirmed by relief of pain after injection of local anesthetic. Treatment options include antiinflammatory medications, rest, coccyx cushion, physical therapy, and massage. If the coccyx is unstable or hypermobile, local injection may be more useful compared with manual stretching.[73] Radiofrequency thermocoagulation, pulsed radiofrequency, cryoneurolysis, and sacral modulation have been promoted.[74] Coccygectomy should be assiduously avoided.

Pelvic floor prolapse
Pelvic prolapse may be noted in as many as 50% of multiparous women. The cause of pelvic prolapse is believed to be a multifactorial combination of aging, trauma, devascularization, changing collagen content, and lowered estrogen levels.[75] Pelvic floor prolapse in young premenopausal patients has been associated with decreased collagen content compared with normal controls.[76] Pop-Q examination and visualization are the gold standard for diagnosis; MRI defecography may be helpful in some situations. Organ prolapse may include the anterior compartment: cystocele, uterine prolapse, and enterocele. Rectocele may cause issues with obstructive defecation. Rectal prolapse can be associated with mucous discharge and incontinence. Surgical treatment has been the gold standard for most gynecologic, urologic, or gastrointestinal prolapse, although use of a pessary may relieve symptoms for anterior pelvic floor prolapse in some patients. The causes and treatment options for rectal prolapse are discussed elsewhere in this issue.

Infectious Causes

Gynecologic diseases, such as chlamydia, gonorrhea, syphilis, HIV-AIDS, trichomoniasis, vaginitis, and genital herpes, may cause pelvic pain.[77] Symptoms include bloody or malodorous vaginal discharge, urinary symptoms, dyspareunia, and cervical motion tenderness on examination. Objective findings may be minimal and reinfection without partner treatment is common. Treatment may be delayed if there is not a high level of suspicion. Chronic infections may contribute to infertility.

Chronic Pain Syndromes

A substantial number of patients with CPP do not demonstrate objective findings. These patients often undergo substantial workup and may have had transient improvements from treatment, but they continue to have recurrent pain. In these patients, Janicki[14] describes a chronic pain syndrome that involves the hypersensitization of nerve cells, increased role of the autonomic nervous system, and "windup" of the pain environment. Once patients experience this phenomenon, even minor pain stimulants can exacerbate or maintain the pain. Howard and colleagues[78] describe pain mapping of the visceral organs using a blunt probe laparoscopically under conscious sedation. Treatment involves injection at pressure points.

TREATMENT OPTIONS FOR PATIENTS WITHOUT DEFINED CAUSE

Patients in whom a specific cause for their pain cannot be identified often undergo a variety of treatments. Predictors of successful treatment include history of other pain syndromes, good family and social support systems, employment status, and beliefs about pain.[7] First-line treatment is generally scheduled NSAIDs to decrease pain and inflammation. Narcotics are not recommended, secondary to concerns for abuse and addiction potential as well as risks of constipation or antimotility side effects. Tricyclic antidepressants and neuropathic medications such as gabapentin lack good quality evidence to demonstrate efficacy, although they may be helpful for some patients.

Neuroablative techniques include radiofrequency thermocoagulation, pulsed radiofrequency, cooled radiofrequency, and cryoneurolysis. Neuroablative techniques are used primarily for neuralgias of the abdominal wall or pelvic floor and may destroy neural tissue directly or alter neuron conduction. Although most techniques have been used with success, side effects including neuroma formation and postprocedural neuritis have been documented.[79–81] Chemical neuroablation has also been used. Traditional techniques involve the use of alcohol, phenol, or hypertonic saline for patients refractory to other techniques.[82] Side effects include flaccid paralysis of injected and surrounding nerves. Botox is a strong neurotoxin that prevents release of acetylcholine at the neuromuscular junction. Analgesic effects last approximately 3 to 5 months longer than muscle relaxant effects.[83] Botox is increasingly used with some success for both pelvic floor muscle spasms and undifferentiated CPP.[84] A 2013 review of literature demonstrated relief in subjects with CPP secondary to pelvic floor muscle spasm; however, a lack of data on optimum dosage, technique, and duration of effect was noted.[85]

Laparoscopy has also been used as both a diagnostic and therapeutic tool. The most common causes of CPP discovered on laparoscopy include adhesions and endometriosis. Up to 58% of gynecologic laparoscopies are associated with pelvic pain, but more than half of patients will have a negative laparoscopy.[86–88] Adhesions are often thought to be a source of CPP; however, a prospective, randomized, clinical trial observed no benefit to surgical lysis of adhesions to treat CPP.[89] A second trial randomized subjects to either diagnostic laparoscopy alone or laparoscopic adhesiolysis. Both groups experienced a significant initial improvement in pain scores, but there was no difference between the groups at 1 year.[90] Only 45% of subjects treated with laparoscopic adhesiolysis experienced improvement in quality-of-life scores at the 2-year follow-up. Additionally, 55% of subjects were noted to have complete relapse of pain following adhesiolysis.[91]

In cases of severe pelvic pain, hysterectomy has been performed. Up to 10% of all hysterectomies are performed for CPP.[92] However, up to 40% of patients will have recurrent pelvic pain after hysterectomy. Risks factors for recurrence include lack of pelvic pathologic diagnosis, lack of commercial insurance, and age younger than 30.[93]

In one study, standard treatment was compared with integrated approach. Subjects in the standard treatment group underwent traditional treatment with root cause analysis and frequent laparoscopy. In the integrated approach, equal attention was devoted to somatic, physiologic, dietary, environmental, and physiotherapeutic factors. The groups were similar in baseline clinical characteristics and pain scores. Evaluation of pain scores at 1 year revealed the superiority of the integrated approach.[89]

CHALLENGES FACING DIAGNOSIS, TREATMENT, AND ELIMINATION OF CPP

CPP is a heterogenous group of disorders that cover a wide range of specialties. Because of the diversity in expertise, diagnosis, and treatment options, facilitating care for these patients can be difficult for the following reasons:

- The patient population is varied, which complicates research in terms of extrapolating findings or treatment success to a broader group of patients.
- There are minimal data from randomized controlled trials to direct treatment.
- Data available in one specialty may not be accessed by other specialties. Data in the gynecologic literature may not be read by gastroenterologists, urologists, or physiatrists, which limits incorporation of new findings.
- Data suggest that multidisciplinary treatment may benefit patients, but there is lack of funding and impetus to create and maintain such collaborative efforts.

REFERENCES

1. Reiter RC. Evidence-based management of chronic pelvic pain. Clin Obstet Gynecol 1998;41(2):422–35.
2. Apte G, Nelson P, Brismée JM, et al. Chronic female pelvic pain—part 1: clinical pathoanatomy and examination of the pelvic region. Pain Pract 2012;12(2): 88–110.
3. Mathias SD, Kuppermann M, Liberman RF, et al. Chronic pelvic pain: prevalence, health-related quality of life, and economic correlates. Obstet Gynecol 1996;87(3):321–7.
4. Zondervan KT, Yudkin PL, Vessey MP, et al. The community prevalence of chronic pelvic pain in women and associated illness behaviour. Br J Gen Pract 2001;51(468):541–7.
5. Grace VM, Zondervan KT. Chronic pelvic pain in New Zealand: prevalence, pain severity, diagnoses and use of the health services. Aust N Z J Public Health 2004;28(4):369–75.
6. Garry R. Diagnosis of endometriosis and pelvic pain. Fertil Steril 2006;86: 1307–9.
7. Reiter RC, Gambone JC. Demographic and historic variables in women with idiopathic chronic pelvic pain. Obstet Gynecol 1990;75(3 Pt 1):428–32.
8. Walling MK, Reiter RC, O'Hara MW, et al. Abuse history and chronic pain in women: I. Prevalences of sexual abuse and physical abuse. Obstet Gynecol 1994;84(2):193–9.
9. Collett BJ, Cordle CJ, Stewart CR, et al. A comparative study of women with chronic pelvic pain, chronic nonpelvic pain and those with no history of pain attending general practitioners. Br J Obstet Gynaecol 1998;105(1):87–92.
10. Ryder RM. Chronic pelvic pain. Am Fam Physician 1996;54:2225–32.

11. International Pelvic Pain Society history and physical form. Available at: http://www.pelvicpain.org/pdf/History_and_Physical_Form/IPPS-H&PformR-MSW.pdf. Accessed May 2013.
12. Steege JF. Office assessment of chronic pelvic pain. Clin Obstet Gynecol 1997; 40(3):554–63.
13. Gunter J. Chronic pelvic pain: an integrated approach to diagnosis and treatment. Obstet Gynecol Surv 2003;58(9):615–23.
14. Janicki TI. Chronic pelvic pain as a form of complex regional pain syndrome. Clin Obstet Gynecol 2003;46(4):797–803.
15. Dwarkasing RS, Schouten WR, Geeraedts TE, et al. Chronic anal and perianal pain resolved with MRI. AJR Am J Roentgenol 2013;200(5): 1034–41.
16. Pearce C, Curtis M. A multidisciplinary approach to self-care in chronic pelvic pain. Br J Nurs 2007;16:82–5.
17. Nelson P, Apte G, Justiz R 3rd, et al. Chronic female pelvic pain—part 2: differential diagnosis and management. Pain Pract 2012;12(2):111–41.
18. Buttram VC Jr. The rationale for use of medical suppressive therapy prior to endoscopic surgery. Ann N Y Acad Sci 1994;734:445–9.
19. Scardapane A, Lorusso F, Bettocchi S, et al. Deep pelvic endometriosis: accuracy of pelvic MRI completed by MR colonography. Radiol Med 2013;118(2): 323–38.
20. Manganaro L, Vittori G, Vinci V, et al. Beyond laparoscopy: 3-T magnetic resonance imaging in the evaluation of posterior cul-de-sac obliteration. Magn Reson Imaging 2012;30(10):1432–8.
21. Reid S, Lu C, Casikar I, et al. Prediction of pouch of Douglas obliteration in women with suspected endometriosis using a new real-time dynamic transvaginal ultrasound technique: the sliding sign. Ultrasound Obstet Gynecol 2013; 41(6):685–91.
22. Macario S, Chassang M, Novellas S, et al. The value of pelvic MRI in the diagnosis of posterior cul-de-sac obliteration in cases of deep pelvic endometriosis. AJR Am J Roentgenol 2012;199(6):1410–5.
23. Hudelist G, Fritzer N, Staettner S, et al. Uterine sliding sign: a simple sonographic predictor for presence of deep infiltrating endometriosis of the rectum. Ultrasound Obstet Gynecol 2013;41(6):692–5.
24. Wayne PM, Kerr CE, Schnyer RN, et al. Japanese-style acupuncture for endometriosis-related pelvic pain in adolescents and young women: results of a randomized sham-controlled trial. J Pediatr Adolesc Gynecol 2008;21(5): 247–57.
25. Highfield ES, Laufer MR, Schnyer RN, et al. Adolescent endometriosis-related pelvic pain treated with acupuncture: two case reports. J Altern Complement Med 2006;12(3):317–22.
26. Proctor ML, Farquhar CM, Sinclair OJ, et al. Surgical interruption of pelvic nerve pathways for primary dysmenorrhea. Cochrane Database Syst Rev 2002;(4):CD001896.
27. Liddle AD, Davies AH. Pelvic congestion syndrome: chronic pelvic pain caused by ovarian and internal iliac varices. Phlebology 2007;22:100–4.
28. Tu FF, Hahn D, Steege JF. Pelvic congestion syndrome-associated pelvic pain: a systematic review of diagnosis and management. Obstet Gynecol Surv 2010; 65(5):332–40.
29. Reed BD. Vulvodynia: diagnosis and management. Am Fam Physician 2006;73: 1231–8.

30. Smart OC, MacLean AB. Vulvodynia. Curr Opin Obstet Gynecol 2003;15(6): 497–500.
31. Krieger JN, Nyberg L Jr, Nickel JC. NIH consensus definition and classification of prostatitis. JAMA 1999;282(3):236–7.
32. Nickel JC, Alexander RB, Schaeffer AJ, et al, Chronic Prostatitis Collaborative Research Network Study Group. Leukocytes and bacteria in men with chronic prostatitis/chronic pelvic pain syndrome compared to asymptomatic controls. J Urol 2003;170(3):818–22.
33. Clemons JL, Arya LA, Myers DL. Diagnosing interstitial cystitis in women with chronic pelvic pain. Obstet Gynecol 2002;100:337–41.
34. Parson CL, Greenberger M, Gabal L, et al. The role of urinary potassium in the pathogenesis and diagnosis of interstitial cystitis. J Urol 1998;159:1862–6.
35. Sant GR, Hanno PM. Interstitial cystitis: current issues and controversies in diagnosis. Urology 2001;57(Suppl 6A):82–8.
36. Moldwin RM, Sant GR. Interstitial cystitis: a pathophysiology and treatment update. Clin Obstet Gynecol 2002;45:259–72, 62.
37. Mulholland SG, Hanno PM, Parsons CL. Pentosan polysulfate sodium for therapy of interstitial cystitis. Urology 1990;35:522–58.
38. Dawson TE, Jamison J. Intravesical treatments for painful bladder syndrome/ interstitial cystitis. Cochrane Database Syst Rev 2007;(4):CD006113.
39. Kuo HC, Chancellor MB. Comparison of intravesical botulinum toxin type A injections plus hydrodistention with hydrodistention alone for the treatment of refractory interstitial cystitis/painful bladder syndrome. BJU Int 2009;104: 657–61.
40. Zabihi N, Mourtzinos A, Maher MG, et al. Short-term results of bilateral S2-S4 sacral neuromodulation for the treatment of refractory interstitial cystitis, painful bladder syndrome, and chronic pelvic pain. Int Urogynecol J Pelvic Floor Dysfunct 2008;19:553–7.
41. Gürel H, Gürel SA, Atilla MK. Urethral syndrome and associated risk factors related to obstetrics and gynecology. Eur J Obstet Gynecol Reprod Biol 1999; 83(1):5–7.
42. Costantini E, Zucchi A, Del Zingaro M, et al. Treatment of urethral syndrome: a prospective randomized study with Nd:YAG laser. Urol Int 2006;76(2):134–8.
43. Longstreth GF, Thompson WG, Chey WD, et al. Functional bowel disorders. Gastroenterology 2006;130:1480–91.
44. Shin JH, Howard FM. Management of chronic pelvic pain. Curr Pain Headache Rep 2011;15:377–85.
45. Hogston P. Irritable bowel syndrome as a cause of chronic pain in women attending a gynaecology clinic. Br Med J (Clin Res Ed) 1987;294(6577):934–5.
46. Pimental M, Lembo A, Chey W, et al. Rifaximin therapy for patients with irritable bowel syndrome without constipation. N Engl J Med 2011;364:22–32.
47. Evans BW, Clark WK, Moore DJ, et al. Tegaserod for the treatment of irritable bowel syndrome and chronic constipation. Cochrane Database Syst Rev 2007;(4):CD003960.
48. Rao SS, Paulson J, Mata M, et al. Clinical trial: effects of botulinum toxin on levator ani syndrome—a double-blind, placebo controlled study. Aliment Pharmacol Ther 2009;29:985–91.
49. Atkin GK, Suliman A, Vaizey CJ. Patient characteristics and treatment outcome in functional anorectal pain. Dis Colon Rectum 2011;54(7):870–5.
50. Baranowski AP. Chronic pelvic pain. Best Pract Res Clin Gastroenterol 2009;23: 593–610.

51. Mazza L, Formento E, Fonda G. Anorectal and perineal pain: new pathophysiological hypothesis. Tech Coloproctol 2004;8:77–83.
52. Rome III diagnostic criteria for functional gastrointestinal disorders. Available at: http://www.romecriteria.org/assets/pdf/19_RomeIII_apA_885–898.pdf. Accessed January 3, 2011.
53. Grimaud JC, Bouvier M, Naudy B, et al. Manometric and radiologic investigations and biofeedback treatment of chronic idiopathic anal pain. Dis Colon Rectum 1991;34:690–5.
54. Pisani R, Stubinski R, Datti R. Entrapment neuropathy of the internal pudendal nerve: report of two cases. Scand J Urol Nephrol 1997;31:407–10.
55. Lowenstein B, Cataldo PA. Treatment of proctalgia fugax with topical nitroglycerin: report of a case. Dis Colon Rectum 1998;41:667–8.
56. Katsinelos P, Kalomenopoulou M, Christodoulou K, et al. Treatment of proctalgia fugax with botulinum A toxin. Eur J Gastroenterol Hepatol 2001;13:1371–3.
57. Takano M. Proctalgia fugax: caused by pudendal neuropathy? Dis Colon Rectum 2005;48:114–20.
58. Gracia Solanas JA, Ramirez Rodriguez JM, Elia Guedea M, et al. Sequential treatment for proctalgia fugax. Mid-term follow-up. Rev Esp Enferm Dig 2005; 97:491–6.
59. Falletto E, Masin A, Lolli P, et al. Is sacral nerve stimulation an effective treatment for chronic idiopathic anal pain? Dis Colon Rectum 2009;52:456–62.
60. Nilsson-Wikmar L, Holm K, Oijerstedt R, et al. Effect of three different physical therapy treatments on pain and activity in pregnant women with pelvic girdle pain: a randomized clinical trial with 3, 6, and 12 months follow-up postpartum. Spine 2005;30:850–6.
61. O'Sullivan PB, Beales DJ. Diagnosis and classification of pelvic girdle pain disorders – part 1: a mechanism based approach within a biopsychosocial framework. Man Ther 2007;12:86–97.
62. Ferreira CW, Alburquerque-Sendín F. Effectiveness of physical therapy for pregnancy-related low back and/or pelvic pain after delivery: a systematic review. Physiother Theory Pract 2013;29(6):419–31.
63. Mens JM, Vleeming A, Snijders CJ, et al. The active straight leg raising test and mobility of the pelvic joints. Eur Spine J 1999;8:468–73.
64. Bollow M, Braun J, Taupitz M, et al. CT-guided intraarticular corticosteroid injection into the sacroiliac joints in patients with spondyloarthropathy: indication and follow-up with contrast-enhanced MRI. J Comput Assist Tomogr 1996;20(4):512–21.
65. Cohen SP, Hurley RW, Buckenmaier CC 3rd, et al. Randomized placebo-controlled study evaluating lateral branch radiofrequency denervation for sacroiliac joint pain. Anesthesiology 2008;109:279–88.
66. Kapural L, Nageeb F, Kapural M, et al. Cooled radiofrequency system for the treatment of chronic pain from sacroiliitis: the first case-series. Pain Pract 2008;8:348–54.
67. Drossman D, Li Z, Andruzzi E, et al. U.S. householder survey of functional gastrointestinal disorders: prevalence, sociodemography, and health impact. Dig Dis Sci 1993;38(9):1569–80.
68. Grant SR, Salvati EP, Rubin RJ. Levator syndrome: an analysis of 316 cases. Dis Colon Rectum 1975;18:161–3.
69. Nicosia JF, Abcarian H. Levator syndrome: a treatment that works. Dis Colon Rectum 1985;28:406–8.
70. Wald A. Functional anorectal and pelvic pain. Gastroenterol Clin North Am 2001; 30:243–51.

71. Thomson AJ, Jarvis SK, Lenart M, et al. The use of botulinum toxin type A (BOTOX) as treatment for intractable chronic pelvic pain associated with spasm of the levator ani muscles. BJOG 2005;112(2):247–9.
72. Gilliland R, Heymen J, Altomare D, et al. Biofeedback for intractable rectal pain. Dis Colon Rectum 1997;40(2):190–6.
73. Maigne JY, Chatellier G, Faou ML, et al. The treatment of chronic coccydynia with intrarectal manipulation: a randomized controlled study. Spine 2006;31: E621–7.
74. Patijn J, Janssen M, Hayek S, et al. Coccygodynia. Pain Pract 2010;10(6):554–9.
75. Tinelli A, Malvasi A, Rahimi S, et al. Age-related pelvic floor modifications and prolapse risk factors in postmenopausal women. Menopause 2010;17: 204–12.
76. Soderberg MW, Falconer C, Bystrom B, et al. Young women with genital prolapse have a low collagen concentration. Acta Obstet Gynecol Scand 2004;83:1193–8.
77. Tarr ME, Gilliam ML. Sexually transmitted infections in adolescent women. Clin Obstet Gynecol 2008;51:306–18.
78. Howard FM, EL-Minawi AM, Sanchez RA. Conscious pain mapping by laparoscopy in women with chronic pelvic pain. Obstet gynecol 2000;96:934–9.
79. Rhame EE, Levey KA, Gharibo CG. Successful treatment of refractory pudendal neuralgia with pulsed radiofrequency. Pain Physician 2009;12:633–8.
80. Vallejo R, Benyamin RM, Kramer J, et al. Pulsed radiofrequency denervation for the treatment of sacroiliac joint syndrome. Pain Med 2006;7:429–34.
81. Mitra R, Zeighami A, Mackey S. Pulsed radiofrequency for the treatment of chronic ilioinguinal neuropathy. Hernia 2007;11:369–71.
82. Chen FP, Soong YK. The efficacy and complications of laparoscopic presacral neurectomy in pelvic pain. Obstet Gynecol 1997;90:974–7.
83. Tsui JK, Eisen A, Stoessl AJ, et al. Double- blind study of botulinum toxin in spasmodic torticollis. Lancet 1986;2:245–6.
84. Abbott JA, Jarvis SK, Lyons SD, et al. Botulinum toxin type A for chronic pain and pelvic floor spasm in women: a randomized controlled trial. Obstet Gynecol 2006;108:915–23.
85. Bhide AA, Puccini F, Khullar V, et al. Botulinum neurotoxin type A injection of the pelvic floor muscle in pain due to spasticity: a review of the current literature. Int Urogynecol J 2013;24(9):1429–34.
86. Howard FM. The role of laparoscopy as a diagnostic tool in chronic pelvic pain. Baillieres Best Pract Res Clin Obstet Gynaecol 2000;14(3):467–94.
87. Peterson HB, Hulka JF, Phillips JM. American Association of Gynecologic Laparoscopists' 1988 membership survey on operative laparoscopy. J Reprod Med 1990;35(6):587–9.
88. Hulka JF, Peterson HB, Phillips JM, et al. Operative laparoscopy. American Association of Gynecologic Laparoscopists 1991 membership survey. J Reprod Med 1993;38(8):569–71.
89. Peters AA, van Dorst E, Jellis B, et al. A randomized clinical trial to compare two different approaches in women with chronic pelvic pain. Obstet Gynecol 1991; 77(5):740–4.
90. Swank DJ, Swank-Bordewijk SC, Hop WC, et al. Laparoscopic adhesiolysis in patients with chronic abdominal pain: a blinded randomised controlled multicentre trial. Lancet 2003;361(9365):1247–51.
91. Dunker MS, Bemelman WA, Vijn A, et al. Long-term outcomes and quality of life after laparoscopic adhesiolysis for chronic abdominal pain. J Am Assoc Gynecol Laparosc 2004;11(1):36–41.

92. Carlson KJ, Nichols DH, Schiff I. Indications for hysterectomy. N Engl J Med 1993;328(12):856–60.
93. Hillis SD, Marchbanks PA, Peterson HB. The effectiveness of hysterectomy for chronic pelvic pain. Obstet Gynecol 1995;86(6):941–5.

Pruritus Ani: Diagnosis and Treatment

Yosef Y. Nasseri, MD[a],*, Marc C. Osborne, MD[b]

KEYWORDS

- Pruritus ani • Primary • Secondary • Diagnosis • Treatment

KEY POINTS

- Pruritus ani is a dermatologic condition characterized by itching or burning in the perianal area.
- Pruritus ani can be either primary (idiopathic) or secondary.
- There are a multitude of different causes of pruritus ani, making diagnosis and treatment options numerous.

INTRODUCTION

Pruritus ani is defined as a dermatologic condition characterized by itching and/or burning in the perianal region.[1] Pruritus ani affects 1% to 5% of the population, is four times more prevalent in men than women, and is most commonly present in the fourth to sixth decades of life.[2,3] Pruritus ani is categorized an either primary (idiopathic) or secondary. Although some papers state that 50% to 90% of pruritus ani cases are idiopathic, others claim that roughly 75% of cases have associated pathology.[4,5] There are nearly 100 different causes for pruritus ani, making differential diagnoses and treatment options vast.[5] This article provides a thorough review of secondary and idiopathic pruritus ani and outlines effective diagnostic and treatment options.

HISTORICAL PERSPECTIVE

The earliest known mention of pruritus ani is in the Chester Beatty Medical Papyrus. This ancient Egyptian papyrus was given to the British Museum by American industrialist Chester Beatty. Ten of its 41 remedies were devoted to management of anal itching and irritation.[6] Because of a lack of understanding of the many conditions that may cause anal itching, pruritus ani was known as a "condition that eludes all attempts at

[a] The Surgery Group of Los Angeles, 8631 West 3rd Street, Suite 200E, Los Angeles, CA 90048, USA; [b] Division of Colon and Rectal Surgery, Department of Surgery, University of Minnesota, 1055 Westgate Drive, Suite 190, St Paul, MN 55114, USA
* Corresponding author.
E-mail address: yossef@hotmail.com

Gastroenterol Clin N Am 42 (2013) 801–813
http://dx.doi.org/10.1016/j.gtc.2013.09.002
0889-8553/13/$ – see front matter © 2013 Elsevier Inc. All rights reserved.

cure."[7] Subsequently, numerous topical and injectable treatments for pruritus ani have been developed or reported. In 1966, Caplan[8] demonstrated the role of soiling and fecal contamination of the skin as a cause of pruritus symptoms. This is generally considered to be the most common cause of symptoms when secondary causes have been ruled out. Anorectal physiology studies also support this theory. They demonstrated that patients with pruritus have a more pronounced accommodation of the internal anal sphincter with rectal distention compared with control subjects and leak sooner on a saline infusion test.[9,10] Thus, most modern treatment protocols focus on eliminating irritants, skin protection, and proper anal hygiene.

ETIOLOGY OF ITCH

Itch is an unpleasant sensation that leads to the desire to scratch and can be categorized into the following groups: cutaneous, neuropathic, neurogenic, and psychogenic.[11] Cutaneous or pruritoceptive itch is caused by inflammation of the skin. Neuropathic itch is caused by damage to the peripheral nervous system and can be present anywhere along the afferent nerve pathway. Neurogenic itch is induced centrally. Lastly, psychogenic itch is caused by delusional states.

The sensation of itch can be brought on by various stimulus modalities including thermal; electrical; mechanical (heat, xerosis, and so forth); and chemical stimuli. Histamine has been studied extensively as a potential neuronal mechanism of itch; however, it is not the only substance that produces itching. Kallikrein, bradykinin, papain, and trypsin are all itch-mediating substances that are not responsive to blockades with classic histamine antagonists, such as diphenhydramine. As a consequence, antihistamines have proved ineffective in treating pruritus in many instances.[12]

Itch is a surface phenomenon initiated by the stimulation of C-fibers in the epidermis and subepidermis. C-fibers are slow-conduction velocity unmylenated fibers with extensive terminal branches and transmit messages that the brain interprets as the sensation of itch. Itch receptors may be located more superficially than pain receptors and consequently, itch is believed to be a subthreshold of pain.[13] The idea that itch receptors are located superficially is supported by the fact that minor mechanical stimuli can create the sensation of itch.

Scratching the affected skin provides inadequate feedback to inhibit itching and prolonged itching can cause damaging excoriations and infections, which provides additional itching stimuli. Thus, scratching results in a vicious cycle of itching and scratching that is difficult to break.

SECONDARY CAUSES

Pruritus ani has been attributed to idiopathic and secondary causes. Secondary pruritus ani, which is pruritus induced by an underlying cause, can be divided into the following categories: inflammatory, nonsexual infectious, systemic, premalignant and malignant, and anorectal causes (**Table 1**). Sexually transmitted causes of perianal itch and pathology is discussed separately elsewhere in this issue. In all of these cases pruritus ani is exacerbated by the scratch–itch cycle, which can lead to infections and further increase the itching frequency.

Inflammatory Diseases

Numerous inflammatory diseases can manifest with perianal symptoms and puritus ani including psoriasis, atopic dermatitis, seborrheic dermatitis, lichen planus, and lichen sclerosis.

Table 1
Causes of secondary pruritus ani

Inflammatory Diseases	Nonsexual Infectious Diseases	Sexually Transmitted Diseases
Psoriasis	Pilonidal disease	Gonorrhea
Atopic dermatitis	Hidradentis suppurativa	Syphilis
Contact dermatitis	Crohn disease	Chancroid
Seborrheic dermatitis	Tinea cruris	Granuloma iguinale
Scleroderma	Herpes zoster	Molluscum contagiosum
Erythema multiforme	Trichomoniasis	Herpes simplex
Pemphigus vulgaris	Bilhartziasis	Condyloma acuminata
Dermatitis herpetiformis	Oxyurasis (pinworm)	Chlamydia
Lichem planus	Larva currens	
Lichen sclerosis et atrophicus	Cimicosis (bed bugs)	
Radiation dermatitis	Pediculosis (lice)	
Darier disease	Scabies	
Premalignant and Malignant Diseases	**Systemic Diseases**	**Anorectal Diseases**
Acanthosis nigricans	Diabetes mellitus	Hemorrhoids
Leukoplakia	Leukemia and lymphoma	Anal creases
Mycosis fungoids	Hepatic diseases	Fistula in ano
Leukemia cutis	Thyroid disorders	Fissures
Squamous cell carcinoma	Renal failure	Rectal prolapse
Basal cell carcinoma	Iron deficiency anemia	
Bowen disease	Vitamin A and D deficiencies	
Melanoma	Aplastic anemia	
Dysplastic nevus		
Paget disease		

Psoriasis

Psoriasis has been shown in numerous studies to be a prevalent underlying cause of pruritus ani. Typical psoriasis presents on the trunk, knees, elbows, and scalp. Psoriasis present in the anus, groin, genitals, and axillae is referred to as "inverse psoriasis" because it presents as the inverse of the normal distribution. Although the exact incidence is unknown, one study found that a significant portion of patients (54%) with inverse psoriasis had involvement of the anus.[14] Typical psoriasis presents as bright red plaquelike lesions, whereas inverse psoriasis is demarcated, paler in color, and has lesions without scales.[15] Psoriasis cannot be cured but can be treated with short-term use of a low-to-mid potency steroid for up to 4 weeks. After the induction of remission the patient should switch to a nonsteroidal topical treatment, such as calcipotriene, for maintenance (**Fig. 1**).[16]

Atopic dermatitis

Atopic dermatitis is a chronic inflammatory, pruritic disease of the skin that is induced by an allergic response. People with atopic dermatitis are also likely to have asthma, eczema, and hay fever. Lesions are nonspecific diffuse erythema, dry and scaly, and often marked by evidence of excoriations. Biopsies are often inconclusive because of the mixed inflammatory infiltrate with eosinophils. Thus, a careful patient history

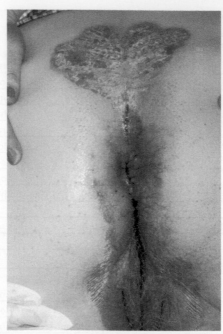

Fig. 1. Inverse psoriasis. (*From* Finne CO, Fenyk JR. Dermatology and pruritus ani. In: Beck DE, Roberts PL, Saclarides TJ, et al, editors. The ASCRS Textbook of Colon and Rectal Surgery. New York: Springer, 2011; with kind permission from Springer Science and Business Media.)

provides the physician with the best chance of making a correct diagnosis. Atopic dermatitis has been shown to be associated with keratosis pilaris (rough, dry bumps) on the arms and thighs; Morgan folds (creases found beneath the eyes); "sniffers" (a crease found across the nose); urticaria; and white dermatographism.[17] Treatment options include the use of strong moisturizing agents, anti-inflammatory agents, and antihistamines.

Seborrheic dermatitis
Seborrheic dermatitis is not a common cause of pruritus ani and is characterized by extensive, moist erythema in the perineum.[18] Seborrheic dermatitis usually presents in the scalp, chest, ears, beard, and suprapubic area and is easily treated with 2% sulfur with 1% hydrocortisone lotion.[15]

Lichen planus
Lichen planus is believed to be caused by an altered cell-mediated immune response to an unidentified source. Patients with lichen planus may also have another disease of altered immunity including myasthenia gravis, alopecia, vitiligo, ulcerative colitis, and lichen sclerosis. Lichen planus can also present in patients with chronic active hepatitis and primary biliary cirrhosis. Widespread lichen sclerosis should be looked for in these patients.[19] Cutaneous lesions are shiny, flat-topped papules that are more darkly pigmented than the surrounding skin. Lesions typically develop on the flexural surfaces of the limbs with a generalized eruption developing after a week and a maximal spreading occurring between 2 and 16 weeks. Genital involvement is common and can be extremely pruritic. Direct immunofluorescence study reveals globular

deposits of IgM. The condition usually resolves itself within 6 (>50%) to 18 months (85%).[19] Treatment options include topical steroids or, for more severe cases, light therapy (narrow-band or broadband UVB therapy).

Lichen sclerosis

Lichen sclerosis, usually appearing as lichen sclerosus et atrophicus in dermatologic literature, is a chronic disease of unknown cause. Lichen sclerosis is five to six times more prevalent in women than men and involves the vulva and extends posteriorly to the perianal region.[15,18] Typical lesions are porcelain-white papules and plaques. In females one should inspect the interlabial sulci, labia minora, clitoral hood, clitoris, and perineal body and in males the prepuce, coronal sulcus, and glans penis.[20] The affected areas typically break down and reveal the underlying, raw tissue that can be extraordinarily painful and pruritic. As the underlying tissue heals, the area is replaced by chronic inflammation, sclerosis, and atrophy.[3] During a physical examination one typically sees white patches in a pattern surrounding the vulva and anus. Squamous cell carcinoma is the most common malignancy described in association with anogenital lichen sclerosus. Women with lichen sclerosis have a 300-fold increased risk of developing cancer compared with those without the disease.[21] Treatment of the condition does not reduce this risk. Short term (6–8 weeks) treatment with a potent topical steroid, such as clobetasol, is highly effective in reducing symptoms.[20] Retinoids, testosterone creams, and tacrolimus ointment have also been described.[22–24] Because of the risk of squamous cell carcinoma, nonresponding patients should have a skin biopsy to rule out malignancy.[5]

Nonsexually Transmitted Infectious Diseases

Although bacterial, fungal, and parasitic infections make up the minority of pruritus ani causes, their contribution must not be underestimated.

Candida

Candida is responsible for 10% to 15% of pruritus ani.[18,25] It is characterized by diffuse, marginated erythematous and many times macerated plaques. These lesions, localized to the inguinal and perianal region, are generally painful and very itchy. Such factors as old age, sweating, obesity, tight-fitting clothing, prolonged use of antibiotics, diabetes, and immunosuppressive therapy can predispose a person to Candida vulvitis or Candida balanitis. One review showed that surgical treatment of anal disorders (hemorrhoids, fissure, spasm, mucosal prolapse) eliminated Candida and dermatophyte infections in 20 out of 23 patients who cultured positive with symptomatic itching before the procedure.[26] Diagnosis can be achieved using a culture or scraping of the lesion. Scrapings can be negative for hyphae if topical steroids were used; however, the use of steroids typically exacerbates dermatophyte growth. Topical and systemic antifungal agents have been used as treatment options.

Numerous nonsexually transmitted bacterial infections have been shown to lead to pruritus ani including Streptococcus, Staphylococcus aureus, and Corynebacterium minutissium. Weismann and colleagues[27] found 19 patients with pruritus over a period of 1 to 20 years who had negative throat and nose cultures but were positive for either β hemolytic streptococci or S aureus in the perianal region. Erythrasma, a skin disease characterized by brown, scaly patches and caused by the bacterium C minutissium, typically presents with itching and can often be found at such sites as the toes and groin. It is best diagnosed with the Wood lamp, which shows a fluorescent coral pink or red color. False-negative results can be produced if the patient has recently showered.[28–35] Erythromycin, tetracycline, and betamethasone lotion have been effective in the treatment of perianal *C minutissium*.[3] *Streptococcus* is treated with amoxicillin, penicillin, and/or topical applications of mupirocin (bactroban). *S aureus* is treated with penicillin, doxycycline, or clindamycin.

Parasitic infections

Parasitic infections, specifically *Enterobius vermicularis* (pinworms), can be a common cause of pruritus ani in children. A cellophane tape test, applied in the early hours of the morning, can identify the adult worms and their eggs and confirm the diagnosis.[18] Treatment is with albendazole or mebendazole. Other common parasites that induce pruritus ani include *Sarcoptes scabei* and *Pediculosis pubis*.

Herpes zoster

Herpes zoster, commonly referred to as shingles, is an infection of the varicella zoster virus. Herpes zoster can only occur in people who were previously infected with the virus and although the disease can occur at any age, it typically presents in patients older than the age of 50. The rash has a unique appearance and can usually be diagnosed visually. Herpes zoster causes a deep red rash with blisters that do not cross the midline of the body. Treatment options include antiviral medications including valacyclovir hydrochloride.

Systemic Diseases

Table 1 lists several systemic diseases associated with pruritus. These conditions are more often associated with generalized pruritus rather than pruritus ani specifically. In a prospective study of 55 patients presenting with generalized pruritus to a dermatology clinic, 12 were found to have a systemic cause of the pruritus.[36] The underling conditions included iron deficiency anemia, hepatitis, uremia, diabetes mellitus, chronic lymphocytic leukemia, and lung cancer. Iron deficiency anemia was the most common diagnosis. Pruritus was the presenting symptom in 5 of the 12 patients.

Uremic pruritus

Uremic pruritus, or itching associated with end-stage renal disease, is a common complaint among patients on dialysis, affecting up to 90% of patients. Transplantation is the only known cure.[37] Several biochemical mediators have been implicated in the pathogenesis this condition. Serotonin was initially thought to be a common cause of uremic and hepatic pruritus. However, several randomized controlled trials failed to find much clinical benefit with treatment of ondansetron, a selective serotonin antagonist.[38] Gabapentin, omega-3 fatty acids, topical baby oil, sertraline, and pregabalin have all been used with some success to treated uremic pruritus.[39–43]

Pruritus from cholestasis is a common condition in patients with liver disease. Cholestyramine, naltrexone, rifampin, and sertraline have all been used with variable success in treating this troublesome problem.[44]

Premalignant and Malignant Diseases

There are numerous premalignant and malignant conditions that can lead to pruritus ani including intraepithelial neoplasia (AIN), or Bowen disease, and Paget disease. Half of patients with perianal Paget disease and perianal Bowen disease have associated itch.[5]

Intraepithelial neoplasia

AIN is a condition associated with human papilloma virus and condylomata and can present inside or outside of the anal canal. AIN can range from low- to high-grade dysplasia, with high-grade dysplasia, also known as Bowen disease, being an intermediate stage toward malignant transformations into squamous cell carcinoma of the anus. Patients present with minor complaints and are usually diagnosed during evaluation of condylomata or pruritus. Patients with low-grade dysplasia can be treated topically. Alternatively, high-grade dysplasia is a premalignant condition. It is typically treated by mapping with punch biopsies and excision. Large amounts of uninvolved tissue may be excised to achieve clear margins. The recurrence rate with wide excision is 23.1% and the cancer rate is below 10% (**Fig. 2**).[45,46]

Paget disease
Paget disease (cutaneous adenocarcinoma in situ) is rare; however, if found it may indicate an underlying carcinoma. As such, flexible sigmoidoscopy is crucial as part of the work-up. The condition typically manifests itself as an erythematous, eczematoid plaque in the perianal region.[3] Paget disease is most common in the seventh decade of life. A wide excision is the treatment of this condition.

Anorectal Causes

Coexisting anal conditions induce pruritus ani by contributing to fecal contamination or increasing moisture in the perianal region. Conditions include hemorrhoids, fissures, fistula in ano, skin tags, and prolapse. Literature suggests that correcting these disorders in select patients is helpful in alleviating itch.[17]

The St. Louis University group found that out of 109 patients with pruritus ani, 52% whose sole complaint was itching had anorectal disease as the cause.[47] Conditions found in this study included hemorrhoids, idiopathic proctitis, fissure, condyloma, ulcerative proctitis, fistula, and abscess. Furthermore, Murie and colleagues,[48] in a study of 82 hemorrhoidal patients, found that pruritus is more common in patients with hemorrhoids than in age- and gender-linked control subjects. They also reported that treatment of hemorrhoids, prolapse, and rectal bleeding reduced the incidence of pain, pruritus, and soiling. Scarborough's[49] study in a proctologic clinic found that out of 275 patients with anorectal disease, 54% complained of anal itching. Additionally, Bowyer and McColl[50] found that out of 200 patients with pruritus ani, 43 had hemorrhoids that were contributory and in 16 cases were the sole cause. Furthermore, in that patient population they observed that fissure treatment in five patients, skin tag

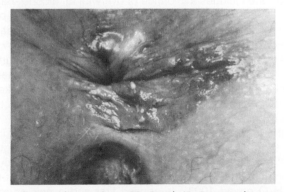

Fig. 2. Anal Bowen disease. (*From* Finne CO, Fenyk JR. Dermatology and pruritus ani. In: Beck DE, Roberts PL, Saclarides TJ, et al, editors. The ASCRS Textbook of Colon and Rectal Surgery. New York: Springer, 2011; with kind permission from Springer Science and Business Media.)

removal in five patients, and treatment of spasm in four patients led to complete relief. They postulated that skin tags may trap fecal matter in the perianal region, which induces the irritant process.

PRIMARY CAUSES

Pruritus ani is considered primary or idiopathic when no other demonstrable cause can be found. Washington Hospital Center has a useful classification system for pruritus ani based on the physical features of the skin as follows: stage 0 is normal skin; stage 1 is erythematous and inflamed skin; stage 2 is lichenified skin; and stage 3 is lichenified, coarse skin often with ulcerations.[15]

Perianal fecal contamination can lead to pruritus ani symptoms, as shown by Caplan's fecal patch test study.[8] By applying autologous feces patch tests to males on both the inner arm and perianal region, Caplan was able to show that perianal skin reacts differently from skin elsewhere on the body. Anal symptoms were present in a third of the men with pruritus ani and 53% of asymptomatic men.[8] Symptoms ceased when the area was washed and did not show allergic reaction.

Any factor that leads the perianal area to become moist, soiled, or irritated has the potential to result in pruritus ani symptoms. Thus, an extensive physical examination and questionnaire should be completed as seen in **Box 1**. Numerous studies have shown that patients with pruritus ani are more likely to have loose stools, drink more water, and have weekly fecal soiling than patients without this condition.[51,52] Exaggerated rectoanal inhibitory reflexes and earlier incontinence were also found in patients with pruritus ani.[9,10,53] The rectoanal inhibitory reflex is the natural relaxation of the internal anal sphincter and concurrent squeeze of the external anal sphincter in response to rectal distention. This exaggerated reflex and leakage seen with infusion of smaller volumes of a saline infusion test in patients with idiopathic pruritus ani provide some evidence for the role of soiling as the cause of idiopathic or primary pruritus ani.

Once a diagnosis of primary pruritus ani has been made, treatment is directed to proper anal hygiene, avoiding moisture in the anal area, removing offending agents, alteration of diet, and protection of skin. Patients are also encouraged to view therapy as control of chronic symptoms rather than a one time treatment. All patients should receive a patient education handout for reference at home.

Optimal anal hygiene includes avoidance of overwiping, alcohol-based wipes, perfumes, dyes, and witch hazel products. Patients should only use plain, white, unscented, toilet paper for wiping the anal area. In severe cases patients should be encouraged to take a bath after a bowel movement or take a shower and cleanse the area with a detachable shower head. The anal area is then pat dried with a towel or dried with a hair dryer on the cool setting. Control of seepage or leakage with either fiber or antidiarrheal agents removes an offending agent and makes anal hygiene easier. The optimal consistency of stool should be soft, but well formed, and easy to clean with one wipe.

After cleaning the anal area, the skin should be protected with a zinc oxide–based barrier ointment, such as Calmoseptine (Calmoseptine, Inc, Huntington Beach, CA). For severe cases, consider weekly office application of Berwick's dye and benzoin. The Berwick's solution (crystal violet 1% + brilliant green 1% + 95% ethanol 50% + distilled H_2O q.s.ad 100%) is applied first and a hair dryer set on cool is used to dry the solution on the skin. Tincture of benzoin is then applied as a sealant and barrier and similarly dried with a hair dryer on cool. The Berwick's solution remains on the skin for up to a week so long as only water is used as a cleanser.

Box 1
Patient history questionnaire

Itching/Burning

When did the itching start?

When is the itching worst?

What type of clothing do you normally wear (ie, tight or loose fitting)?

When you itch do you scratch the area?

Is itching associated with bowel movements?

Is the anal area typically moist, either with sweat or fecal seepage?

Diet

Do you notice that when you eat certain foods the itching gets worst?

Have you kept a food diary?

Do you have any existing food allergies?

What is your typical fluid intake?

Cleansing Techniques

How do you cleanse the affected area (ie, with soap or just water)?

How often do you cleanse the area?

Bowel Movements

How frequently do you have a bowel movement?

Are you normally constipated?

How often do you have diarrhea?

Do your bowel movements vary in frequency and consistency?

Has there been a recent change in your bowel movements?

Do you use or do the following: laxatives, fiber supplements, and/or enemas?

Sexual History

Do you have sex with men, women, or both?

Have you ever had an STD test?

Do you have anal sex?

What is your method of protection?

How many partners have you had within the last year?

For women

Is your menstrual cycle regular?

Have you ever been pregnant, if so, how many live births have you had?

Medical History

Have you ever had surgery for an anorectal condition?

Do you have diabetes or another chronic systemic disease?

Have you ever had any injury or surgery for a condition of the peripheral or central nervous system?

Have you experienced significant weight gain or weight loss recently?

Table 2	
Foods and local irritants associated with pruritus ani	
Foods	**Local Irritants**
Coffee	Soaps
Tomatoes	Perfumes
Beer	Fecal contamination or moisture
Cola	Tight clothing
Tea	Topical or systemic medications
Peanuts	
Milk products	
Citrus	
Chocolate	
Lemon or lemon juice	
Grapes	

Diet changes include avoiding the "Cs": coffee (and tea); cola; chocolate; citrus (to-matoes); and calcium (dairy products). **Table 2** contains a full list of food implicated in pruritus ani. A high-fiber diet also helps stool consistency, and thus minimizes fecal soiling.

Tight-fitting clothing promotes moisture in the anal area and should be avoided. Underwear should be cotton rather than nylon. Athlete's foot powder instead of a barrier cream may be used in patients who have significant perspiration to treat moisture.

Topical steroids are effective in breaking the itch-injury cycle and may be necessary to provide symptoms relief when starting therapy. The adverse effects of steroids include skin atrophy, ulceration, rebound symptoms after withdrawal, striae, spontaneous bleeding, and may be themselves a cause of itching. When initiating therapy, 1% hydrocortisone for a limited period of time and then a change to a barrier ointment is a generally safe strategy. Patients who have received excessive or potent steroids should be tapered down slowly.

Anal tattooing has been advocated as a therapy for patients who have failed multiple other regimens. The technique involves intradermal injection of a solution of 1% methylene blue, bupivacaine, and lidocaine. Eusebio and coworkers[54] reported complete relief or improvement in 21 of 23 patients. Skin necrosis is a known complication.

Psychological factors associated with itching have been described.[18] Patients may describe an intense desire to itch despite adequate empiric treatment of primary pruritis ani or no other secondary cause. In these cases use of central-acting medications including doxepin, amitryptiline, nortyptiline, gabapentin, and cimetidine may be useful.[17] Socks placed over the hands at night may also prevent nocturnal itching.

SUMMARY

Pruritus ani is a common condition with multiple causes and therefore effective therapy may be elusive at first. Primary causes are thought to be fecal soiling or food irritants. Secondary causes include malignancy, infections including sexually transmitted diseases, benign anorectal diseases, systemic diseases, and inflammatory conditions. Therapy is directed at the underlying cause when identified. A broad differential diagnosis must be considered and reassessment of therapy is paramount. In the absence of an obvious secondary cause, empiric treatment is directed at improved anal hygiene, removal of common irritants, and protection of the anal skin.

ACKNOWLEDGMENTS

Karinne Van Groningen, BS, worked closely with Drs Nasseri and Osborne on drafting this paper and conducting the research.

REFERENCES

1. Billingham RP, Isler JT, Kimmins MH, et al. The diagnosis and management of common anorectal disorders. Curr Probl Surg 2004;33(7):586–645.
2. Chaudhry V, Bastawrous A. Idiopathic pruritus ani. Semin Colon Rectal Surg 2003;14:196–202.
3. Markell K, Billingham R. Pruritus ani: etiology and management. Surg Clin North Am 2010;90(1):125–35.
4. Metcalf A. Anorectal disorders. Five common causes of pain, itching, and bleeding. Postgrad Med 1995;98(5):81–4, 87–9, 92–4.
5. Siddiqi S, Vijay V, Ward M, et al. Pruritus ani. Ann R Coll Surg Engl 2008;90(6): 457–63.
6. Banov L Jr. Pruritis ani and anal hygiene. J S C Med Assoc 1985;81:557.
7. Corman ML. Colon and rectal surgery. 5th edition. Philadelphia: Lippincott Williams & Wilkins; 2005. p. 606–7.
8. Caplan RM. The irritant role of feces in the genesis of perianal itch. Gastroenterology 1966;50:19–23.
9. Allan A, Ambrose NS, Silverman S, et al. Physiological study of pruritus ani. Br J Surg 1987;74:576–9.
10. Farouk R, Duthie GS, Pryde A, et al. Abnormal transient internal sphincter relaxation in idiopathic pruritus ani: physiological evidence from ambulatory monitoring. Br J Surg 1994;81:603–6.
11. Twycross R, Greaves MW, Handwerker H, et al. Itch: scratching more than the surface. QJM 2003;96:7–26.
12. Ringkamp M, Schepers R, Schimada S, et al. A role for nociceptive myelinated nerve fibers in itch sensation. J Neurosci 2011;31(42):14841–9.
13. Keele C. Chemical causes of pain and itch. Proc R Soc Med 1957;50(7):477–84.
14. Wang G, Li C, Gao T, et al. Clinical analysis of 48 cases of inverse psoriasis: a hospital-based study. Eur J Dermatol 2005;15:176–8.
15. Gordon PH, Nivatvongs S. Perianal dermatologic disease. In: Gordon PH, editor. Principles and practice of surgery for the colon, rectum, and anus. 3rd edition. New York: Informa Healthcare; 2007. p. 247–73.
16. Kalb RE, Bagel J, Korman NJ, et al. Treatment of intertriginous psoriasis: from the Medical Board of the National Psoriasis Foundation. J Am Acad Dermatol 2009;60:120–4.
17. Finne C, Fenyk J. Dermatology and pruritus ani. In: Beck DE, Roberts PL, Saclarides TJ, et al, editors. The ASCRS textbook of colon and rectal surgery. 2nd edition. Springer Science+Business Media, LLC; 2011. p. 277–94.
18. Zuccati G, Lotti T, Mastrolorenzo A, et al. Pruritus ani. Dermatol Ther 2005;18(4): 355–62.
19. Chuang TY, Stitle L. Lichen planus. Emedicine website. Available at: http:// emedicine.medscape.com/article/1123213-overview. Accessed February 25, 2013.
20. Neill SM, Tatnall FM, Cox NH. Guidelines for the management of lichen sclerosus. Br J Dermatol 2002;147:640–9.

21. Carli P, Cuttaneo A, De Magnis A, et al. Squamous cell carcinoma arising in the vulval lichen sclerosus: a longitudinal cohort study. Eur J Cancer Prev 1995;4: 491–5.
22. Sheth S, Schechtman AD. Itchy perianal erythema. J Fam Pract 2007;56(12): 1025–7.
23. Meffert J. Lichen sclerosus et atrophicus. In: Emedicine website. 2009. Available at: http://emedicine.medscape.com/article/1123316-overview. Accessed April 28, 2012.
24. Assman T, Becker-Wegerich P, Grewe M, et al. Tacrolimus ointment for the treatment of vulvar lichen sclerosus. J Am Acad Dermatol 2003;48:935–7.
25. Verbov J. Pruritus ani and its management: a study and reappraisal. Clin Exp Dermatol 1984;9:46–52.
26. Pirone E, Infantino A, Masin A, et al. Can proctological procedures resolve perianal pruritus and mycosis? A prospective study of 23 cases. Int J Colorectal Dis 1992;127:8–20.
27. Weismann K, Petersen C, Roder B. Pruritus ani caused by beta-haemolytic streptococci. Acta Derm Venereol 1996;76:415.
28. Asgeirsson T, Nunoo R, Luchtefeld M. Hidradenitis suppurativa and pruritus ani. Clin Colon Rectal Surg 2001;24(1):71–80.
29. Jacobs E. Anal infections caused by herpes simplex virus. Dis Colon Rectum 1976;19(2):151–7.
30. Whitlow C. Bacterial sexually transmitted diseases. Clin Colon Rectal Surg 2004; 17(4):209–14.
31. Centers for Disease Control and Prevention. Sexually transmitted diseases treatment guidelines 2002. MMWR Recomm Rep 2002;51(RR-6):1–78.
32. O'Farrell N. Donovanosis. Sex Transm Infect 2002;78:452–7.
33. Cates W. Estimates of the incidence and prevalence of sexually transmitted diseases in the United States. American Social Health Association Panel. Sex Transm Dis 1999;26(Suppl 4):S2–7.
34. Chang G, Welton M. Human papillomavirus, condylomata acuminata, and anal neoplasia. Clin Colon Rectal Surg 2004;17(4):221–30.
35. Sohn N, Robilotti JG. The gay bowel syndrome. A review of colonic and rectal conditions in 200 male homosexuals. Am J Gastroenterol 1977;67:478–84.
36. Polat M, Oztas P, Ilhan MN, et al. Generalized pruritus: a prospective study concerning etiology. Am J Clin Dermatol 2008;9(1):39–44.
37. Kfoury LW, Jurdi MA. Uremic pruritus. J Nephrol 2012;25(5):644–52.
38. To TH, Clark K, Lam L, et al. The role of ondansetron in the management of cholestatic or uremic pruritus: a systematic review. J Pain Symptom Manage 2012;44(5):725–30.
39. Anand S. Gabapentin for pruritus in palliative care. Am J Hosp Palliat Care 2013; 30(2):192–6.
40. Lin TC, Lai YH, Guo SE, et al. Baby oil therapy for uremic pruritus in haemodialysis patients. J Clin Nurs 2012;21(1–2):139–48.
41. Ghanei E, Zeinali J, Borghei M, et al. Efficacy of omega-3 fatty acids supplementation in treatment of uremic pruritus in hemodialysis patients: a double-blind randomized controlled trial. Iran Red Crescent Med J 2012;14(9): 515–22.
42. Shakiba M, Sanadgol H, Azmoude HR, et al. Effect of sertraline on uremic pruritus improvement in ESRD patients. Int J Nephrol 2012;2012:363901.
43. Shavit L, Grenader T, Lifschitz M, et al. Use of pregabalin in the management of chronic uremic pruritus. J Pain Symptom Manage 2013;45(4):776–81.

44. Gossard AA. Care of the cholestatic patient. Clin Liver Dis 2013;17(2):331–44.
45. Marchesa P, Fazio VW, Oliart S, et al. Perianal Bowen's disease: a clinicopathologic study of 47 patients. Dis Colon Rectum 1997;40:1286–93.
46. Marfing TE, Abel ME, Gallagher DM. Perianal Bowen's disease and associated malignancies. Results of a survey. Dis Colon Rectum 1987;30:782–5.
47. Daniel GL, Longo WE, Vernava AM III. Pruritus ani causes and concerns. Dis Colon Rectum 1994;37:670–4.
48. Murie JA, Sim AJ, Mackenzie I. The importance of pain, pruritus and soiling as symptoms of haemorrhoids and their response to haemorrhoidectomy or rubber band ligation. Br J Surg 1981;68:247–9.
49. Scarborough R. Pruritus ani: its etiology and treatment. Ann Surg 1933;98(6): 1039–45.
50. Bowyer A, McColl I. A study of 200 patients with pruritus ani. Proc R Soc Med 1970;63(Suppl):96–8.
51. Friend WG. The cause and treatment of idiopathic pruritus ani. Dis Colon Rectum 1977;20:40–2.
52. Smith LE, Henrichs D, McCullah RD. Prospective studies on the etiology and treatment of pruritus ani. Dis Colon Rectum 1982;25:358–63.
53. Eyers AA, Thomson JP. Pruritus ani: is anal sphincter dysfunction important in aetiology? BMJ 1979;2:1549–51.
54. Eusebio EB, Graham J, Mody N. Treatment of intractable pruritis ani. Dis Colon Rectum 1991;34:289.

Surgical Management of Fecal Incontinence

Joshua I.S. Bleier, MD[a],*, Brian R. Kann, MD[b]

KEYWORDS

- Fecal incontinence • Surgical • Management • Sphincteroplasty
- Sacral neuromodulation • Bulking agents • Sphincter

KEY POINTS

- Fecal incontinence is a very prevalent but likely underreported disorder.
- Appropriate history and physical examination, including obstetric history, is important to determine the cause of incontinence.
- Medical management is the appropriate first-line treatment, but when this fails surgery is the next approach.
- The most common current surgical approaches include sphincteroplasty, anal canal bulking agents, and sacral nerve stimulation.
- More complex approaches include stimulated graciloplasty, artificial bowel sphincter, tibial nerve stimulation, magnetic anal sphincter, radiofrequency ablation, and antegrade continence enema; however, these approaches tend to have a higher morbidity.

INTRODUCTION

Fecal incontinence is an embarrassing and socially paralyzing condition that affects up to 18% of the population and as many as 50% of nursing home residents.[1] The maintenance of fecal continence is an extremely intricate process that involves the coordinated efforts and interaction of several different neuronal pathways and the musculature of the pelvic floor and anorectum. Several additional factors, including systemic disease, bowel motility, stool consistency, sphincter integrity, and patient emotion, play important roles in regulating continence. This article outlines the numerous causes of fecal incontinence, details the evaluation of patients complaining of altered fecal continence, briefly describes nonsurgical modalities for treatment, and focuses on the surgical methods of treating this debilitating condition that occurs much more frequently than most realize.

[a] Division of Colon and Rectal Surgery, Pennsylvania Hospital/Hospital of the University of Pennsylvania, University of Pennsylvania, 800 Walnut Street, 20th Floor, Philadelphia, PA 19106, USA; [b] Division of Colon and Rectal Surgery, Penn Presbyterian Medical Center, University of Pennsylvania, 51 North 39th Street, Suite W266, Philadelphia, PA 19104, USA
* Corresponding author.
E-mail address: Joshua.bleier@uphs.upenn.edu

Gastroenterol Clin N Am 42 (2013) 815–836
http://dx.doi.org/10.1016/j.gtc.2013.09.006
0889-8553/13/$ – see front matter © 2013 Elsevier Inc. All rights reserved.

gastro.theclinics.com

ETIOLOGY

The most common causes of fecal incontinence seen by colorectal surgeons is anal sphincter injury, with obstetric injury being the most frequently cited cause in women.[2] Overt anal sphincter disruption accompanies as many as 10% of vaginal deliveries, whereas sonographic evidence of occult sphincter damage can be seen in as many as 30% of first vaginal deliveries.[3,4] The obstetric-related disturbance is affected by not just the direct sphincter injury but also other risk factors, such as forceps delivery, occipitoposterior position, and prolonged labor, which can lead to pelvic denervation injury.[4] In fact, 60% of patients with an obstetric injury will also have evidence of pudendal nerve damage.[5,6] Although a small percentage of women will experience altered continence because of a direct sphincter injury in the immediate postpartum period, most will not present with symptoms until later in life, when the supporting pelvic floor musculature begins to weaken and compensatory mechanisms are lost.

Traumatic injury to the anal sphincter, both accidental and nonaccidental, can also result in altered fecal continence. Perineal impalement injuries, although rare, can be devastating, because they are often associated with not just a direct sphincter injury but also injuries to the rectum and pelvic innervation; they frequently require a temporary diverting stoma, and long-term continence after stoma closure in these patients is often difficult to achieve. Traumatic injuries to the anal sphincter may also occur in conjunction with sexual abuse, voluntary anoreceptive intercourse, or insertion of foreign bodies.

Iatrogenic injury to the anal sphincter may occur in several settings, the most common of which is after surgical intervention for various anorectal disorders. A recent systematic review showed an overall continence disturbance rate of 14% after lateral internal anal sphincterotomy for anal fissure; incontinence to flatus was seen in 9%, soilage/seepage in 6%, incontinence to liquid stool in 0.67%, and incontinence to solid stool in 0.83%.[7] Incontinence after hemorrhoidectomy should occur infrequently, although patients with preexisting altered continence are more likely to show further deterioration in their continence postoperatively,[8] a fact that should be taken into consideration when contemplating excisional hemorrhoidectomy. Fecal incontinence after anal fistulotomy has long been the bane of the procedure; minor alterations in continence can be seen in as many as 18% to 52% of patients, and major changes can occur in 35% to 45% of patients.[9] Long-term fecal soiling can be seen in up to 43% of patients after endoanal advancement flaps for fistula in ano.[10] In a database review of patients with alterations in fecal continence after anorectal surgery, Lindsey and colleagues[11] showed that a common factor was the presence of an internal sphincter injury, resulting in reversal of the normal resting pressure gradient of the anal canal. Another iatrogenic cause of fecal incontinence is pelvic radiotherapy, which can directly affect anal sphincter function and also decrease rectal compliance.[12]

Anorectal disease not managed surgically may also be an independent risk factor for developing altered fecal continence. Rectal prolapse may stent the anus open or chronically dilate the sphincters. Prolapsing internal hemorrhoids may also stent the anal canal open, allowing for fecal seepage. Patients with large external hemorrhoids may have difficulty with perianal hygiene after defecation, leading to chronic soiling, which is often perceived as incontinence by the patient. Chronic rectal inflammation or decreased compliance to drug therapy for inflammatory bowel disease or infectious proctitis may also lead to alterations in continence. Distal rectal cancer can cause proximal impaction and overflow incontinence, and direct sphincter or neural invasion.

Although obstetric trauma is a common cause of pelvic denervation injury, other neurologic causes of altered fecal continence exist. Patients who have multiple sclerosis or other central nervous system–related disorders may experience altered fecal continence as their disease progresses. Patients with longstanding diabetes are prone to autonomic neuropathies, including pudendal neuropathy. Patients with congenital malformations such as spina bifida, meningomyelocele, and imperforate anus often have derangements in pelvic floor and anal sphincter function.

Lastly, simple factors such as the senescent process of aging may affect fecal continence as muscles lose bulk and strength over time. Senile dementia and psychiatric illness may also play a role in altered fecal continence because of patient's lack of awareness of the call to defecate.

EVALUATION
History

Obtaining a detailed history may be difficult, because patients are often embarrassed and hesitant to offer details of their incontinence unless they are approached with a direct line of questioning. It is important to create as comfortable an environment as possible during the history and physical examination. A thorough obstetric history in women in essential, including number of pregnancies and deliveries, means of delivery (eg, vaginal, cesarean, forceps-assisted, vacuum-assisted), obstetric injury from perineal laceration or episiotomy, and episodes of prolonged labor. Timing of onset and progression of symptoms can provide meaningful information regarding the cause and potential efficacy of therapy. Neurologic causes should be considered and investigated in appropriate patients.

Questioning should clarify whether the patient exhibits incontinence to solid stool, liquid stool, or flatus, or a combination thereof. A determination should also be made regarding whether the patient has active or passive incontinence. Active incontinence, or urge incontinence, describes the loss of stool despite efforts by the patient to control it. This condition typically suggests an intact sensory mechanism with the loss of function or integrity of the external anal sphincter. Passive incontinence is the loss of stool without the patient sensing it, and typically suggests a neurologic origin of the patient's complaints.

Quantifying the degree of incontinence is important, especially in establishing a baseline score that can then be compared with posttreatment scores and used to measure the effect imparted by a particular management scheme. Numerous scoring systems are available for use. The Wexner (Cleveland Clinic Florida) Fecal Incontinence Score (CCF-FIS) is an independently validated tool that is easy to use for the patient and the physician, and incorporates a quality of life component.[13] The Fecal Incontinence Quality of Life questionnaire is another useful tool for quantifying a patient's degree of incontinence and its impact on quality of life.[9]

Physical Examination

The physical examination should start with the patient in a comfortable position, typically the Sims (left lateral decubitus) position. The perineum should be inspected, looking particularly for scars from prior surgeries or trauma (obstetric or otherwise). Other findings may include fistulae in ano, skin excoriation from chronic soiling, rectal prolapse, and prolapsing hemorrhoids. The bulk of the perineal body should be assessed. At rest, the anal verge should be closed and not patulous. The patient should be asked to perform a Valsalva maneuver to evaluate for prolapse. Perianal sensation to pinprick should be evaluated, as should the anocutaneous "wink" reflex to light tough, which can be thought of as a "poor man's assessment" of neurologic function.

Digital rectal examination should be performed to subjectively determine the patient's resting sphincter tone and voluntary squeeze pressures. Palpation for rectal masses or fecal impaction should be performed. The experienced examiner may appreciate a large anterior sphincter defect or motion abnormality if present. Visualization of the anorectal mucosa should also be performed, either through anoscopy or rigid proctosigmoidoscopy to evaluate for mucosal abnormalities, which might suggest inflammatory bowel disease, infectious proctitis, or a neoplastic process.

Diagnostic Studies

Endoanal ultrasound

The primary means of imaging the anatomy of the anal canal, including the anal sphincters, has become endoanal ultrasonography. The test is easily performed in an office-based setting, without sedation, and is very well tolerated by most patients. Ultrasonographically, the external anal sphincter appears hyperechoic, the internal anal sphincter appears hypoechoic (**Fig. 1**), and scar tissue shows mixed echogenicity. Anatomic sphincter defects can be easily identified and the degree of the defect can be measured (**Fig. 2**). The thickness of the perineal body can also be measured.

Anorectal manometry

Anorectal manometry can provide valuable information regarding the functional status of the anal sphincters and the distal rectum in the evaluation of the patient with fecal incontinence. This technique also is a well-tolerated, office-based procedure that is easy to perform, but requires dedicated equipment and trained personnel. Several commercially available systems are available; some utilize multi-channel water-perfused catheters, whereas others use direct microtransducers to record resistance.

Several measurements can be obtained from manometry studies. The mean resting pressure of the anal sphincters is normally 40 to 70 mm Hg, most of which is generated by the internal anal sphincter,[14] which is in a continuous state of maximal contraction. Low resting pressures may be seen in patients with altered fecal continence from disturbances in the function of the internal anal sphincter. The maximal squeeze pressure is typically 2 to 3 times the baseline resting pressure; it is generated mostly by voluntary contraction of the external anal sphincter. Defects of the external anal sphincter

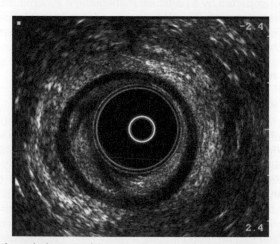

Fig. 1. Normal endoanal ultrasound (EAUS). The internal anal sphincter (IAS) appears as an unbroken hypoechoic ring. The external anal sphincter (EAS) appears as a hyperechoic ring.

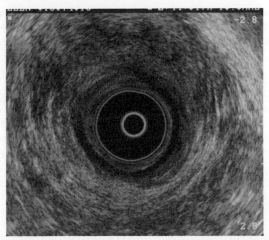

Fig. 2. EAUS of mixed sphincter defect. Discontinuity in the ultrasonographic appearance represent defects in both the internal and external sphincter.

muscle from trauma (eg, surgical, obstetric) may result in decreased maximal squeeze pressures. The high-pressure zone is the length of the internal anal sphincter through which pressures are greater than half of the maximal resting pressure; it measures approximately 2.0 to 3.0 cm in women and 2.5 to 3.5 cm in men.[15]

The rectoanal inhibitory reflex (RAIR) is represented by initial contraction of the external anal sphincter followed by a pronounced internal anal sphincter relaxation in response to rectal distension. This reflex enables the sensory mucosa of the anal canal to "sample" the contents of the distal rectum and help distinguish between gas, liquid, and solid stool. The RAIR is altered in patients with Hirschsprung disease, scleroderma, and Chagas disease. Rectal sensation can be measured by incrementally instilling a balloon placed in the rectum with small aliquots of air; normal sensation usually occurs with 40 mL of insufflation. Decreased rectal sensation can lead to fecal impaction with subsequent overflow incontinence. Lastly, rectal compliance can be measured as the change in pressure associated with a change in volume. A poorly compliant rectum is not able to readily accommodate the stool it receives and may contribute to fecal incontinence. Inflammatory conditions or external beam radiation may lead to decreased rectal compliance.

Pudendal nerve terminal motor latency
Determination of pudendal nerve terminal motor latency (PNTML) is an important component in the evaluation of patients with fecal incontinence, because pudendal neuropathy can often lead to alterations in fecal control. A disposable electrode is attached to the examiner's finger, which is directed toward the Alcock canal within the rectum. An impulse is delivered to the pudendal nerve, and a more distal sensory electrode determines how long it takes for the external anal sphincter to contract. Normal values are less than 2.0 ± 0.2 ms. Prolonged PNTML may be seen as a result of obstetric trauma to the pudendal nerves or with systemic diseases, such as diabetes.

Electromyography
Electromyography uses needles placed into the sphincter muscles to record electrical activity; it can be used to map the external anal sphincter and identify neuromuscular

integrity. Alternatively, an intra-anal sponge or surface electrode can be used. Because of the discomfort and expertise required, single-fiber electromyography never gained universal acceptance.

Defecography

Defecography, or a defecating proctography, involves instillation of contrast material into the rectum, after which the patient evacuates the material under direct fluoroscopic visualization. Although the test is often uncomfortable and embarrassing for patients, it provides extremely useful dynamic images of the rectum and pelvic floor during the act of defecation. In the evaluation of the patient with fecal incontinence, defecography may show incomplete evacuation of the rectum, leading to overflow incontinence. It may also show lack of rectal distention, indicating decreased rectal compliance. Dynamic magnetic resonance imaging defecography is a more recently described alternative to fluoroscopic defecography.[16]

Colonoscopy

Endoscopic evaluation of the colonic mucosa should be considered essential in patients with fecal incontinence. A stricture or mass may cause partial obstruction, allowing for overflow incontinence. Various inflammatory conditions of the colon and rectum may also lead to looser stools or loss of rectal compliance, predisposing to incontinence. A large villous lesion may cause excessive mucous production, often leading to soilage.

MEDICAL MANAGEMENT

The most important initial step in managing fecal incontinence is determining the underlying cause. Certain causes, such as chronic diarrhea or constipation, neurologic conditions, and systemic illnesses, may be best managed by medical means. Unfortunately, published data are lacking regarding the true efficacy of medical management, as evidenced by a Cochrane review evaluating this topic.[17] Initial management should center on a conservative approach that aims to change the consistency and frequency of stools by avoiding laxatives, starting or increasing the use of stool bulking agents, changing dietary habits, and starting antimotility drugs. The goal should be bulkier, more solid stools that are evacuated completely and the establishment of a regular, predictable bowel pattern.

Fiber supplements serve to add bulk to stool and absorb fluid, creating a more solid stool. Both natural and synthetic products are available, and no one product has been shown to have a benefit over the others. Commercially available products include Metamucil, Benefiber, Citrucel, Konsyl, and Fibercon. Patients should be educated regarding a high-fiber diet, aiming for 25 to 30 g of fiber per day.

Up to 50% of patients with chronic diarrhea also have fecal incontinence.[18] Therefore, constipating agents may play a key role in managing these patients' symptoms. Constipating agents, such as loperamide, diphenoxylate-atropine, codeine, and amitriptyline, can be particularly helpful in this group of patients. Loperamide is a synthetic opioid that inhibits bowel motility via mu receptors in the gut; it also has been shown to increase resting internal anal sphincter pressures.[19]

Regular use of enemas to maintain an empty rectum may also be of benefit to several patients. In a study of patients with spina bifida, fecal continence was able to be achieved in 76% of children and 60% of adults with the use of a scheduled regimen of enemas.[20] In elderly patients with constipation and overflow incontinence, a combination of 30 g of lactulose along with daily glycerin suppositories and weekly tap water enemas was shown to reduce fecal incontinence episodes by 35%.[21]

BIOFEEDBACK

Biofeedback is a "retraining" program that aims to provide strength, sensory, and co-ordination training for patients with pelvic floor disorders, including fecal incontinence. The goal is to help patients relearn how to defecate completely, regularly, and effectively. Patients are educated regarding pelvic floor coordination and recognition of sensory thresholds.

This specialized physical therapy can be performed in several different ways, but it most often uses the placement of a pressure-sensitive probe into the anal canal to monitor the strength and coordination of the anal sphincter and pelvic floor musculature. Through transmitting data from the probe to a monitor, patients are able to visualize the effect of their efforts. Through a series of exercises and visual feedback, improvements can be made in pelvic muscle control, rectal sensory threshold, and overall defecatory control.[22]

Several studies have shown the effectiveness of biofeedback in improving fecal incontinence, with success rates ranging from 50% to 90%.[23] In a study comparing biofeedback with pelvic floor exercises alone, 44% of patients in the biofeedback group were able to achieve complete continence, versus 21% in the pelvic floor exercise group ($P = .008$).[24]

Unfortunately, many trials lack adequate control groups, and several factors that may have an impact on success, such as the motivation of the patient and the effect of the individual therapist, are difficult to control for. Biofeedback is time-consuming and labor-intensive, and requires a motivated patient. Several methods are described using varying schedules, exercises, and means of feedback. A Cochrane review evaluating the efficacy of biofeedback concluded that no one method has shown superiority over the others; it also concluded that the limited number of trials together with methodological weaknesses do not allow for a definitive assessment of the role of biofeedback in the management of fecal incontinence, although some suggestion was seen that the addition of electrical stimulation may enhance the outcome over biofeedback alone.[25] Regardless, it is an entirely safe technique that offers potential benefit and should be considered first-line therapy in the highly motivated patient for whom traditional medical management has failed.[26]

SURGICAL MANAGEMENT

When medical management of fecal incontinence is inadequate, the next step in management requires surgical intervention, which is the thrust of this article. The next section provides a thorough, but certainly not exhaustive, overview of the most common means of surgical management of fecal incontinence.

Sphincteroplasty

Overlapping sphincteroplasty has traditionally been the most common operation performed for the direct repair of an anatomic sphincter defect associated with fecal incontinence. Through a curvilinear incision anterior to the anus (**Fig. 3**), the sphincter and associated scar are mobilized (**Fig. 4**) and reapproximated in an overlapping fashion (**Fig. 5**), preserving the scar to provide extra bulk and strength to the repair (**Fig. 6**). Care should be taken not to extend the mobilization too far posterolaterally, to avoid inadvertent pudendal nerve injury. An anterior levatorplasty is often performed in conjunction with the sphincter repair. Outcomes after a direct end-to-end repair are typically inferior to those after an overlapping repair.[27]

Short-term outcomes suggest good to excellent results with overlapping sphincteroplasty in 31% to 83% of patients.[26] However, several studies have shown

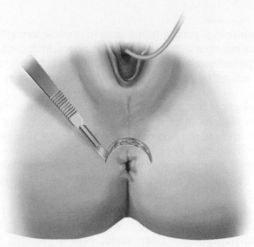

Fig. 3. A curvilinear incision through the perineum. (*From* Wexner SD, Fleshman J. Colon and rectal surgery: anorectal operations. Philadelphia: Wolters Kluwer Health, 2011; with permission.)

deterioration in the benefits of sphincteroplasty with regard to fecal continence over time.[2,28,29] A recent systematic review evaluating the long-term outcomes of anal sphincter repair reviewed studies with a minimum follow-up of 60 months and found that the initially "good" subjective outcomes with sphincteroplasty deteriorated over time. Despite this, however, most patients remained satisfied with their surgical outcomes and quality of life.[30]

The effect of preexisting pudendal neuropathy on the outcome of overlapping sphincteroplasty is somewhat controversial. Gilliland and colleagues[31] found that bilateral normal pudendal nerve terminal motor latencies were predictive of long-term success after overlapping sphincteroplasty; 62% of 59 patients with bilaterally normal pudendal nerve terminal motor latencies had successful outcomes, compared

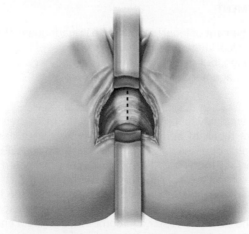

Fig. 4. Sphincter scar is encountered, and left intact. (*From* Wexner SD, Fleshman J. Colon and rectal surgery: anorectal operations. Philadelphia: Wolters Kluwer Health, 2011; with permission.)

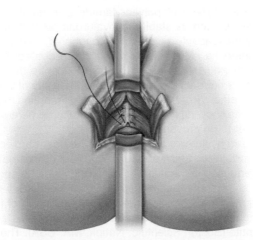

Fig. 5. The internal anal sphincter is imbricated during overlapping repair. (*From* Wexner SD, Fleshman J. Colon and rectal surgery: anorectal operations. Philadelphia: Wolters Kluwer Health, 2011; with permission.)

with only 16.7% of 12 patients with unilateral or bilateral prolonged pudendal nerve terminal motor latencies ($P<.01$). Conversely, Chen and colleagues[32] reported significant improvements in continence in patients with unilateral or bilateral prolonged pudendal nerve terminal motor latency.

Injectable Bulking Agents

One of the newest modalities to be applied to the surgical management of fecal incontinence is injectable bulking agents. These materials are injected into the anal canal to physically augment the area and provide an enhanced occlusive mechanical barrier to fecal loss. Several materials have been brought to market, including autologous fat,

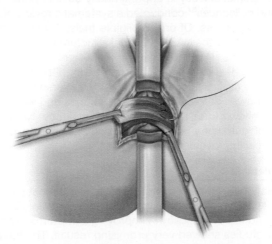

Fig. 6. The external sphincter is overlapped and repaired. (*From* Wexner SD, Fleshman J. Colon and rectal surgery: anorectal operations. Philadelphia: Wolters Kluwer Health, 2011; with permission.)

collagen, hydrogel cross-linked with polyacrylamide, polydimethylsiloxane elastomer, bioabsorbable materials such as stabilized hyaluronic acid (NASHA Dx), injectable synthetic calcium hydroxyapatite ceramic microspheres, silicone biospheres (PTQ, Uroplasty Inc, Minnetonka, MN, USA), and carbon-coated beads (Durasphere, Carbon Medical Technologies, St Paul, MN, USA). Despite the myriad of materials and attempts, debate remains as to the most appropriate site of injection (submucosal vs intramuscular) and efficacy of the procedure, which remains modest, with approximately 50% of patients showing mild to moderate improvement of symptoms. Long-term durability has yet to be proven.

NASHA Dx (stabilized hyaluronic acid) is one of the best-studied materials studied. A double-blinded, randomized trial reported that 52% of those treated with NASHA Dx had 50% or more reduction in the number of incontinence episodes compared with 31% who received sham treatment. Adverse events included 1 rectal abscess and 1 prostatic abscess.[33] In a systematic review of a large group of injectable implants, Hussain and colleagues[34] found that short-term success was associated with the use of PTQ or Coaptite (Boston Scientific, Natick, MA, USA). The use of local anesthetic and failure to use laxatives in the postoperative period was associated with a lower likelihood of success. Watson and colleagues[35] performed a review of a large group of agents and similarly found that most published studies showed improvement in at least 50% of subjects with little reported morbidity, and concluded that anal bulking agents may play a role in alleviating symptoms of fecal seepage or soilage rather than treating more severe incontinence to solid stool. From a prospectively maintained database evaluating the use of collagen injection into the internal anal sphincter, Maslekar and colleagues[36] conducted a retrospective cohort study aimed at looking at medium-term efficacy with a minimum of 36 months of follow-up. They found that in a cohort of 100 patients, 56% reported an improvement in fecal incontinence scores from a mean of 14 to a mean of 8. Among patients overall, 68% reported improvement; however, 38% required a repeat injection, whereas another 15% required a third injection. The median interval between first and final injection was 12 months. No morbidity was reported. They concluded that injection of collagen into the internal anal sphincter is safe and effective in patients with passive fecal incontinence, but repeat treatment may be needed for optimal efficacy in approximately 50% of patients.

Finally, Maeda and colleagues[37] conducted a systematic review of all controlled trials of injectable bulking agents. Of only 5 eligible trials, 4 were at high risk for bias based on methodology. Only the NASHA Dx trial structure was truly methodologically sound. As stated earlier, the NASHA Dx trial showed a significant reduction in the number of incontinent episodes, whereas a trial comparing PTQ versus sham was too small to reliably show a clinical benefit. In a trial of PTQ versus carbon-coated beads (Durasphere), PTQ showed some short-term advantages and was safer. Ultrasound-guided delivery was shown to be safer than digital guidance. No study incorporated patient evaluation of outcomes, so objective continence scores were difficult to compare with practical improvements in daily life.

Sacral Nerve Stimulation

Sacral nerve stimulation (SNS) has emerged as one of the most promising modalities for treating severe fecal incontinence. Initially used to treat urinary incontinence, it was also anecdotally found to have efficacy in improving symptoms associated with fecal incontinence. Initial studies showed very promising results. The therapy involves implantation of an electrode adjacent to the S3 nerve root through the sacral foramen, and subsequent delivery of regular electrical impulses (**Fig. 7**). The implantation of the device involves an initial test phase to determine efficacy, followed by implant of

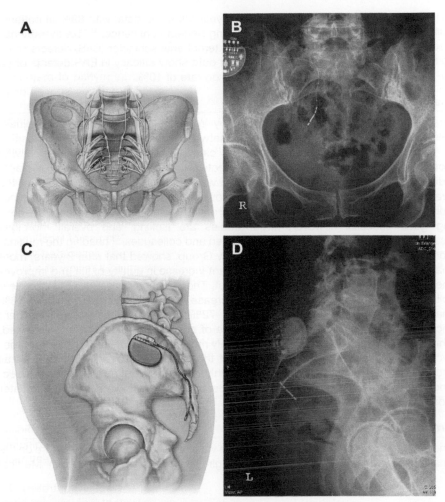

Fig. 7. Radiographic and schematic view showing appropriately placed sacral nerve stimulator. (*A*) Anterior anatomic view, (*B*) AP pelvic radiograph, (*C*) Lateral anatomic view, (*D*) Lateral radiograph. (*From* Wexner SD, Fleshman J. Colon and rectal surgery: anorectal operations. Philadelphia: Wolters Kluwer Health, 2011; with permission.)

the permanent stimulator in those with improvement. Tjandra and colleagues[38] performed the earliest prospective trial, comparing SNS to best medical therapy in patients with and without external sphincter defects of up to 120°. In this study of 120 patients (60 in SNS group, 60 in the control group), 90% of patients in the SNS group reported success (defined as at least a 50% improvement in the number of incontinent episodes); perfect continence was achieved in 47.2%. The control group showed no appreciable improvement.

The largest multi-institutional international trial conducted by the SNS study group found an initial 90% success rate with test stimulation. At 3-year follow-up, 83% of patient reported a 50% or greater reduction in the number of weekly incontinent episodes, with a mean decrease in the number of episodes per week from 9.4 to 1.7. Importantly, 40% of patients reported durable, perfect continence.[39] A recent follow-up to this seminal study reported 5-year follow-up data, with 89% of patients still reporting success and 36% still reporting perfect continence.[40] This therapy has been shown to be effective in trials with external anal sphincter (EAS) defects of up to 60%; however, European and Australian data show efficacy in EAS defects of up to 120°.[38] Adverse events include an infection rate of 10%.

Gracioplasty

Gracioplasty was recently reintroduced by Williams in 1989,[41] but was originally described more than 100 years ago by Chetwood,[42] and involves the transposition of the gracilis muscle to encircle the anal canal. The procedure is described with both native functioning muscle, which effectively functions as a biologic cerclage, but is more commonly used in association with continuous pulse stimulation of the gracilis muscle to convert the muscle to provide more appropriate slow-twitch functioning (**Fig. 8**). This procedure is technically difficult, with high-volume centers reporting good success; however, large studies are lacking, and overall morbidity associated with the procedure is high. Baeten and colleagues,[43] heading the multinational Dynamic Gracioplasty Therapy Study Group, showed that after 2 years, more than 60% of patients maintained a significant increase in quality of life and improvement of incontinence symptoms. In contrast, Thornton and colleagues,[44] in a 5-year follow-up study, showed a significant decrease in overall success, with only 16% maintaining good continence. More than 72% of patients had some significant morbidity in the donor site, and a 50% rate of obstructed defecation was reported. This procedure remains an option in the highly motivated patient, especially after proctectomy and reconstruction, but in light of the high complication rates and overall morbidity and the current list of other highly successful options, it is rarely used, and is best performed in specialty centers. Because of the withdrawal of the stimulator from the market, this procedure is currently not available in the United States.

Artificial Bowel Sphincter

The artificial bowel sphincter (ABS) operates via generation of external pressure on the anal canal to maintain tonic closure. Originally developed by American Medical

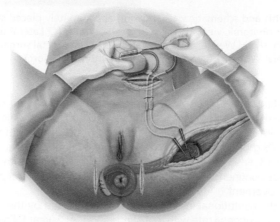

Fig. 8. The appearance of the tunneled gracilis, encircling the anus, stimulated with 2 electrodes. (*From* Wexner SD, Fleshman J. Colon and rectal surgery: anorectal operations. Philadelphia: Wolters Kluwer Health, 2011; with permission.)

Systems (Minnetonka, MN, USA), the device consists of an inflatable cuff that is surgically implanted to encircle the anal canal, a control pump, and a pressure-regulating balloon implanted anterior to the bladder (**Fig. 9**). The control pump is typically implanted into the labia or scrotum. The cuff is maintained in a chronically filled state until the patient manually pumps the fluid out of the cuff, into the reservoir, which allows the cuff to deflate. Over a period of several minutes, the cuff gradually refills (**Fig. 10**). Christiansen first described the use of this device in 1987,[45] and in a systematic review published by Mundy and colleagues[46] in 2004, up to 66% of patients reported maintenance of function. The long-term use of the ABS has been plagued with complications, including infection rates of greater than 20% and explantation rates approximating 50%, mainly because of dysfunction and erosion of the device. A more recent publication by Darnis and colleagues[47] reported a consecutive series of 21 patients receiving the ABS. All patients reported at least one morbidity, and infections or ulcerations occurred in 76% of patients, with one-third having perineal pain or evacuation disorders. Seventeen patients (81%) underwent explantation of the device. Nevertheless, in those who maintained a functioning device at 1 year, continued satisfactory continence was reported.

In contrast, Wong and colleagues[48] reported a series of 52 patients who underwent ABS implantation with a mean follow-up of greater than 5 years. They noted that 50% of patients required revision, and only 27% required explantation. In more than two-thirds of patients with an active device, significant improvements in Wexner score and quality of life indices were reported. In 2009, Wexner and colleagues[49] reported on a consecutive series of 51 patients who received an ABS over a 9-year period in order to determine factors associated with failure. In this series, 23 (41.2%) patients experienced device infections, most of which were early-stage (18/23); 5 of 23 experienced late-stage infections. Multivariate analysis showed that a history of prior perineal sepsis and time between implantation and first bowel movement were independent risk

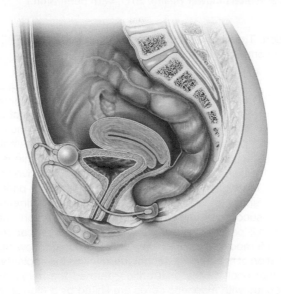

Fig. 9. A lateral view showing the placement of the artificial bowel sphincter in a woman. (*From* Wexner SD, Fleshman J. Colon and rectal surgery: anorectal operations. Philadelphia: Wolters Kluwer Health, 2011; with permission.)

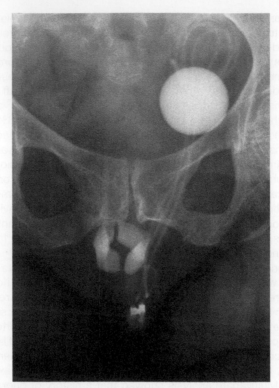

Fig. 10. Abdominal X-ray showing artificial bowel sphincter in place, bladder inflated with radiopaque liquid. (*From* Wexner SD, Fleshman J. Colon and rectal surgery: anorectal operations. Philadelphia: Wolters Kluwer Health, 2011; with permission.)

factors for infection. These data support effective results of the ABS, but show an almost prohibitive complication rate.

Anal Cerclage

In the late 1800s, Thiersch described the anal cerclage for treating rectal procidentia. This procedure involved anal encirclement with sutures to obstruct the anal aperture and prevent prolapse. This paradigm has also been modified for the treatment of fecal incontinence. In 2013, Devesa and colleagues[50] reported on the implantation of a silicone band as a prosthetic sling using a modified Thiersch technique in a series of 33 patients. In all but 1 patient, success was reported with objective assessment using the Wexner scores. Morbidity was significant, however, with 2 patients having early infections, and 2 reporting late infections or erosions. Thirteen patients were explanted, with 10 successful reimplantations. In 1986, Larach and Vazquez[51] reported a series of 12 patients who underwent a similar procedure with a silastic mesh implant, with 9 reporting excellent results at 2.5-year follow-up.

A novel modification of the cerclage technique involves the implantation of a string of magnetic beads that occlude the anal orifice, termed the *magnetic anal sphincter* (MAS). Titanium beads with magnetic cores are linked by a titanium wire and remain closed at rest, preventing fecal loss. The force generated by a Valsalva maneuver during defecation forces the beads apart, allowing passage of stool. Mantoo and colleagues[52] reported their short-term results in 2012, showing significant improvement in Fecal Incontinence Quality of Life scores. Wong and colleagues[53] reported on a non-randomized comparison study between the MAS (n = 16) and SNS (n = 12). Mean follow-up in the MAS and SNS groups were 18 and 22 months, respectively. One patient in each group required device explant. Four patients in the MAS group experienced complications, but a significant improvement in continence was reported in both groups. Long-term results using the MAS have yet to be reported, but this modality remains a promising option.

Tibial Nerve Stimulation

Tibial nerve stimulation (TNS), like SNS, was first performed for urinary incontinence and described by Nakamura and colleagues[54] in 1983. It was also found to have efficacy in patients with concomitant fecal incontinence, as Shafik and colleagues[55] reported in 2003 in a series of patients undergoing percutaneous TNS. Queralto and colleagues[56] further modified the technique and reported on transcutaneous TNS in 2006. In a preliminary study of 10 patients, 8 showed a mean improvement in their incontinence scores after 4 weeks. In the first randomized controlled trial of its kind, Leroi and colleagues[57] reported on 144 patients who were randomized to TNS or sham. Among those who received active treatment, 47% showed at least a 30% decrease in continence scores compared with 27% of patients in the sham group, but this result did not achieve statistical significance. Nonetheless, the authors believed that active treatment was more effective than sham. Only 1 adverse event (a sensation of burning in the test leg) in the test group was reported. Of the 66 patients in the test group, only 6 reported perfect continence. Thomas and colleagues[58] recently published a systematic review of all reports on TNS for fecal incontinence. They identified 13 studies, most of which were of poor quality. However, in a total of 273 patients who received treatment, at least a 50% improvement in the number of incontinent episodes was seen in 63% to 82% of patients. These investigators found that patients with urge and mixed incontinence experienced more improvement than those with passive incontinence. Follow-up was highly variable, ranging from 1 to 30 months. Overall, this appears to be a safe and somewhat effective modality, but good-quality, long-term results are generally lacking. The procedure is not currently available for open-label use in the United States.

Secca Procedure

Radiofrequency ablation is a modality that has also been used to treat fecal incontinence, and is known as the *Secca procedure* (Curon Medical, Inc, Fremont, CA, USA). It is based on the scarification that results from controlled heating of tissue and subsequent cicatrization from collagen denaturation.[59] The technique was originally described as the *Stretta procedure*, and is used clinically to treat gastroesophageal reflux disease through scarring of the distal esophagus.[60] This paradigm was applied to the anal canal based on the premise that a controlled stricturing of the anal canal would result in a functional partial obstruction akin to the cerclage techniques. Initial results were promising. Efron and colleagues[61] reported on 50 patients enrolled in a multicenter trial; 43 women and 7 men underwent the procedure. Cleveland Clinic Faecal Incontinence Score (CCFIS) improved from a mean of 14.5 to 11.1 at 6 months. Quality-of-life parameters, such as coping, embarrassment, and depression, were all improved. Only 2 minor complications were reported. Takahashi and colleagues[62] treated 10 patients, all women, who experienced a significant improvement in median Wexner score from 13.5 to 5.0 at 12 months. Corresponding improvement was also seen in all quality-of-life indicators. Notably, but not surprisingly, pelvic floor testing did show a significant reduction in rectal compliance; however, anoscopic examination was grossly normal. In a follow-up publication, Takahashi and colleagues[63] reported that results were durable at 2 years. At 5 years, mean fecal incontinence scores had improved from 14.37 to 8.26, with almost 85% showing a greater than 50% improvement.[64] All quality-of-life scores also continued to show significant improvement. Later, Ruiz and colleagues[65] reported more modest results in 24 patients treated with the Secca procedure. Among the 16 patients available for 12-month follow-up, mean CCFIS showed improvement from a baseline of 15.6 to 12.9. No significant long-term complications were reported. Short-term complications included 3 episodes of self-limited bleeding. Similarly, Lefebure and colleagues[66] conducted a single-center nonrandomized trial involving 15 patients. At 12 months, mean incontinence scores improved from 14.07 to 12.33. The only quality-of-life indicator that showed improvement was the depression score. This modality certainly seems to have some efficacy, but may not be as effective as other less-invasive approaches.

Gluteoplasty

Gluteoplasty is a procedure initially described at the turn of the century. Like graciloplasty, it is based on the premise of wrapping functional muscle around the anal canal. It has the advantage of being a locally based, well-vascularized flap that is activated during normal walking, and thus contracts during normal daily activity. This procedure is infrequently performed. Devesa and colleagues[67] published one of the largest studies involving 20 patients who underwent bilateral gluteoplasty. More than 50% showed a significant improvement in functional pressures of the pelvic floor. However, quality-of-life data were not presented, and continence improvements were limited primarily to control of solid stool, with little improvement in control of liquid stool and gas.

In a retrospective series of 25 patients with fecal incontinence of varying origins who underwent unilateral gluteoplasty, Hultman and colleagues[68] found that continence was restored in more than 70%. However, morbidity was significant: 64% of patients had significant donor-site and perirectal complications. Mean length of follow-up was more than 20 months, and no gait or hip dysfunction was reported. However, because of the variability of success, complexity, and high morbidity rate, this procedure is still infrequently performed.

Antegrade Continence Enema

Another option for patients with intractable fecal incontinence is the antegrade continence enema (ACE), first described by Malone and colleagues[69] in 1990. The initial description of this procedure involved amputating the appendix from the cecum, reversing it, and reimplanting the distal end into the cecum through a submucosal tunnel, thus creating a flap valve to prevent reflux of fecal contents through the conduit. The end of the appendiceal conduit was then brought out through a small trephination in the right lower quadrant abdominal wall as a continent appendicostomy. Antegrade colonic enemas through this stoma could then be used to flush and empty the colon, thus helping to minimize episodes of fecal incontinence. The procedure was initially performed in children with myelomeningocele and anorectal malformations, often in conjunction with reconstructive bladder surgery. The procedure has subsequently been used successfully in adults for the management of refractory fecal incontinence and refractory constipation.

Several technical modifications to ACE have been introduced since its initial description. Many surgeons who perform this procedure now believe that it is not necessary to amputate and reverse the appendix, because a cecal wrap around the base of the in situ appendix can also create a valve mechanism and prevent reflux of stool. More recently controversy has occurred regarding whether any continence maneuver is necessary at all, and some authors now advocate simply bringing the distal end of the appendix through the abdominal wall, amputating the tip, and maturing the appendicostomy. Complications of the ACE procedure include stomal stenosis in up to 30% of patients, reflux through the conduit, fecal impaction in the conduit, and stomal prolapse.[70,71] Appendicitis in the conduit has also been described.[72]

In patients who have undergone previous appendectomy, a cecal tube can be fashioned using a linear stapler, which is then exteriorized as a cecostomy. Castellan and colleagues[73] found no differences in functional outcomes between appendiceal and cecal conduits. Another alternative is to create a conduit from the terminal ileum, which has the advantage of maintaining continence via the ileocecal valve.

Worsøe and colleagues[74] reviewed the long-term functional results of ACE in a series of 80 adult patients and found that treatment was deemed successful in 74% of patients over a mean follow-up of 75 months, as judged by patient questionnaires. Chéreau and colleagues[71] also reported a success rate of 86% in a series of 64 patients with a median follow-up of 48 months. In this series, the Wexner score improved from a median of 14.3 preoperatively to 3.4 postoperatively (P<.0001).

An interesting use of the ACE procedure in is conjunction with a perineal colostomy for patients requiring abdominoperineal resection (APR) as a means to avoid a permanent abdominal colostomy. Portier and colleagues[75] described this technique in a series of 18 patients who underwent APR with creation of a perineal colostomy in conjunction with an ACE procedure. The patients then performed antegrade enemas every 24 to 48 hours and reported acceptable continence scores and quality-of-life scores.

With the advent of laparoscopic surgery and the lack of a need for an antireflux procedure, the laparoscopic ACE procedure has gained popularity. Lynch and colleagues[76] compared their experiences with open and laparoscopic approaches to ACE and found the laparoscopic approach to be easier to perform. Thomas and Bassuini[77] described a laparoscopic approach to the cecodivision ACE procedure in patients who had undergone prior appendectomy. Another minimally invasive option described more recently is the use of a percutaneous endoscopic sigmoid colostomy tube for antegrade irrigation of the distal colon, which has been shown to be safe and effective in select patients.[78]

Stoma

For a small number of patients, the aforementioned means of managing symptoms of fecal incontinence are either impractical or ineffective. For these patients, a fairly radical but effective means of controlling their symptoms and restoring quality of life is the creation of a stoma.[26] Although a stoma is typically effective at controlling symptoms related to fecal incontinence, it may be associated with significant psychological issues, social stigmata (real or self-imposed), and risk of complications, such as stomal prolapse, problems with stoma pouching, and parastomal hernia. Although literature regarding the use of a permanent stoma for the management of fecal incontinence is fairly limited, a group for whom it seems particularly well suited is those with spinal cord injury.[79,80] Because these patients are typically bedridden or immobile, proper stoma siting preoperatively is essential to minimize complications related to stoma pouching.

In patients with severe incontinence for whom other alternative methods have failed, a stoma will typically improve patients' quality of life and allow them to resume fairly normal daily activities. Norton and colleagues[81] reported the results of survey of 69 patients who had undergone creation of a colostomy for the management of fecal incontinence. When asked to rate the ability to live with a stoma on a scale of 0 to 10, the median response was 8 and satisfaction with the stoma was given a median rating of 9. Of the respondents, 83% believed that the stoma restricted their life "a little bit" or "not at all," and 84% would "probably" or "definitely" choose to have the stoma again.

SUMMARY

No one correct solution exists for all types of incontinence and the informed colorectal surgeon needs to evaluate each patient's needs and anatomic issues uniquely. The fact that so many modalities exist speaks not only to the prevalence and impact of this problem but also to the fact that an optimum solution has yet to be devised. Sacral nerve stimulation seems to currently hold the most promise and is backed by not only a high success rate but also an excellent long-term track record. Despite the enormity of this problem, the multitude of available options provides a great deal of hope for patients with this devastating affliction.

REFERENCES

1. Brown HW, Wexner SD, Segall MM, et al. Accidental bowel leakage in the mature women's health study: prevalence and predictors. Int J Clin Pract 2012;66(11):1101–8.
2. Madoff RD, Parker SC, Varma MG, et al. Faecal incontinence in adults. Lancet 2004;364(9434):621–32.
3. Sultan AH, Kamm MA, Hudson CN, et al. Anal-sphincter disruption during vaginal delivery. N Engl J Med 1993;329(26):1905–11.
4. Warshaw J. Obstetric anal sphincter injury: incidence, risk factors, and repair. Semin Colon Rectal Surg 2001;12:90.
5. Snooks SJ, Henry MM, Swash M. Faecal incontinence due to external anal sphincter division in childbirth is associated with damage to the innervation of the pelvic floor musculature: a double pathology. Br J Obstet Gynaecol 1985; 92(8):824–8.
6. Jacobs PP, Scheuer M, Kuijpers JH, et al. Obstetric fecal incontinence. Role of pelvic floor denervation and results of delayed sphincter repair. Dis Colon Rectum 1990;33(6):494–7.
7. Garg P, Garg M, Menon GR. Long-term continence disturbance after lateral internal sphincterotomy for chronic anal fissure: a systematic review and meta-analysis. Colorectal Dis 2013;15(3):e104–17.
8. Li YD, Xu JH, Lin JJ, et al. Excisional hemorrhoidal surgery and its effect on anal continence. World J Gastroenterol 2012;18(30):4059–63.
9. Wolff BG, Fleshman JW, Beck DE, et al. The ASCRS textbook of colon and rectal surgery. New York: Springer Science + Business media, LLC; 2007.
10. van Koperen PJ, Wind J, Bemelman WA, et al. Long-term functional outcome and risk factors for recurrence after surgical treatment for low and high perianal fistulas of cryptoglandular origin. Dis Colon Rectum 2008;51(10):1475–81.
11. Lindsey I, Jones OM, Smilgin-Humphreys MM, et al. Patterns of fecal incontinence after anal surgery. Dis Colon Rectum 2004;47(10):1643–9.
12. Birnbaum EH, Myerson RJ, Fry RD, et al. Chronic effects of pelvic radiation therapy on anorectal function. Dis Colon Rectum 1994;37(9):909–15.
13. Jorge JM, Wexner SD. Etiology and management of fecal incontinence. Dis Colon Rectum 1993;36(1):77–97.

14. Lestar B, Penninckx F, Kerremans R. The composition of anal basal pressure. An in vivo and in vitro study in man. Int J Colorectal Dis 1989;4(2):118–22.
15. Roberts PL. Principles of monometry. Semin Colon Rectal Surg 1992;3:64.
16. Brandao AC, Ianez P. MR imaging of the pelvic floor: defecography. Magn Reson Imaging Clin N Am 2013;21(2):427–45.
17. Cheetham M, Brazzelli M, Norton C, et al. Drug treatment for faecal incontinence in adults. Cochrane Database Syst Rev 2003;(3):CD002116.
18. Goode PS, Burgio KL, Halli AD, et al. Prevalence and correlates of fecal incontinence in community-dwelling older adults. J Am Geriatr Soc 2005;53(4):629–35.
19. Sun WM, Read NW, Verlinden M. Effects of loperamide oxide on gastrointestinal transit time and anorectal function in patients with chronic diarrhoea and faecal incontinence. Scand J Gastroenterol 1997;32(1):34–8.
20. Vande Velde S, Van Biervliet S, Van Laecke E, et al. Colon enemas for fecal incontinence in patients with spina bifida. J Urol 2013;189(1):300–4.
21. Chassagne P, Jego A, Gloc P, et al. Does treatment of constipation improve faecal incontinence in institutionalized elderly patients? Age Ageing 2000; 29(2):159–64.
22. Mellgren A. Fecal incontinence. Surg Clin North Am 2010;90(1):185–94 [table of contents].
23. Hayden DM, Weiss EG. Fecal incontinence: etiology, evaluation, and treatment. Clin Colon Rectal Surg 2011;24(1):64–70.
24. Heymen S, Scarlett Y, Jones K, et al. Randomized controlled trial shows biofeedback to be superior to pelvic floor exercises for fecal incontinence. Dis Colon Rectum 2009;52(10):1730–7.
25. Norton C, Cody JD. Biofeedback and/or sphincter exercises for the treatment of faecal incontinence in adults. Cochrane Database Syst Rev 2012;(7):CD002111.
26. Tjandra JJ, Dykes SL, Kumar RR, et al. Practice parameters for the treatment of fecal incontinence. Dis Colon Rectum 2007;50(10):1497–507.
27. Tjandra JJ, Han WR, Goh J, et al. Direct repair vs. overlapping sphincter repair: a randomized, controlled trial. Dis Colon Rectum 2003;46(7):937–42 [discussion: 942–3].
28. Malouf AJ, Norton CS, Engel AF, et al. Long-term results of overlapping anterior anal-sphincter repair for obstetric trauma. Lancet 2000;355(9200):260–5.
29. Engel AF, Kamm MA, Sultan AH, et al. Anterior anal sphincter repair in patients with obstetric trauma. Br J Surg 1994;81(8):1231–4.
30. Glasgow SC, Lowry AC. Long-term outcomes of anal sphincter repair for fecal incontinence: a systematic review. Dis Colon Rectum 2012;55(4):482–90.
31. Gilliland R, Altomare DF, Moreira H Jr, et al. Pudendal neuropathy is predictive of failure following anterior overlapping sphincteroplasty. Dis Colon Rectum 1998; 41(12):1516–22.
32. Chen AS, Luchtefeld MA, Senagore AJ, et al. Pudendal nerve latency. Does it predict outcome of anal sphincter repair? Dis Colon Rectum 1998;41(8):1005–9.
33. Graf W, Mellgren A, Matzel KE, et al. Efficacy of dextranomer in stabilised hyaluronic acid for treatment of faecal incontinence: a randomised, sham-controlled trial. Lancet 2011;377(9770):997–1003.
34. Hussain ZI, Lim M, Stojkovic SG. Systematic review of perianal implants in the treatment of faecal incontinence. Br J Surg 2011;98(11):1526–36.
35. Watson NF, Koshy A, Sagar PM. Anal bulking agents for faecal incontinence. Colorectal Dis 2012;14(Suppl 3):29–33.
36. Maslekar S, Smith K, Harji D, et al. Injectable collagen for the treatment of fecal incontinence: long-term results. Dis Colon Rectum 2013;56(3):354–9.

37. Maeda Y, Laurberg S, Norton C. Perianal injectable bulking agents as treatment for faecal incontinence in adults. Cochrane Database Syst Rev 2013;(2):CD007959.
38. Tjandra JJ, Chan MK, Yeh CH, et al. Sacral nerve stimulation is more effective than optimal medical therapy for severe fecal incontinence: a randomized, controlled study. Dis Colon Rectum 2008;51(5):494–502.
39. Mellgren A, Wexner SD, Coller JA, et al. Long-term efficacy and safety of sacral nerve stimulation for fecal incontinence. Dis Colon Rectum 2011;54(9):1065–75.
40. Hull T, Giese C, Wexner SD, et al. Long-term durability of sacral nerve stimulation therapy for chronic fecal incontinence. Dis Colon Rectum 2013;56(2):234–45.
41. Williams NS, Hallan RI, Koeze TH, et al. Construction of a neorectum and neoanal sphincter following previous proctocolectomy. Br J Surg 1989;76(11): 1191–4.
42. Chetwood CH. Plastic operation for restoration of the sphincter ani with a report of a case. Med Rec 1902;61:529.
43. Baeten CG, Bailey HR, Bakka A, et al. Safety and efficacy of dynamic graciloplasty for fecal incontinence: report of a prospective, multicenter trial. Dynamic Graciloplasty Therapy Study Group. Dis Colon Rectum 2000;43(6):743–51.
44. Thornton MJ, Kennedy ML, Lubowski DZ, et al. Long-term follow-up of dynamic graciloplasty for faecal incontinence. Colorectal Dis 2004;6(6):470–6.
45. Christiansen J, Lorentzen M. Implantation of artificial sphincter for anal incontinence. Lancet 1987;2(8553):244–5.
46. Mundy L, Merlin TL, Maddern GJ, et al. Systematic review of safety and effectiveness of an artificial bowel sphincter for faecal incontinence. Br J Surg 2004;91(6):665–72.
47. Darnis B, Faucheron JL, Damon H, et al. Technical and functional results of the artificial bowel sphincter for treatment of severe fecal incontinence: is there any benefit for the patient? Dis Colon Rectum 2013;56(4):505–10.
48. Wong MT, Meurette G, Wyart V, et al. The artificial bowel sphincter: a single institution experience over a decade. Ann Surg 2011;254(6):951–6.
49. Wexner SD, Jin HY, Weiss EG, et al. Factors associated with failure of the artificial bowel sphincter: a study of over 50 cases from Cleveland Clinic Florida. Dis Colon Rectum 2009;52(9):1550–7.
50. Devesa JM, Hervas PL, Vicente R, et al. Anal encirclement with a simple prosthetic sling for faecal incontinence. Tech Coloproctol 2011;15(1):17–22.
51. Larach SW, Vazquez B. Modified Thiersch procedure with silastic mesh implant: a simple solution for fecal incontinence and severe prolapse. South Med J 1986; 79(3):307–9.
52. Mantoo S, Meurette G, Podevin J, et al. The magnetic anal sphincter: a new device in the management of severe fecal incontinence. Expert Rev Med Devices 2012;9(5):483–90.
53. Wong MT, Meurette G, Stangherlin P, et al. The magnetic anal sphincter versus the artificial bowel sphincter: a comparison of 2 treatments for fecal incontinence. Dis Colon Rectum 2011;54(7):773–9.
54. Nakamura M, Sakurai T, Tsujimoto Y, et al. Transcutaneous electrical stimulation for the control of frequency and urge incontinence. Hinyokika Kiyo 1983;29(9): 1053–9.
55. Shafik A, Ahmed I, El-Sibai O, et al. Percutaneous peripheral neuromodulation in the treatment of fecal incontinence. Eur Surg Res 2003;35(2):103–7.
56. Queralto M, Portier G, Cabarrot PH, et al. Preliminary results of peripheral transcutaneous neuromodulation in the treatment of idiopathic fecal incontinence. Int J Colorectal Dis 2006;21(7):670–2.

57. Leroi AM, Siproudhis L, Etienney I, et al. Transcutaneous electrical tibial nerve stimulation in the treatment of fecal incontinence: a randomized trial (CONSORT 1a). Am J Gastroenterol 2012;107(12):1888–96.
58. Thomas GP, Dudding TC, Rahbour G, et al. A review of posterior tibial nerve stimulation for faecal incontinence. Colorectal Dis 2013;15(5):519–26.
59. Margolin DA. New options for the treatment of fecal incontinence. Ochsner J 2008;8(1):18–24.
60. McClusky DA 3rd, Khaitan L, Swafford VA, et al. Radiofrequency energy delivery to the lower esophageal sphincter (Stretta procedure) in patients with recurrent reflux after antireflux surgery: can surgery be avoided? Surg Endosc 2007; 21(7):1207–11.
61. Efron JE, Corman ML, Fleshman J, et al. Safety and effectiveness of temperature-controlled radio-frequency energy delivery to the anal canal (Secca procedure) for the treatment of fecal incontinence. Dis Colon Rectum 2003;46(12):1606–16 [discussion: 1616–8].
62. Takahashi T, Garcia-Osogobio S, Valdovinos MA, et al. Radio-frequency energy delivery to the anal canal for the treatment of fecal incontinence. Dis Colon Rectum 2002;45(7):915–22.
63. Takahashi T, Garcia-Osogobio S, Valdovinos MA, et al. Extended two-year results of radio-frequency energy delivery for the treatment of fecal incontinence (the Secca procedure). Dis Colon Rectum 2003;46(6):711–5.
64. Takahashi-Monroy T, Morales M, Garcia-Osogobio S, et al. SECCA procedure for the treatment of fecal incontinence: results of five-year follow-up. Dis Colon Rectum 2008;51(3):355–9.
65. Ruiz D, Pinto RA, Hull TL, et al. Does the radiofrequency procedure for fecal incontinence improve quality of life and incontinence at 1-year follow-up? Dis Colon Rectum 2010;53(7):1041–6.
66. Lefebure B, Tuech JJ, Bridoux V, et al. Temperature-controlled radio frequency energy delivery (Secca procedure) for the treatment of fecal incontinence: results of a prospective study. Int J Colorectal Dis 2008;23(10): 993–7.
67. Devesa JM, Madrid JM, Gallego BR, et al. Bilateral gluteoplasty for fecal incontinence. Dis Colon Rectum 1997;40(8):883–8.
68. Hultman CS, Zenn MR, Agarwal T, et al. Restoration of fecal continence after functional gluteoplasty: long-term results, technical refinements, and donor-site morbidity. Ann Plast Surg 2006;56(1):65–70 [discussion: 70–1].
69. Malone PS, Ransley PG, Kiely EM. Preliminary report: the antegrade continence enema. Lancet 1990;336(8725):1217–8.
70. Malone PS. The antegrade continence enema procedure. BJU Int 2004;93(3): 248–9.
71. Chéreau N, Lefevre JH, Shields C, et al. Antegrade colonic enema for faecal incontinence in adults: long-term results of 75 patients. Colorectal Dis 2011; 13(8):e238–42.
72. McAndrew HF, Griffiths DM, Pai KP. A new complication of the Malone antegrade continence enema. J Pediatr Surg 2002;37(8):1216.
73. Castellan MA, Gosalbez R, Labbie A, et al. Outcomes of continent catheterizable stomas for urinary and fecal incontinence: comparison among different tissue options. BJU Int 2005;95(7):1053–7.
74. Worsøe J, Christensen P, Krogh K, et al. Long-term results of antegrade colonic enema in adult patients: assessment of functional results. Dis Colon Rectum 2008;51(10):1523–8.

75. Portier G, Bonhomme N, Platonoff I, et al. Use of Malone antegrade continence enema in patients with perineal colostomy after rectal resection. Dis Colon Rectum 2005;48(3):499–503.

76. Lynch AC, Beasley SW, Robertson RW, et al. Comparison of results of laparoscopic and open antegrade continence enema procedures. Pediatr Surg Int 1999;15(5–6):343–6.

77. Thomas K, Bassuini M. Laparoscopic caecodivision ACE (antegrade continence enema) procedure. Tech Coloproctol 2008;12(1):65–7.

78. Ramwell A, Rice-Oxley M, Bond A, et al. Percutaneous endoscopic sigmoid colostomy for irrigation in the management of bowel dysfunction of adults with central neurologic disease. Surg Endosc 2011;25(10):3253–9.

79. Saltzstein RJ, Romano J. The efficacy of colostomy as a bowel management alternative in selected spinal cord injury patients. J Am Paraplegia Soc 1990; 13(2):9–13.

80. Stone JM, Wolfe VA, Nino-Murcia M, et al. Colostomy as treatment for complications of spinal cord injury. Arch Phys Med Rehabil 1990;71(7):514–8.

81. Norton C, Burch J, Kamm MA. Patients' views of a colostomy for fecal incontinence. Dis Colon Rectum 2005;48(5):1062–9.

Rectal Prolapse and Intussusception

Quinton Hatch, MD[a], Scott R. Steele, MD[b],*

KEYWORDS

- Rectal prolapse • Internal intussusception • Rectopexy • Resection rectopexy
- Perineal rectosigmoidectomy • Altemeier procedure • Delorme procedure • STARR

KEY POINTS

- Rectal prolapse affects patients of both genders and all ages.
- A detailed history and physical examination is paramount, with attention on risk factors for underlying disease, functional problems with fecal incontinence or constipation, as well as a complete evaluation for concomitant defects that may need to be addressed at the time or following repair of the prolapse.
- Adjunctive testing is not often required, other than in patients with significant constipation or incontinence, and those with risk factors for other diseases (ie, colonoscopy in an appropriate patient).
- The mainstay of operative therapy involves both transabdominal and perineal techniques (via open and minimally invasive approaches), and may include fixation through sutures, tacks, or mesh. In general, transabdominal repairs are associated with lower recurrence rates, and transperineal ones are reserved for those at high risk with multiple comorbidities.
- Patients should be counseled that their functional problems may or may not improve, even following successful repair.

 A video of robotic assisted rectopexy accompanies this article at http://www.gastro.theclinics.com

Rectal prolapse (ie, procidentia) is the full-thickness intussusception of the rectum through the anus (**Fig. 1**).[1] This condition is distinguished from internal intussusception in that it is more akin to telescoping of the bowel on itself without expression through

Disclosures: The authors have adhered to the policies for protection of human subjects as prescribed in 45 CFR 46. The views expressed are those of the author(s) and do not reflect the official policy of the Department of the Army, the Department of Defense or the US Government. Financial Disclaimer: The authors have no financial disclosures relevant to this article and have received no compensation, funding, or outside editorial assistance.
[a] Department of Surgery, Madigan Army Medical Center, 9040A Fitzsimmons Drive, Fort Lewis, WA 98431, USA; [b] Division of Colon and Rectal Surgery, Madigan Army Medical Center, 9040A Fitzsimmons Drive, Fort Lewis, WA 98431, USA
* Corresponding author.
E-mail address: harkersteele@mac.com

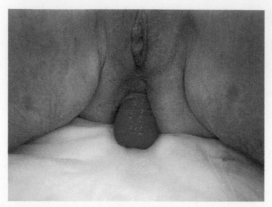

Fig. 1. Full-thickness rectal prolapse. (*Courtesy of* Philip Y. Pearson, MD, Philadelphia, PA.)

the anal verge. In addition, it is delineated from mucosal prolapse, in which only the mucosa prolapses through the anal canal, classically with visualization of the radial folds. Full-thickness rectal prolapse is a socially debilitating condition that is associated with bleeding, constipation, fecal soilage, and incontinence.[2,3] It is part of the spectrum of disorders caused by weakening of the pelvic floor, and often occurs in conjunction with one or more of the other disorders in the spectrum. Despite the multitude of operations described through the years for this common condition, surgical repair is still often plagued by higher than expected recurrence rates and wide-ranging improvements in functional outcomes. This article reviews the data for the operative repair of full-thickness rectal prolapse.

EPIDEMIOLOGY

Although rectal prolapse is thought by many to be a disease of the elderly, procidentia has a bimodal age distribution with peaks at the extremes of age.[1,4,5] It can occur at any stage in life. In children it is most commonly diagnosed before 3 years, and is seen more often in boys. Rectal prolapse in adults generally occurs after the fifth decade and is associated with the female gender 80% to 90% of the time.[1,4,5] The condition occurs infrequently, with an incidence in adults between 0.25 and 0.42% and a prevalence of 1% in adults more than 65 years of age.[2,6,7] Despite this seemingly low number, it is a common condition evaluated by health care providers of all specialties, and especially those treating colorectal disease.

CAUSES

In children it is thought that rectal prolapse results from the lack of the natural sacral curve rather than a weakening of the pelvic floor.[2] Without the sacral curve there is little or no anorectal angulation, which means the two structures lie in the same vertical plane. Increases in intra-abdominal pressure caused by diarrhea, vomiting, cough, or constipation therefore lead directly to increases in anorectal pressure and secondary rectal prolapse. Because this is a disorder of increased abdominal pressure rather than a weakened pelvic floor (as in adults), treatment involves relieving constipation and improving bowel habits rather than surgical repair.[2] The remainder of this article focuses on adult procidentia.

Competing theories as to the cause of adult rectal prolapse have existed since the twentieth century. Moschcowitz[8] proposed that the clinical picture was caused by an anterior sliding herniation of the pouch of Douglas secondary to a pelvic floor defect. However, the use of defecography by Broden and Snellman[9] in 1968 showed that the disorder was a true full-thickness intussusception of the rectum through the anus, with a lead point approximately 6 to 8 cm from the anal verge. Nevertheless, it is widely thought that pouch of Douglas herniation is an early stage of the rectal prolapse process and, when combined with the loss of posterior rectal fixation, this inevitably leads to full-thickness rectal prolapse.[10]

To develop procidentia patients must typically possess certain physiologic or anatomic abnormalities, which include the presence of an abnormally deep pouch of Douglas[5,9,11–13]; lax and atonic condition of the muscles of the pelvic floor and anal canal[5,9,12]; weakness of both internal and external anal sphincters, often with evidence of pudendal nerve neuropathy[5,12,13]; and the lack of normal fixation of the rectum, which results in a mobile mesorectum and lax lateral ligaments.[5,12–14] There is debate as to what comes first. As the rectum chronically prolapses through the sphincteric complex, this inevitably leads to the muscles becoming more dilated/patulous, as well as to repeated trauma on the nerves. This ends in conditions ripe for a worsened pelvic floor state, which leads to more frequent prolapse, and the cycle continues.

Other risk factors associated with the development of adult procidentia are the same as those that predispose patients to a weak pelvic floor. These risk factors include age more than 40 years, female gender, multiparity, large birth weight of vaginally delivered babies, prior pelvic surgery, increased body mass index, chronic straining, chronic diarrhea, chronic constipation, cystic fibrosis, neurologic diseases that lead to denervation of the pelvic floor (ie, cauda equina syndrome, spinal cord lesions), connective tissue disorders (ie, Marfan syndrome, Ehlers-Danlos syndrome), dementia, and stroke.[2,5,15,16] Even more than in routine patients, rectal prolapse in this cohort is often seen in conjunction with other pelvic floor defects.[2,5,15,16] In rare cases, the immunologic myopathy of schistosomiasis has been linked to pelvic floor weakening and rectal prolapse.[17]

COMPLICATIONS FROM UNTREATED PROLAPSE

Untreated rectal prolapse can result in several complications, including progressive problems with incontinence from chronic stretching and neuropathy, as well as constipation from obstructed defecation.[18] Although some may consider these as more functional issues associated with the prolapse, rather than true complications, they can be progressive and debilitating. Long-standing prolapse can have second-order effects as well. The straining from constipation may lead to an anterior solitary rectal ulcer from repeated mucosal trauma. These ulcers are almost always associated with rectal prolapse or internal intussusception,[19] and in severe cases may result in gastrointestinal hemorrhage and chronic pain.[2,5,20] An infrequent acute complication is incarceration or strangulation of the prolapsed rectum, which is a surgical emergency (Fig. 2).[2] Complete prolapse is also associated with a ~4-fold increase in relative risk of colorectal malignancy, although there is likely no causative effect, but it highlights the need for screening in appropriate patients.[21] For these reasons, it is important to accurately diagnose and appropriately evaluate and manage these patients.

CLINICAL EVALUATION

First and foremost, the diagnosis of rectal prolapse is a clinical diagnosis based on history and physical examination. Patients generally present complaining of an anal mass with defecation that may or may not spontaneously reduce. In some cases, this can occur with simple abdominal pressure (ie, Valsalva) or even bending or squatting.

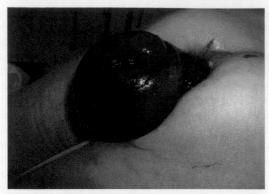

Fig. 2. Incarcerated rectal prolapse. (*Courtesy of* Isaac Felemovicious, MD, Minneapolis, MN.)

Associated symptoms include fecal or mucous soilage, incomplete bowel evacuation, and abdominal/pelvic discomfort.[22,23] Pain is usually not an associated symptom. Furthermore, up to 75% of patients with procidentia report incontinence, whereas 15% to 65% report constipation.[22–25]

The hallmark physical examination finding of complete rectal prolapse is concentric rectal rings protruding through the anus (see **Fig. 1**). Unless severe disease exists, eliciting the prolapse may prove difficult in the clinical setting. It is important to examine the patient during Valsalva, because this often reproduces the prolapse and allows assessment of puborectalis function. It may be necessary to examine the patient in the squatting position or even on the commode to simulate defecation. An enema may be used to help induce the prolapse in the clinic for patients with a strong history but whose conditions are difficult to visualize on initial examination. Although many colorectal surgeons use prone-jackknife position for routine evaluations, this may fail to show even a moderately sized prolapse.

Digital rectal examination should be performed, paying specific attention to the identification of masses or concomitant pelvic floor disorders such as cystocele, enterocele, or rectocele. Poor sphincter tone is almost universal in patients with rectal prolapse, and should be gauged both at rest and with squeeze. The function of the pelvic floor muscles, and particularly the puborectalis, may be assessed by asking the patient to Valsalva during the digital inspection. A lack of posterior relaxation of the muscular sling during Valsalva may indicate a nonrelaxing or paradoxic puborectalis muscle.

DIFFERENTIAL DIAGNOSIS

Several conditions can mimic rectal prolapse, both in terms of symptoms and clinical examination. For example, acute hemorrhoidal prolapse is common and is frequently confused with procidentia. This condition can be differentiated from rectal prolapse by the presence of radial rather than concentric folds as well as an everted and posterior anus rather than a normal, central anatomic anus.[2] Rectal mucosal prolapse involves intussusception of only the mucosal layer through the anus, and therefore does not represent a complete, or full-thickness, rectal prolapse. It generally consists of a prolapse of less than 5 cm of tissue, whereas complete prolapse usually presents with more than 5 cm.[2] Complete prolapse may be further differentiated from mucosal prolapse by palpating for a sulcus between the anal sphincter complex and the prolapsed tissue. A sulcus presents with complete prolapse, but is absent in mucosal prolapse.[2]

A sigmoidocele, or pouch of Douglas hernia, may represent the earliest stage of rectal prolapse, and generally presents as an anterior rectal bulge. Solitary rectal ulcers may present as a polypoid mass that is sometimes confused with rectal prolapse. Although these ulcers are almost always associated with rectal prolapse, they are a separate disorder caused by repeated mucosal trauma.[26] In rare cases, a neoplasm (ie, malignant or pedunculated polyp) can present as rectal prolapse or be the lead point for prolapsing tissue.

CLASSIFICATION

No commonly accepted classification scheme exists to grade the extent of prolapse. Altemeier and colleagues[27] initially categorized procidentia in terms of layer of prolapse (ie, mucosal vs full thickness) and their relationship to hemorrhoids and cul-de-sac sliding hernia. A more recent practical system was proposed by Beahrs and colleagues[28] in 1972. This system is based on completeness of prolapse. Type I procidentia is defined as incomplete mucosal prolapse (partial prolapse). Type II procidentia is prolapse of full-thickness rectal layers (complete prolapse). Type II is further broken down into first-degree, second-degree, and third-degree prolapse, which correspond with high or concealed (internal intussusception or occult), externally visible with straining, and externally visible at all times, respectively.

ANCILLARY STUDIES

Although rectal prolapse is diagnosed on physical examination alone, it is difficult to determine the extent of pelvic floor dysfunction in certain patients without further studies. The presence of other concomitant pelvic floor abnormalities such as cystocele, enterocele, rectocele, sigmoidocele, or vaginal vault prolapse may necessitate complex pelvic floor repair rather than simply addressing the rectal prolapse (**Fig. 3**). As such, further diagnostic studies should strongly be considered in this cohort. In addition, those patients due for routine screening examinations or who have worrisome symptoms (ie, bleeding, changes in bowel habits, systemic symptoms) may require further evaluation.

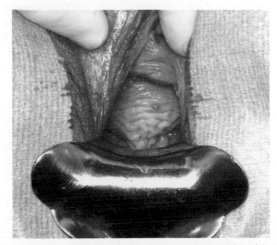

Fig. 3. Cystocele. Note the use of the single-blade retractor to aid in the examination. (*Courtesy of* Ann Lowry, MD, Minneapolis, MN.)

Colonoscopy

Although the results of colonoscopy rarely influence the management of rectal procidentia, it is an important study to rule out other disorders, particularly neoplasm.[29,30] Therefore, if a patient is of average risk and is current on recommended colorectal cancer screening, colonoscopy is not necessary for planning further management.[18] For those patients with concerning symptoms or who are due for an examination, a colonoscopy to clear the colon is important before any prolapse repair. Colonoscopic findings often seen in rectal prolapse include anterior erythema and inflammation.[2] Biopsy of these areas may show colitis cystic profunda, which is a benign finding that may be mistaken for adenocarcinoma. Solitary rectal ulcers may also be present, and are usually seen on the anterior wall at 4 to 12 cm from the anal verge.[2] Ulceration and colitis cystic profunda may contribute significantly to the symptoms associated with procidentia.[2] In addition, rectal inflammation with rectal granulomas can also be visualized and may signify occult procidentia (type II, first degree).[2]

Ultrasound

Ultrasound is not required for diagnosing the prolapse; it is more useful in patients with significant fecal incontinence with questionable sphincter defects. In this setting, endoanal ultrasound is up to 90% sensitive and specific for detecting internal and external anal sphincter defects,[31,32] which are present in approximately 70% of patients with complete prolapse.[33] The addition of three-dimensional (3D) and four-dimensional technology allows real-time assessment of the pelvic floor during Valsalva, rest, and squeeze. Pelvic organ prolapse and avulsion of the puborectalis muscle during strain have both been reported using 3D ultrasound.[34,35] However, the benefit of ultrasound examination for identifying and classifying pelvic organ prolapse remains in question. Deitz and colleagues[36] showed that translabial ultrasound of patients with organ prolapse correlated well with clinical staging in all 3 compartments; however, a more recent study showed poor agreement between translabial ultrasound and evacuation studies in patients with obstructed defecation with rectocele or rectal prolapse.[37] The use of ultrasound as part of the work-up for clinically diagnosed rectal prolapse is likely of minimal benefit, because sphincter defects are rarely addressed at the time of surgery for the prolapse. Furthermore, the narrow field of view and poor correlation with evacuation studies indicate that ultrasound is an inferior study for assessing global pelvic floor function. It is often best to repair the prolapse and pursue the sphincter evaluation only as needed after determining the functional response following repair.

Fluoroscopy

Cinedefecography allows the assessment of obstructed defecation (pelvic floor descent, anorectal angle, and percent of contrast evacuation) as well as rectal prolapse and internal intussusception.[38] Physiologic and anatomic defects can be identified using fluoroscopy in up to 80% of patients with obstructed defecation.[16] However, perhaps the most important aspect is the ability of fluoroscopy to identify concomitant pelvic floor disorders such as cystocele, rectocele, sigmoidocele, or enterocele,[39–41] which are present in 15% to 30% of patients with rectal prolapse.[42] These disorders may contribute to an increased recurrence rate after surgery if not addressed. Therefore, they should be identified before surgery and either repaired or discussed with the patient regarding the possibility of a need for subsequent repair.[42] Preoperative defecography has been shown to affect management strategy in up to 40% of patients.[43] Cinedefecography is therefore recommended for patients in whom concomitant complex pelvic floor anomalies are suspected.

Dynamic Pelvic Magnetic Resonance Imaging

The benefit of magnetic resonance imaging (MRI) compared with fluoroscopy or ultrasound is that it is noninvasive, provides simultaneous dynamic evaluation of all pelvic organs in multiple plains, and allows visualization of pelvic floor support structures. It has been shown to correlate well with fluoroscopic studies in the identification of pelvic organ prolapse, and frequently alters the surgical approach.[44–47] This finding is highlighted in one study showing that dynamic MRI changed the operative approach in 67% of patients with fecal incontinence.[45] It has not been specifically studied in the rectal prolapse population; however, patients with the potential for concomitant pelvic floor disorder may benefit from a dynamic study to determine whether a complex pelvic floor reconstruction is necessary. Dynamic MRI accomplishes this with 1 noninvasive test, rather than multiple fluoroscopic studies that separately assess for cystocele, sigmoidocele, rectocele, or enterocele.

Colonic Transit Marker Studies

Transit studies are an important element in the work-up for chronic constipation, but they have limited usefulness in the specific evaluation of rectal prolapse. Although 1 small study showed a slightly prolonged colonic transit time in full-thickness prolapse compared with internal intussusception, there was no significant difference from idiopathic constipation.[48] In another study addressing transit times before and after Ripstein rectopexy, the investigators showed that prolonged preoperative transit times correlated with evacuation difficulties after surgery.[49] Other investigators have shown decreased colonic transit times in patients with prolapse after resection rectopexy versus controls or rectopexy alone.[50,51] Thus, it may be that the main potential benefit of transit studies is the preoperative identification of patients who are best suited for a resection,[52] especially for those patients who may be under consideration for a total abdominal colectomy versus a sigmoid resection (standard resection rectopexy) because of underlying colonic inertia.

Anorectal Manometry

The use of anorectal manometry in patients with procidentia commonly shows a decreased anal resting pressure, normal or decreased squeeze pressure, and a dampened anorectal inhibitory reflex.[53,54] There are differing data regarding the ability of preoperative manometry to predict postoperative continence. One prospective study of 23 patients showed higher rates of postoperative continence in patients with higher preoperative resting and maximum squeeze anal pressures.[55] However, a larger retrospective study identified only preoperative maximum squeeze pressure greater than 60 mm Hg as predicting lower rates of postoperative incontinence.[56] The same study found no association between degree of incontinence and manometry findings. Regardless of the ability of manometry to accurately predict postoperative incontinence, its use rarely (if ever) changes the operative strategy, because nearly all patients have improvements in anorectal pressures after surgery.[55] Therefore, it is likely better to await the changes in function after surgery before using these tests outside limited indications.

Pudendal Nerve Terminal Motor Latency

Pudendal nerve terminal motor latency (PNTML) can be used to test the nerve function of the external sphincter, which is generally prolonged in those with procidentia.[57] Although postoperative unilateral or bilateral pudendal neuropathy has been associated with higher rates of postoperative incontinence,[57] no studies have shown the ability of preoperative PNTML to predict postoperative functional outcome.[58–60] In addition, the neuropathy that is characteristic of the repetitive trauma use with chronic prolapse is likely to lead to prolonged PNTML in a large percentage of cases.

Electromyography

Electromyogram (EMG) has also been used to assess the functionality of the sphincter complex. One study looking at EMG results in patients with fecal incontinence and/or rectal prolapse found that abnormal results are almost always seen in patients with fecal incontinence, either with or without concomitant rectal prolapse. However, in patients with rectal prolapse and no incontinence, the results of EMG are usually normal. Based on these results, there may be a difference in the pathophysiology of rectal prolapse in patients with and without fecal incontinence.[61] Either way, there seems to be little or no role for preoperative EMG in patients with straightforward rectal prolapse, because the results have no impact on management.

MANAGEMENT
Nonoperative Therapy

Although surgical management is the gold standard for treating complete prolapse, several nonoperative therapies have also been described. For patients with incomplete prolapse, minimally symptomatic prolapse, or who are poor surgical candidates, conservative measures may provide some benefit. Because rectal prolapse is associated with alterations in bowel habits, initial nonoperative interventions should be directed at minimizing these alterations to the greatest extent possible. All patients should therefore take in 25 to 30 g of fiber per day in addition to drinking 1 to 2 L of water.[62] Biofeedback and pelvic floor exercises (ie, Kegel) have shown benefit in patients with incontinence and obstructed defecation, and should strongly be considered in such patients who present with rectal prolapse.[63,64] As a last-line therapy, a perineal pad may be placed to act as a sort of truss. Conservative measures do not fully reverse or correct a prolapsed pelvic organ, and these serve as temporizing or palliative procedures in most cases.

Operative Repair

Primary indications for operative repair of procidentia include the sensation of an anal mass, fecal incontinence, or chronic constipation. However, the presence of rectal prolapse can be considered an indication for surgery, because the disorder is progressive and may lead to rectal incarceration/strangulation.[3] Although the goals of surgical therapy are to improve or restore fecal continence, and to correct functional constipation from outlet dysfunction or obstructed defecation, these results are widely variable. The major objective is to resolve/reduce the prolapse.[5,12,14] Several operations have been described for the treatment of rectal prolapse, and, as with most disorders that have multiple described surgical approaches, no single, ideal operation exists. Nevertheless, all operative techniques use one or both of the basic principles of rectal prolapse repair: rectal fixation to the sacrum and resection or plication of redundant bowel.[5,12,14] The finer details regarding the degree of rectal dissection in each plane, whether or not to divide the lateral ligaments, the use of mesh, and the surgical approach (transabdominal vs perineal, laparoscopic vs open vs robotic) are all heavily debated points of contention.[3,5]

Abdominal versus perineal

The 2 broad categories of operative approach are abdominal and perineal. The benefit of the perineal approach is that it can be performed under regional, or even local, anesthesia. As such, it is ideally suited for older, sicker patients who cannot tolerate general anesthesia. Based on several observational and retrospective studies, it is commonly thought that surgery via a perineal approach is associated with higher rates of recurrence.[58,65,66] Madiba and associates[5] performed the most extensive review of the literature and determined that abdominal approaches have decreased recurrence rates (0%–12%) compared with perineal approaches (0%–38%), although improvement in functional outcomes seemed similar. Overall mortality remained low (0%–6%) for all procedures. Only 1 randomized, prospective study has directly compared perineal proctosigmoidectomy and pelvic floor repair (levatorplasty) with abdominal rectopexy and pelvic floor repair.[67] Recurrence rates were similar in both arms, although functional outcomes were significantly improved in the abdominal rectopexy group. Fecal incontinence, maximum anal resting pressure, rectal compliance, and frequency of bowel movements were all improved in patients who underwent abdominal rectopexy relative to patients who underwent a perineal surgery. Although these differences were statistically significant, it is difficult to draw strong conclusions because the study only included 10 patients per group. The largest prospective, randomized trial to date, the PROSPER trial (prolapse surgery; perineal or rectopexy), has finished recruiting patients but has yet to publish any long-term results.[68] This study will enhance understanding of differential outcomes between perineal and abdominal approaches.

Perineal approaches

Perineal approaches include perineal proctosigmoidectomy (Altemeier procedure), mucosal sleeve resection (Delorme procedure), and anal encirclement (Thiersch procedure) (**Tables 1** and **2**). Perineal rectosigmoidectomy involves the full-thickness excision of the rectum and a portion of the sigmoid colon followed by a low anastomosis just proximal to the levators (**Fig. 4**). The procedure is associated with high rates of postoperative morbidity (up to ~35%, in part caused by patient selection) and recurrence (up to 26% with prolonged follow-up).[25,27,58,69–76] Of particular concern are the poor functional outcomes that include high rates of incontinence, soilage, and urgency, largely caused by the loss of the compliant rectum along with a reduction in resting anal sphincter pressure.[5,58,67,77,78] For this reason, many surgeons recommend a levatorplasty in conjunction with the rectosigmoidectomy,[79–83] which recreates the anorectal angle.[82] The addition of levatorplasty to rectosigmoidectomy improves both the recurrence rate and functional outcomes, to include continence and frequency of defecation.[81] There are some data to suggest that rectosigmoidectomy with concomitant levatorplasty is associated with the longest recurrence-free interval, the lowest overall recurrence rate, and the best functional outcomes of all the perineal procedures.[81] The downside to levator repair mainly relates to an increased rate of dyspareunia in women.

The Delorme procedure involves stripping the mucosa of the prolapsing rectum from the sphincters and muscularis propria, followed by plication of the muscularis propria and reanastomosis of the mucosal ring. Recurrence rates are high, ranging from 4% to 38%; however, the addition of posterior levatorplasty and sphincter repair has been shown to significantly decrease recurrence rates and improve functional outcomes in patients with concomitant severe pelvic floor disorders.[84] Pescatori and colleagues[85] added sphincteroplasty to the Delorme procedure in their series, and likewise noted improvements in continence and constipation compared with the

Table 1
Outcomes of Delorme procedure for procidentia

Study	N	Delorme Procedure Follow-up (mo)	Recurrence, No. (%)	Constipation (%)	Continence (%)
Monson et al,[146] 1986	27	35	2 (7)	NS	NS
Graf et al,[143] 1992	14	18	3 (21)	NS	55 (+)
Senapati et al,[107] 1994	32	21	4 (12.5)	50 (+)	46 (+)
Oliver et al,[147] 1994	41	47	8 (22)	NS	58 (+)
Tobin and Scott,[108] 1994	43	20	11	NA	50 (+)
Lechaux et al,[84] 1995	85	33	11 (14)	100 (+)	45 (+)
Kling et al,[144] 1996	6	11	1 (17)	100 (+)	67 (+)
Agachan et al,[81] 1997	8	24	3 (38)	NS	(+)
Pescatori et al,[85] 1998	33	39	6 (18)	44 (+)	(+)
Yakut et al,[14] 1998	27	38	4 (4.2)	NS	NS
Watts and Thompson,[148] 2000	101	36	30 (27)	13 (+)	25 (+)
Liberman et al,[145] 2000	34	43	0	88 (+)	32 (+)
Lieberth et al,[140] 2009	76	43	14.5	7 (+)	79 (+)
Youseff et al,[141] 2013	82	12	8.5 (7)	18 (−)	85 (+)

Abbreviations: (+), improvement; (−), worsening; NA, not applicable; NS, not stated.
Data from Madiba T, Baig M, Wexner S. Surgical management of rectal prolapse. Arch Surg 2005;140:63–73.

Table 2
Outcomes of perineal rectosigmoidectomy for procidentia

Study	N	Perineal Rectosigmoidectomy Follow-up (mo)	Recurrence, No. (%)	Constipation (%)	Continence (%)
Theuerkauf et al,[149] 1970	13	NS	38.5	NS	33.3 (+)
Altemeier et al,[27] 1971	106	228	3 (3)	NS	NS
Friedman et al,[71] 1983	20	12–204	7 (35)	NS	30 (+); 20 (−)
Gopal et al,[72] 1984	18	NS	1 (5.6)	NS	NS
Watts et al,[65] 1985	33	23	0	NS	6 (+); 22 (−)
Prasad et al,[83] 1986	25	NS	0	NS	88 (+)
Williams et al,[73] 1992	56	12	6 (6)	NS	46 (+); 0 (−)
Williams et al,[73] 1992	11	12	0	NS	91 (+)
Takesue et al,[80] 1999	10	42	0	NS	(+)
Johansen et al,[58] 1993	20	26	0	NS	21 (+)
Ramanujam et al,[82] 1994	72	120	4 (6)	NS	67 (+)
Deen et al,[67] 1994	10	18	1 (10)	NS	80
Agachan et al,[81] 1997	32	30	4 (13)	NC	(+)
Agachan et al,[81] 1997	21	30	1 (5)	NC	(+)
Kim et al,[25] 1999	183	47	29 (16)	61 (+)	53 (+)
Glasgow et al,[75] 2008	45	44	4 (8.9)	12 (+)	19 (+)
Lee et al,[69] 2011	123	13	14 (11.4)	NS	NS

Abbreviation: NC, no change.
Data from Madiba T, Baig M, Wexner S. Surgical management of rectal prolapse. Arch Surg 2005;140:63–73.

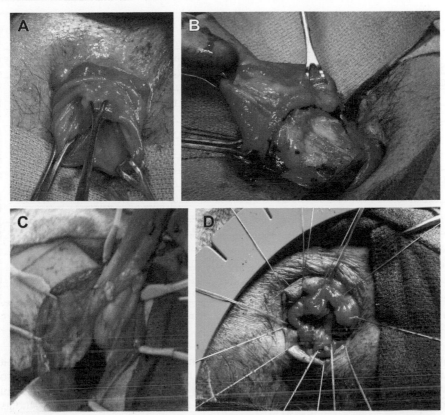

Fig. 4. (*A*) Perineal rectosigmoidectomy. Prolapsing the rectum to identify the initial point of dissection. (*B*) Initial dissection point 2 cm proximal to the dentate line. (*C*) Entering the peritoneal cavity with full-thickness dissection. (*D*) Completed full-thickness anastomosis with sutures in place. Note the use of the Lone Star Retractor. (*Courtesy of Scott R. Steele, MD, Olympia, WA.*)

Delorme procedure alone. The Delorme procedure is especially prone to failure in cases of proximal procidentia with rectosacral separation on defecography, fecal incontinence, chronic diarrhea, or perineal descent greater than or equal to 9 cm on straining, and should therefore generally be avoided in these patients.[86]

The Thiersch procedure involves encircling the external anal sphincter with either a silver wire or some other prosthetic material. This procedure does not directly address the prolapsing tissue, but prevents further descent by tightening the anal sphincter. With recurrence rates of 33% to 44% and improvements in modern anesthesia, there is limited or no role for its use.[1,4,5,12,87,88] More recent technical variants of the traditional Thiersch procedure that have shown promise include the use of a magnetic ring for patients with fecal incontinence, but these have not been described specifically for rectal prolapse.

Abdominal procedures
Suture rectopexy Abdominal procedures include suture rectopexy, posterior prosthetic or mesh rectopexy, anterior sling rectopexy (Ripstein procedure), and ventral rectopexy (**Table 3**). For suture rectopexy, the rectum is thoroughly mobilized and

Table 3
Outcomes of suture rectopexy for procidentia

Study	N	Follow-up (mo)	Recurrence, No. (%)	Constipation (%)	Continence (%)
Open Suture Rectopexy					
Carter,[90] 1983	32	144	1 (3)	NS	NS
Novell et al,[91] 1994	32	47	1 (3)	31 (−)	15 (+)
Graf et al,[92] 1996	53	97	5 (9)	30 (+) 27 (−)	36 (+) 12 (−)
Khanna et al,[93] 1996	65	65	0	83 (+)	75 (+)
Briel et al,[89] 1997	24	67	0	NS	67 (+)
Laparoscopic Suture Rectopexy					
Kessler et al,[150] 1999	32	48	2 (6)	NS	NS
Bruch et al,[151] 1999	32	30	0	76 (+)	64 (+)
Kellokumpu et al,[122] 2000	17	24	2 (7)	70 (+)	82 (+)
Heah et al,[152] 2000	25	26	NS	14 (+)	50 (+)
Benoist et al,[99] 2001	18	NS	NS	11 (−)	77 (+)
Lee et al,[69] 2011	8	6.9	1 (12.5)	NS	NS
Wilson et al,[153] 2011	59	48	6 (9)	17 (−)	NS

Data from Madiba T, Baig M, Wexner S. Surgical management of rectal prolapse. Arch Surg 2005;140:63–73.

sutured or tacked to the sacral fascia. Although the sutures/tacks hold this in place, it is the adhesions and fibrosis resulting from the dissection that secure the rectum to the presacral fascia, which prevents recurrence by protecting from the descent of redundant tissue.[1] Recurrence rates range from 0% to 27%, although most studies report rates from 0% to 3%.[89–93] The procedure is associated with considerable variation in postoperative constipation. In part this is secondary to the degree of rectal mobilization. Although most repairs carry the posterior dissection down to the pelvic floor, the anterior and lateral dissections are variable. Division of the lateral attachments has been shown to be associated with lower rates of recurrence at the cost of increased constipation.[94] However, fecal incontinence is most often improved by suture rectopexy, likely from simple avoidance of the mass protruding through the sphincters.[5]

Mesh repairs Insertion of a mesh or a prosthetic, either posterior to the rectum (posterior mesh rectopexy) or as an anterior sling secured posteriorly to the sacral promontory (Ripstein procedure), theoretically promotes a more vigorous fibrotic reaction than suture rectopexy alone (**Tables 4** and **5**).[12] Recurrence rates for posterior mesh rectopexy are reported at 3%.[5,91,95–97] As with suture rectopexy, posterior mesh rectopexy has variable impacts on postoperative constipation, whereas continence rates are often improved.[91,95,97–101] Proponents of the anterior sling rectopexy claim this restores the normal rectal anatomy by providing a firm anterior fascial support, while recreating the posterior rectal curve. Recurrence rates after anterior sling rectopexy range from 0% to 13%, and there is a trend toward improvement in fecal incontinence. As with other procedures, postoperative constipation rates are variable.[98,102–108] In recent years prosthetic material has largely fallen out of favor because of the risk of mesh erosion with resultant stenosis and fistula formation.[12] Furthermore, at least one study failed to show significant mesh-associated fibrosis in patients who required a reoperation.[12]

Table 4
Outcomes of posterior mesh rectopexy for procidentia

Study	N	Follow-up (mo)	Recurrence, No. (%)	Constipation (%)	Continence (%)
Open Posterior Mesh Rectopexy					
Penfold and Hawley,[96] 1972	101	48	3 (3)	NS	22 (+)
Morgan et al,[97] 1972	150	36	3 (3)	58 (+)	42 (+)
Notaras,[154] 1973	19	84	0	NS	NS
Keighley and Shouler,[23] 1984	100	24	0	NS	64 (+)
Mann and Hoffman,[95] 1988	59	NS	NS	39 (−)	25 (+)
Sayfan et al,[100] 1990	16	NS	NS	NC 75; 25 (−)	75 (+)
Luukkonen et al,[112] 1992	15	NS	0	100	53 (+)
Winde et al,[104] 1993	47	51	0	NS	17 (+)
Novell et al,[91] 1994	31	47	2 (3)	48 (−)	3 (+)
Scaglia et al,[103] 1994	16	12	0	14 (−)	19 (+)
Galili and Rabau,[113] 1997	37	44	1 (3)	NS	(+)
Yakut et al,[14] 1998	48	38	0	NC	(+)
Aitola et al,[98] 1999	96	78	6 (6)	24 (+)	26 (+)
Mollen et al,[101] 2000	18	42	0	NC 75	NS
Laparoscopic Posterior Mesh Rectopexy					
Darzi et al,[87] 1995	29	8	0	NS	NS
Himpens et al,[114] 1999	37	26	0	38 (−)	92 (+)
Boccasanta et al,[155] 1999	10	30	0	0	(+)
Zittel et al,[156] 2000	29	22	1	NC	76 (+)
Benoist et al,[99] 2001	14	NS	NS	21 (−)	10 (+)
Kariv et al,[142] 2006	42	60	9.3	74 (+)	48 (+)

Data from Madiba T, Baig M, Wexner S. Surgical management of rectal prolapse. Arch Surg 2005;140.63–73.

Table 5
Outcomes of Ripstein procedure for procidentia

Study	N	Ripstein Procedure			
		Follow-up (mo)	Recurrence, No. (%)	Constipation (%)	Continence (%)
Launer et al,[157] 1982	54	64	6 (12)	10 (−)	41 (+); 10 (−)
Holmström et al,[158] 1986	108	83	4 (4)	17 (−)	37 (+)
Roberts et al,[159] 1988	135	41	13 (10)	69 (+)	78 (+)
Winde et al,[104] 1993	47	51	0	17 (+)	23 (+)
Tjandra et al,[102] 1993	142	50	10 (7)	NC	18 (+)
Scaglia et al,[103] 1994	16	12	0	NC	23 (+)
Schultz et al,[160] 1996	24	NS	NS	NS	64 (+)
Schultz et al,[106] 2000	69	82	1 (2)	37 (+); 8 (−)	20 (+); 8 (−)

Data from Madiba T, Baig M, Wexner S. Surgical management of rectal prolapse. Arch Surg 2005;140:63–73.

Resection rectopexy (Frykman-Goldberg procedure) First described in the 1960s,[109] the addition of rectosigmoid resection to rectopexy offers several potential benefits (**Table 6**). The anastomotic suture or staple line causes a dense fibrosis that fixes the proximal rectum to the sacral promontory.[12] Furthermore, the removal of the redundant sigmoid colon corrects the altered angle of the rectum and creates a short, straight tract from the fixed splenic flexure to the rectum, which may play a role in correcting obstructed defecation.[1,12,109–111] Most studies of resection rectopexy (Frykman-Goldberg procedure) support this assertion, reporting lower rates of post-operative constipation and equivocal rates of fecal continence compared with recto-pexy alone.[14,25,50,67,112–114] Recurrence rates are also low following resection rectopexy, ranging from 0% to 5%.[14,25,50,67,112–114] Patients with chronic constipation before surgery are most likely to benefit from a resectional operation.[25,115–117] How-ever, only 2 small, prospective, randomized studies have addressed resection rectopexy, both of which confirmed significantly lower rates of postoperative constipation.[112,118]

Ventral rectopexy Ventral rectopexy involves mobilization of the anterior rectum, with no or minimal posterior dissection (Orr-Loygue procedure), followed by anterior mesh placement and sacral fixation (**Table 7**). The procedure was devised because of a desire to spare the patient from the problematic autonomic complications that are often associated with complete rectal mobilization. It is used most commonly for inter-nal intussusception (discussed later), but has been used for grade 2 and 3 complete rectal prolapse as well. Recurrence rates are similar to other abdominal procedures (0%–15%).[119] In D'Hoore and colleagues'[120] series of 42 patients with a median follow-up of 5 years, the recurrence rate was 5%. This procedure is subject to the

Table 6
Outcomes of resection rectopexy for procidentia

Study	N	Follow-up (mo)	Recurrence, No. (%)	Constipation (%)	Continence (%)
Open Resection Rectopexy					
Frykman and Goldberg,[109] 1969	80	NS	0	NS	NS
Watts et al,[65] 1985	138	48	2 (2)	NS	78 (+)
Sayfan et al,[100] 1990	13	NS	NS	80 (+)	66 (+)
Luukkonen et al,[112] 1992	15	NS	0	60 (+)	33 (+)
Tjandra et al,[102] 1993	18	50	NS	56 (+)	11 (+)
Deen et al,[67] 1994	10	17	0	NS	90
Huber et al,[50] 1995	42	54	0	18 (+)	44 (+)
Yakut et al,[14] 1998	19	38	0	(+)	(+)
Kim et al,[25] 1999	176	98	9 (5)	43 (+)	55 (+)
Johnson et al,[115] 2007	5	17	NS	25 (−)	65 (+)
Laparoscopic Resection Rectopexy					
Stevenson et al,[111] 1998	34	18	0	64 (+)	70 (+)
Xynos et al,[161] 1999	10	12	NS	NA	100 (+)
Benoist et al,[99] 2001	16	NS	NS	0	100 (+)
Ashari et al,[116] 2005	117	62	2 (1.7)	69 (+); 0 (−)	33 (+)
Lee et al,[69] 2011	8	7	1 (12.5)	NS	NS

Data from Madiba T, Baig M, Wexner S. Surgical management of rectal prolapse. Arch Surg 2005;140:63–73.

Table 7
Outcomes of ventral rectopexy for procidentia

	Ventral Rectopexy				
Study	N	Follow-up (mo)	Recurrence, No. (%)	Constipation (%)	Continence (%)
Detry et al,[162] 1984	20	24	0	NS	27 (+)
Loygue et al,[163] 1984	257	<60 in 53%; >60 in 47%	9 (3.5)	NS	39 (+)
Douard et al,[166] 2003	31	28	0	10 (−)	26 (+)
D'Hoore et al,[120] 2004	42	61	2 (5)	33 (+)	52 (+)
Marchal et al,[167] 2005	49	106	2 (4)	6 (+)	33 (+)
Marceau et al,[15] 2005	22	25	2 (9)	14 (−)	14 (+)
Verdaasdonk et al,[165] 2006	13	7	2 (15)	15 (+)	31 (+)
Portier et al,[164] 2006	73	27	3 (4)	29 (+)	60 (+)
Cristaldi et al,[169] 2007	58	3	1 (2)	48 (+)	67 (+)
Collinson et al,[168] 2007	30	3	NS	83 (+)	73 (+)
Slawik et al,[121] 2008	80	6	0	21 (+)	49 (+)

Data from Samaranayake C, Luo C, Plank A, et al. Systematic review on ventral rectopexy for rectal prolapse and intussusception. Colorectal Dis 2010;12:504–12.

same complications as other pelvic surgeries, which include wound infections, hematomas, and urinary tract infections[119]; however, the biggest fear specific to this procedure is mesh erosion caused by placement of mesh directly on the bowel. This fear has not been borne out in the literature, with only 1 case of mesh erosion reported among all series.[121]

Minimally invasive approaches Over the last decade, the role of minimally invasive approaches in colon and rectal surgery has increased greatly. Both laparoscopic and robotic techniques have been attempted for all of the currently used transabdominal rectal prolapse operations. Laparoscopic rectopexy is associated with reduced pain, shortened hospital stay, earlier recovery, and earlier return to work compared with the traditional open approach (**Fig. 5**).[122] Prolapse recurrence rates, as well as

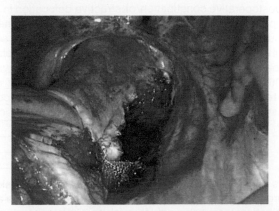

Fig. 5. Laparoscopic mesh resection rectopexy. Mesh is attached to the sacral promontory with absorbable tacks and sutured to mesorectum after mobilization. (*Courtesy of* Bradley J. Champagne, MD, Cleveland, OH.)

postoperative constipation and incontinence, are no different between laparoscopic and open operations.[111,122–124]

The latest trend in colon and rectal surgery is toward robotic surgery. Although no randomized studies have been performed for robotic rectal prolapse surgery, case series have shown similar functional outcomes, but higher recurrence rates compared with laparoscopy.[125] As yet, robotic surgery requires more time, is more costly,[126] and has not yielded superior results.[125] As with all new technology, there is a learning curve that must take place before potential benefits can be elucidated (Video 1).

Internal Intussusception

Internal intussusception is generally discovered during the work-up for obstructed defecation. Although it is technically a full-thickness (type II), grade 1 prolapse, it should be considered separately from grade 2 and 3 complete prolapse for management purposes. Surgical options have traditionally been avoided because of the high postoperative rate of persistent symptoms. Furthermore occult prolapse is rarely progressive and more than 50% of patients experience improvement in constipation with conservative measures alone.[127] As such, increased fiber and water intake, minimization of straining, pelvic floor exercises, and biofeedback should be first-line therapy.[20,64,128–130] However, in refractory or especially debilitating cases of obstructive defecation caused by occult rectal prolapse, several surgical procedures have been described. Among these are stapled transanal rectal resection (STARR), traditional suture rectopexy, and ventral rectopexy.

STARR has gained popularity for the treatment of obstructed defecation, particularly in patients with rectocele or occult/internal rectal intussusception. Concomitant enterocele is a relative contraindication for STARR.[131] For this procedure a circular stapler is advanced transanally. A double-staple technique is then used to remove a circumferential portion of mucosa and reinforce the anterior wall of the anorectal junction. This is thought to correct the structural abnormalities associated with obstructed defecation. Studies of patients with obstructed defecation, in addition to internal intussusception or rectocele, show that most experience symptomatic improvement after the STARR procedure compared with nonoperative management.[132–135] However, high rates of reoperation, recurrence, and postoperative complications[132–135] have led many surgeons to abandon this procedure.

Traditional suture rectopexy with or without resection has shown variably poor results in terms of postoperative constipation/obstructive defecation in patients with internal intussusception.[121,136–138] In contrast, ventral rectopexy may be emerging as the preferred surgery for refractory obstructed defecation in the setting of internal prolapse, although longer-term follow-up and data are awaited before final recommendations can be made. Although limited long-term results are available, it seems that more than 80% of such patients achieve symptomatic relief or improvement following ventral rectopexy. Furthermore, recurrence rates are acceptably low and the patient is spared from the morbidity associated with complete rectal dissection.[121,136,139]

SUMMARY

Rectal prolapse is an infrequent but socially, emotionally, and physically debilitating condition. The surgical management options are numerous, and the appropriate procedure for a given patient is revealed only through careful preoperative work-up. However, no perfect solution exists and functional outcomes are variable with any rectal prolapse repair. It may be that new technologies, such as robotic surgery, hold the key to improved outcomes; however, until that comes to fruition, patients and physicians must have a thorough understanding of both the treatment options and the likelihood of functional recovery.

SUPPLEMENTARY DATA

A video related to this article can be found online at http://dx.doi.org/10.1016/j.gtc.2013.08.002.

REFERENCES

1. Jacobs L, Lin Y, Orkin B. The best operation for rectal prolapse. Surg Clin North Am 1997;77:49–70.
2. Stein E, Stein DE. Rectal procidentia: diagnosis and management. Gastrointest Endosc Clin North Am 2006;16:189–201.
3. Tou S, Brown S, Malik A, et al. Surgery for complete rectal prolapse in adults. Cochrane Database Syst Rev 2008;(4):CD001758.
4. Wassef R, Rothenberger D, Goldberg S. Rectal prolapse. Curr Probl Surg 1986; 23:397–451.
5. Madiba T, Baig M, Wexner S. Surgical management of rectal prolapse. Arch Surg 2005;140:63–73.
6. Kairaluoma M, Kellokumpu I. Epidemiologic aspects of complete rectal prolapse. Scand J Surg 2005;94:207.
7. Patel S, Lembo A. Constipation: rectal prolapse and solitary rectal ulcer syndrome. In: Feldman M, editor. Sleisenger and Fordtran's gastrointestinal and liver disease, vol. 1, 8th edition. Philadelphia: Saunders Elsevier; 2006. p. 230.
8. Moschcowitz A. The pathogenesis, anatomy and cure of prolapse of the rectum. Surg Gynecol Obstet 1912;15:7–21.
9. Broden B, Snellman B. Procidentia of the rectum studied with cineradiography: a contribution to the discussion of causative mechanism. Dis Colon Rectum 1968;11:330–47.
10. Gordon P. Rectal procidentia. In: Gordon PH, Nivatvongs S, editors. Principles and practice of surgery for the colon, rectum, and anus. 2nd edition. St Louis (MO): Quality Medical Publishing; 1999. p. 503–40.
11. Roig J, Buch E, Alós R, et al. Anorectal function in patients with complete rectal prolapse: differences between continent and incontinent individuals. Rev Esp Enferm Dig 1998;90:794–805.
12. Kuijpers H. Treatment of complete rectal prolapse: to narrow, to wrap, to suspend, to fix, to encircle, to plicate or to resect? World J Surg 1992;16:826–30.
13. Nicholls R. Rectal prolapse and the solitary ulcer syndrome. Ann Ital Chir 1994; 65:157–62.
14. Yakut M, Kaymakciioglu N, Simsek A, et al. Surgical treatment of rectal prolapse: a retrospective analysis of 94 cases. Int Surg 1998;83:53–5.
15. Marceau C, Parc Y, Debroux E, et al. Complete rectal prolapse in young patients: psychiatric disease a risk factor of poor outcome. Colorectal Dis 2005; 7:360.
16. Mellgren A, Bremmer S, Johansson C, et al. Defecography. Results of investigations in 2,816 patients. Dis Colon Rectum 1994;37:1133.
17. Blumberg D, Wald A. Other diseases of the colon and rectum. In: Feldman M, Friedman LS, Sleisenger MH, editors. Sleisenger and Fordtran's gastrointestinal and liver disease. 7th edition. Philadelphia: WB Saunders; 2002. p. 2294–5.

18. Steele S, Goldberg J. Rectal prolapse: evidence-based outcomes. In: Cohn S, editor. Acute care surgery and trauma: evidence based practice. 1st edition. New York: Informa Healthcare; 2009. p. 356–67.
19. Schweiger M, Alexander-Williams J. Solitary ulcer syndrome of the rectum: its association with occult rectal prolapse. Lancet 1977;1:1970–1.
20. Felt-Bersma R, Stella M, Cuesta M. Rectal prolapse, rectal intussusception, rectocele, solitary rectal ulcer syndrome, and enterocele. Gastroenterol Clin North Am 2008;37(3):645–68.
21. Rashid Z, Basson M. Association of rectal prolapse with colorectal cancer surgery. Surgery 1996;119:51–5.
22. Hiltunen K, Matikainen M, Auvinen O, et al. Clinical and manometric evaluation of anal sphincter function in patients with rectal prolapse. Am J Surg 1986;151:489.
23. Keighley M, Fielding J, Alexander-Williams J. Results of Marlex mesh abdominal rectopexy for rectal prolapse in 100 consecutive patients. Br J Surg 1983;70:229.
24. Madoff R, Mellgren A. One hundred years of rectal prolapse surgery. Dis Colon Rectum 1999;42:441.
25. Kim D, Tsang C, Wong W, et al. Complete rectal prolapse: evolution of management and results. Dis Colon Rectum 1999;42(4):460–6 [discussion: 466–9].
26. Felt-Bersma R, Cuesta M. Rectal prolapse, rectal intussusception, rectocele, and solitary rectal ulcer syndrome. Gastroenterol Clin North Am 2001;30:199–222.
27. Altemeier W, Culbertson W, Schowengerdt C, et al. Nineteen years' experience with the one-stage perineal repair of rectal prolapse. Ann Surg 1971;173(6):993–1006.
28. Beahrs O, Theurkauf F, Hill J. Procidentia: surgical treatment. Dis Colon Rectum 1972;15:337–46.
29. Winawer S, Zauber AH, Ho MN, et al. Prevention of colorectal cancer by colonoscopic polypectomy. The National Polyp Study Workgroup. N Engl J Med 1993;329:1977–81.
30. Citarda F, Tomaselli G, Capocaccia R, et al, Italian Multicentre Study Group. Efficacy in standard clinical practice of colonoscopic polypectomy in reducing colorectal cancer incidence. Gut 2001;48:812–5.
31. Deen K, Kumar D, Williams J, et al. The prevalence of anal sphincter defects in faecal incontinence: a prospective endoscopic study. Gut 1993;34:685–8.
32. Dobben A, Terra M, Slors J, et al. External anal sphincter defects in patients with fecal incontinence: comparison of endoanal MR imaging and endoanal US. Radiology 2007;242:463–71.
33. Woods R, Voyvodic F, Schloithe A, et al. Anal sphincter tears in patients with rectal prolapse and faecal incontinence. Colorectal Dis 2003;5:544–8.
34. Örnö A, Herbst A, Marsál K. Sonographic characteristics of rectal sensations in healthy females. Dis Colon Rectum 2007;50:64–8.
35. Majida M, Braekken I, Umek W, et al. Interobserver repeatability of three- and four-dimensional transperineal ultrasound assessment of pelvic floor muscle anatomy and function. Ultrasound Obstet Gynecol 2009;33:567–73.
36. Dietz H, Haylen B, Broome J. Ultrasound in the quantification of female pelvic organ prolapse. Ultrasound Obstet Gynecol 2001;18:511–4.
37. Perniola G, Shek C, Chong C, et al. Defecation proctography and translabial ultrasound in the investigation of defecatory disorders. Ultrasound Obstet Gynecol 2008;31:567–71.
38. Woodfield C, Krishnamoorthy S, Hampton B, et al. Imaging pelvic floor disorders: trend toward comprehensive MRI. AJR Am J Roentgenol 2010;194:1640–9.

39. Pomerri F, Zuliani M, Mazza C, et al. Defecographic measurements of rectal intussusception and prolapse in patients and in asymptomatic subjects. AJR Am J Roentgenol 2001;176:641–5.
40. Altringer W, Saclarides T, Dominguez J, et al. Four-contrast defecography: pelvic "floor-oscopy". Dis Colon Rectum 1995;38:696–9.
41. Kelvin F, Hale D, Maglinte D, et al. Female pelvic organ prolapse: diagnostic contribution of dynamic cystoproctography and comparison with physical examination. AJR Am J Roentgenol 1999;173:31–7.
42. Altman D, Zetterstrom J, Schultz I, et al. Pelvic organ prolapse and urinary incontinence in women with surgically managed rectal prolapse: a population-based case-control study. Dis Colon Rectum 2006;49:28–35.
43. Harvey C, Halligan S, Bartram C, et al. Evacuation proctography: a prospective study of diagnostic and therapeutic effects. Radiology 1999;211:223–37.
44. Kelvin F, Maglinte D, Hale D, et al. Female pelvic organ prolapse: a comparison of triphasic dynamic MR imaging and triphasic fluoroscopic cystocolpoproctography. AJR Am J Roentgenol 2000;174:81–8.
45. Hetzer F, Andreisek G, Tsagari C, et al. MR defecography in patients with fecal incontinence: imaging findings and their effect on surgical management. Radiology 2006;240:449–57.
46. Gufler H, Laubenberger J, DeGregorio G, et al. Pelvic floor descent: MR imaging using a half-Fourier RARE sequence. J Magn Reson Imaging 1999;9:378–83.
47. Kaufman H, Buller J, Thompson J, et al. Dynamic pelvic magnetic resonance imaging and cystocolpoproctography alter surgical management of pelvic floor disorders. Dis Colon Rectum 2001;44:1575–83.
48. Prokesch R, Breitenseher M, Kettenbach J, et al. Assessment of chronic constipation: colon transit time versus defecography. Eur J Radiol 1999;32:197–203.
49. Schultz I, Mellgren A, Oberg M, et al. Whole gut transit is prolonged after Ripstein rectopexy. Eur J Surg 1999;165:242–7.
50. Huber F, Stein H, Siewert J. Functional results after treatment of rectal prolapse with rectopexy and sigmoid resection. World J Surg 1995;19:138–43.
51. Brown A, Nicol L, Anderson J, et al. Prospective study of the effect of rectopexy on colonic motility in patients with rectal prolapse. Br J Surg 2005;92:1417–22.
52. Safar B, Vernava A. Abdominal approaches for rectal prolapse. Clin Colon Rectal Surg 2008;21:94–9.
53. Parks A, Swash M, Urich H. Sphincter denervation in anorectal incontinence and rectal prolapse. Gut 1977;18:656–65.
54. Spencer R. Manometric studies in rectal prolapse. Dis Colon Rectum 1984;27:523–5.
55. Williams J, Wong W, Jensen L, et al. Incontinence and rectal prolapse: a prospective manometric study. Dis Colon Rectum 1991;34:209–16.
56. Glasgow S, Birnbaum E, Kodner I, et al. Preoperative anal manometry predicts continence after perineal proctectomy for rectal prolapse. Dis Colon Rectum 2006;49:1052–8.
57. Birnbaum E, Stamm L, Rafferty J, et al. Pudendal nerve terminal motor latency influences surgical outcome in treatment of rectal prolapse. Dis Colon Rectum 1996;39:1215–21.
58. Johansen O, Wexner S, Daniel L, et al. Perineal rectosigmoidectomy in the elderly. Dis Colon Rectum 1993;36:767–72.
59. Sainio A, Voutilainen P, Husa A. Recovery of anal sphincter function following transabdominal repair of rectal prolapse: cause of improved continence? Dis Colon Rectum 1991;34:816–21.

60. Schultz I, Mellgren A, Nilsson B, et al. Preoperative electrophysiologic assessment cannot predict continence after rectopexy. Dis Colon Rectum 1998;41: 1392–8.
61. Neill M, Parks A, Swash M. Physiological studies of the anal sphincter musculature in faecal incontinence and rectal prolapse. Br J Surg 1981;68(8):531–6.
62. Ternent C, Bastawrous A, Morin N, et al. Practice parameters for the evaluation and management of constipation. Dis Colon Rectum 2007;50:2013.
63. Jorge J, Habr-Gama A, Wexner SD. Biofeedback therapy in the colon and rectal practice. Appl Psychophysiol Biofeedback 2003;28:47–61.
64. Khaikin M, Wexner S. Treatment strategies in obstructed defecation and fecal incontinence. World J Gastroenterol 2006;12(20):3168–73.
65. Watts J, Rothenberger D, Buls J, et al. The management of procidentia. 30 years' experience. Dis Colon Rectum 1985;28(2):96–102.
66. Swinton N, Palmer T. The management of rectal prolapse and procidentia. Am J Surg 1960;99:144–51.
67. Deen K, Grant E, Billingham C, et al. Abdominal resection rectopexy with pelvic floor repair versus perineal rectosigmoidectomy and pelvic floor repair for full-thickness rectal prolapse. Br J Surg 1994;81(2):302–4.
68. Available at: http://www.prosper.bham.ac.uk/index. TPTWAa, shtml. Accessed February 27, 2013.
69. Lee S, Lakhtaria P, Canedo J, et al. Outcome of laparoscopic rectopexy versus perineal rectosigmoidectomy for full-thickness rectal prolapse in elderly patients. Surg Endosc 2011;25(8):2699–702.
70. Fleming F, Kim M, Gunzler D, et al. It's the procedure not the patient: the operative approach is independently associated with an increased risk of complications after rectal prolapse repair. Colorectal Dis 2011;14(3):362–8.
71. Friedman R, Muggia-Sulam M, Freund H. Experience with the one-stage perineal repair of rectal prolapse. Dis Colon Rectum 1983;26(12):789–91.
72. Gopal K, Amshel A, Shonberg I, et al. Rectal procidentia in elderly and debilitated patients. Experience with the Altemeier procedure. Dis Colon Rectum 1984;27(6):376–81.
73. Williams J, Rothenberger D, Madoff R, et al. Treatment of rectal prolapse in the elderly by perineal rectosigmoidectomy. Dis Colon Rectum 1992;35(9):830–4.
74. Azimuddin K, Khubchandani I, Rosen L, et al. Rectal prolapse: a search for the "best" operation. Am Surg 2001;67(7):622–7.
75. Glasgow S, Birnbaum E, Kodner I, et al. Recurrence and quality of life following perineal proctectomy for rectal prolapse. J Gastrointest Surg 2008;12(8):1446–51.
76. Riansuwan W, Hull T, Bast J, et al. Comparison of perineal operations with abdominal operations for full-thickness rectal prolapse. World J Surg 2010; 34(5):1116–22.
77. Cutait D. Sacro-promontory fixation of the rectum for complete rectal prolapse. Proc R Soc Med 1959;52(Suppl):105.
78. Yoshioka K, Ogunbiyi O, Keighley M. Pouch perineal rectosigmoidectomy gives better functional results than conventional rectosigmoidectomy in elderly patients with rectal prolapse. Br J Surg 1998;85:1525–6.
79. Keighley M, Shouler P. Abnormalities of colonic function in patients with rectal prolapse and faecal incontinence. Br J Surg 1984;71:892–5.
80. Takesue Y, Yokoyama T, Murakami Y, et al. The effectiveness of perineal rectosigmoidectomy for the treatment of rectal prolapse. Surg Today 1999;29:290–3.
81. Agachan F, Reissman P, Pfeifer J, et al. Comparison of three perineal procedures for the treatment of rectal prolapse. South Med J 1997;90:925–32.

82. Ramanujam P, Vankatesh K, Fietz M. Perineal excision of rectal procidentia in elderly high-risk patients: a ten-year experience. Dis Colon Rectum 1994;37:1027–30.
83. Prasad M, Pearl R, Abcarian H, et al. Perineal proctectomy, posterior rectopexy and postanal levator repair for the treatment of rectal prolapse. Dis Colon Rectum 1986;29:547–52.
84. Lechaux J, Lechaux D, Perez M. Results of Delorme's procedure for rectal prolapse: advantages of a modified technique. Dis Colon Rectum 1995;38:301–7.
85. Pescatori M, Interisano A, Stolfi V, et al. Delorme's operation and sphincteroplasty for rectal prolapse and fecal incontinence. Int J Colorectal Dis 1998;13:223–7.
86. Sielezneff I, Malouf A, Cesari J, et al. Selection criteria for internal rectal prolapse repair by Delorme's transrectal excision. Dis Colon Rectum 1999;42:367–73.
87. Darzi A, Henry M, Guillou P, et al. Stapled laparoscopic rectopexy for rectal prolapse. Surg Endosc 1995;9:301–3.
88. Dietzen C, Pemberton J. Perineal approaches for the treatment of complete rectal prolapse. Neth J Surg 1989;41:140–4.
89. Briel J, Schouten W, Boerma M. Long-term results of suture rectopexy in patients with fecal incontinence associated with incomplete rectal prolapse. Dis Colon Rectum 1997;40:1228–32.
90. Carter A. Rectosacral suture fixation for complete prolapse in the elderly, the frail and the demented. Br J Surg 1983;70:522–3.
91. Novell J, Osborne M, Winslet M, et al. Prospective randomised trial of Ivalon sponge versus sutured rectopexy for full-thickness rectal prolapse. Br J Surg 1994;81:904–6.
92. Graf W, Karlbom U, Påhlman L, et al. Functional results after abdominal suture rectopexy for rectal prolapse or intussusception. Eur J Surg 1996;162:905–11.
93. Khanna A, Misra M, Kumar K. Simplified sutured sacral rectopexy for complete rectal prolapse in adults. Eur J Surg 1996;162:143–6.
94. Speakman C, Madden M, Nicholls R, et al. Lateral ligament division during rectopexy causes constipation but prevents recurrence: results of a prospective randomized study. Br J Surg 1991;78(12):1431–3.
95. Mann C, Hoffman C. Complete rectal prolapse: the anatomical and functional results of treatment by an extended abdominal rectopexy. Br J Surg 1988;75:34–7.
96. Penfold J, Hawley P. Experiences of Ivalon sponge implant for complete rectal prolapse at St Mark's Hospital. Br J Surg 1972;59:846–8.
97. Morgan C, Porter N, Klugman D. Ivalon sponge in the repair of complete rectal prolapse. Br J Surg 1972;59:841–6.
98. Aitola P, Hiltunen K, Matikainen M. Functional results of operative treatment of rectal prolapse over an 11-year period: emphasis on transabdominal approach. Dis Colon Rectum 1999;42:655–60.
99. Benoist S, Taffinder N, Gould S, et al. Functional results two years after laparoscopic rectopexy. Am J Surg 2001;182:168–73.
100. Sayfan J, Pinho M, Alexander-Williams J, et al. Sutured posterior abdominal rectopexy with sigmoidectomy compared with Marlex rectopexy rectal prolapse. Br J Surg 1990;77:143–5.
101. Mollen R, Kuijpers H, van Hoek F. Effects of rectal mobilization and lateral ligaments division on colonic and anorectal function. Dis Colon Rectum 2000;43:1283–7.
102. Tjandra J, Fazio V, Church J, et al. Ripstein procedure is an effective treatment for rectal prolapse without constipation. Dis Colon Rectum 1993;36:501–7.
103. Scaglia M, Fasth S, Hallgren T, et al. Abdominal rectopexy for rectal prolapse: influence of surgical technique on functional outcome. Dis Colon Rectum 1994;37:805–13.

104. Winde G, Reers H, Nottberg H, et al. Clinical and functional results of abdominal rectopexy with absorbable mesh-graft for treatment of complete rectal prolapse. Eur J Surg 1993;159:301–5.

105. Athanasiadis S, Weyand G, Heiligers J, et al. The risk of infection of three synthetic materials used in rectopexy with or without colonic resection for rectal prolapse. Int J Colorectal Dis 1996;11:42–4.

106. Schultz I, Mellgren A, Dolk A, et al. Long-term results and functional outcome after Ripstein rectopexy. Dis Colon Rectum 2000;43:35–43.

107. Senapati A, Nichols R, Thomson J, et al. Results of Delorme's procedure for rectal prolapse. Dis Colon Rectum 1994;37:456–60.

108. Tobin S, Scott I. Delorme operation for rectal prolapse. Br J Surg 1994;81:1681–4.

109. Frykman H, Goldberg S. The surgical treatment of rectal procidentia. Surg Gynecol Obstet 1969;129(6):1225–30.

110. Solla J, Rotheberger D, Goldberg S. Colonic resection in the treatment of complete rectal prolapse. Neth J Surg 1989;41:132–5.

111. Stevenson A, Stitz R, Lumley J. Laparoscopic assisted resection rectopexy for rectal prolapse: early and medium follow-up. Dis Colon Rectum 1998;41:46–54.

112. Luukkonen P, Mikkonen U, Järvinen H. Abdominal rectopexy with sigmoidectomy vs rectopexy alone for rectal prolapse: a prospective, randomized study. Int J Colorectal Dis 1992;7:219–22.

113. Galili Y, Rabau M. Comparison of polyglycolic acid and polypropylene mesh for rectopexy in the treatment of rectal prolapse. Eur J Surg 1997;163:445–8.

114. Himpens J, Cadière G, Bruyns J, et al. Laparoscopic rectopexy according to Wells. Surg Endosc 1999;13:139–41.

115. Johnson E, Stangeland A, Johannessen H, et al. Resection rectopexy for external rectal prolapse reduces constipation and anal incontinence. Scand J Surg 2007;96(1):56–61.

116. Ashari L, Lumley J, Stevenson A, et al. Laparoscopically-assisted resection rectopexy for rectal prolapse: ten years' experience. Dis Colon Rectum 2005; 48:982–7.

117. Brown A, Anderson J, McKee R, et al. Strategy for selection of type of operation for rectal prolapse based on clinical criteria. Dis Colon Rectum 2004;47:103–7.

118. McKee R, Lauder J, Poon F, et al. A prospective randomized study of abdominal rectopexy with and without sigmoidectomy in rectal prolapse. Surg Gynecol Obstet 1992;174:145–8.

119. Samaranayake C, Luo C, Plank A, et al. Systematic review on ventral rectopexy for rectal prolapse and intussusception. Colorectal Dis 2010;12(6):504–12.

120. D'Hoore A, Cadoni R, Penninckx F. Long-term outcome of laparoscopic ventral rectopexy for total rectal prolapse. Br J Surg 2004;91(11):1500–5.

121. Slawik S, Soulsby R, Carter H, et al. Laparoscopic ventral rectopexy, posterior colporrhaphy and vaginal sacrocolpopexy for the treatment of recto-genital prolapse and mechanical outlet obstruction. Colorectal Dis 2008;10(2):138–43.

122. Kellokumpu I, Virozen J, Scheinin T. Laparoscopic repair of rectal prolapse: a prospective study evaluating surgical outcome and changes in symptoms and bowel function. Surg Endosc 2000;14:634–40.

123. Solomon M, Young C, Eyers A, et al. Randomised clinical trial of laparoscopic versus open abdominal rectopexy for rectal prolapse. Br J Surg 2002;89:35–9.

124. Baker R, Senagore A, Luchtefeld M. Laparoscopic assisted vs open resection: rectopexy offers excellent results. Dis Colon Rectum 1995;38:199–201.

125. De Hoog D, Heemskerk J, Nieman F, et al. Recurrence and functional results after open versus conventional laparoscopic versus robot-assisted laparoscopic

rectopexy for rectal prolapse: a case-control study. Int J Colorectal Dis 2007;24: 1201–6.

126. Heemskerk J, de Hoog D, van Gemert W, et al. Robot-assisted vs. conventional laparoscopic rectopexy for rectal prolapse: a comparative study on costs and time. Dis Colon Rectum 2007;40(11):1825–30.

127. Hwang Y, Person B, Choi JS, et al. Biofeedback therapy for rectal intussusception. Tech Coloproctol 2006;10(1):11–5.

128. Christiansen J, Zhu BW, Rasmussen OO, et al. Internal rectal intussusception: results of surgical repair. Dis Colon Rectum 1992;35(11):1026–8.

129. Steele S, Mellgren A. Constipation and obstructed defecation. Clin Colon Rectal Surg 2007;20(2):110–7.

130. Choi J, Hwang YH, Salum MR, et al. Outcome and management of patients with large rectoanal intussusception. Am J Gastroenterol 2001;96(3):740–4.

131. Farouk R, Bhardwaj R, Phillips R. Stapled transanal resection of the rectum (STARR) for the obstructed defaecation syndrome. Ann R Coll Surg Engl 2009;91(4):287–91.

132. Lehur P, Stuto A, Fantoli M, et al. Outcomes of stapled transanal rectal resection vs. biofeedback for the treatment of outlet obstruction associated with rectal intussusception and rectocele: a multicenter, randomized, controlled trial. Dis Colon Rectum 2008;51(11):1611–8.

133. Ommer A, Rolfs T, Walz M. Long-term results of stapled transanal rectal resection (STARR) for obstructive defecation syndrome. Int J Colorectal Dis 2010; 25(11):1287–92.

134. Goede A, Glancy D, Carter H, et al. Medium-term results of stapled transanal rectal resection (STARR) for obstructed defecation and symptomatic rectal-anal intussusception. Colorectal Dis 2011;13(9):1052–7.

135. Gagliardi G, Pescatori M, Altomare DF, et al. Results, outcome predictors, and complications after stapled transanal rectal resection for obstructed defecation. Dis Colon Rectum 2008;51(2):186–95.

136. Collinson R, Wijffels N, Cunningham C, et al. Laparoscopic ventral rectopexy for internal rectal prolapse: short-term functional results. Colorectal Dis 2010;12(2): 97–104.

137. Johnson E, Carlsen E, Mjåland O, et al. Resection rectopexy for internal rectal intussusception reduces constipation and incomplete evacuation of stool. Eur J Surg Suppl 2003;588:51–6.

138. Orrom WJ, Bartolo DC, Miller R, et al. Rectopexy is an ineffective treatment for obstructed defecation. Dis Colon Rectum 1991;34(1):41–6.

139. Sileri P, Franceschilli L, de Luca E, et al. Laparoscopic ventral rectopexy for internal rectal prolapse using biological mesh: postoperative and short-term functional results. J Gastrointest Surg 2012;16(3):622–8.

140. Lieberth M, Kondylis LA, Reilly JC, et al. The Delorme repair for full-thickness rectal prolapse: a retrospective review. Am J Surg 2009;197(3):418–23.

141. Youssef M, Thabet W, Nakeeb A, et al. Comparative study between Delorme operation with or without postanal repair and levateroplasty in treatment of complete rectal prolapse. Int J Surg 2013;11:52–8.

142. Kariv Y, Delaney CP, Casillas S, et al. Long-term outcome after laparoscopic and open surgery for rectal prolapse: a case-control study. Surg Endosc 2006;20(1):35–42.

143. Graf W, Ejerblad S, Krog M, et al. Delorme's operation for rectal prolapse in elderly or unfit patients. Eur J Surg 1992;158(10):555–7.

144. Kling K, Rongione A, Evans B, et al. The Delorme procedure: a useful operation for complicated rectal prolapse in the elderly. Am Surg 1996;62:857–60.

145. Liberman H, Hughes C, Dippolito A. Evaluation and outcome of the Delorme procedure in the treatment of rectal outlet obstruction. Dis Colon Rectum 2000;43: 188–92.
146. Monson J, Jones N, Vowden P, et al. Delorme's operation: the first choice in complete rectal prolapse? Ann R Coll Surg Engl 1986;68(3):143–6.
147. Oliver G, Vachon D, Eisenstat T, et al. Delorme's procedure for complete rectal prolapse in severely debilitated patients: an analysis of 41 patients. Dis Colon Rectum 1994;37:461–7.
148. Watts A, Thompson M. Evaluation of Delorme's procedure as a treatment for full-thickness rectal prolapse. Br J Surg 2000;87:218–22.
149. Theuerkauf FJ, Beahrs O, Hill J. Rectal prolapse: causation and surgical treatment. Ann Surg 1970;171:819–35.
150. Kessler H, Jerby B, Milsom J. Successful treatment of rectal prolapse by laparoscopic suture rectopexy. Surg Endosc 1999;13:858–61.
151. Bruch H, Herold A, Schiedeck T, et al. Laparoscopic surgery for rectal prolapse and outlet obstruction. Dis Colon Rectum 1999;42:1189–94.
152. Heah S, Hartely J, Hurley J, et al. Laparoscopic suture rectopexy without resection is effective treatment for full-thickness rectal prolapse. Dis Colon Rectum 2000;43:638–43.
153. Wilson J, Engledow A, Crosbie J, et al. Laparoscopic nonresectional suture rectopexy in the management of full-thickness rectal prolapse: substantive retrospective series. Surg Endosc 2011;25(4):1062–4.
154. Notaras M. The use of Mersilene mesh in rectal prolapse repair. Proc R Soc Med 1973;66:684–6.
155. Boccasanta P, Venturi M, Reitano M, et al. Laparotomic vs laparoscopic rectopexy in complete rectal prolapse. Dig Surg 1999;16:415–9.
156. Zittel T, Manncke K, Haug S, et al. Functional results after laparoscopic rectopexy for rectal prolapse. J Gastrointest Surg 2000;4:632–41.
157. Launer D, Fazio V, Weakley F, et al. The Ripstein procedure: a 16-year experience. Dis Colon Rectum 1982;25:41–5.
158. Holmström B, Brodén G, Dolk A. Results of the Ripstein operation in the treatment of rectal prolapse and internal rectal procidentia. Dis Colon Rectum 1986;29: 845–8.
159. Roberts P, Schoetz D, Coller J, et al. Ripstein procedure: Lahey Clinic experience: 1963–1985. Arch Surg 1988;123:554–7.
160. Schultz I, Madoff R, Dolk A, et al. Continence is improved after the Ripstein rectopexy: different mechanisms in rectal prolapse and rectal intussusception? Dis Colon Rectum 1996;39:300–6.
161. Xynos E, Chrysos J, Tsiaoussis J, et al. Resection rectopexy for rectal prolapse: the laparoscopic approach. Surg Endosc 1999;13:862–4.
162. Detry R, Vanheuverzwijn R, Mahieu P, et al. The use of prosthetic material in rectopexies. Int Surg 1984;69:301–4.
163. Loygue J, Nordlinger B, Cunci O, et al. Rectopexy to the promontory for the treatment of rectal prolapse. Report of 257 cases. Dis Colon Rectum 1984;27(6): 356–9.
164. Portier G, Iovino F, Lazorthes F. Surgery for rectal prolapse: Orr-Loygue ventral rectopexy with limited dissection prevents postoperative-induced constipation without increasing recurrence. Dis Colon Rectum 2006;49:1136–40.
165. Verdaasdonk E, Bueno de Mesquita J, Stassen L. Laparoscopic rectovaginopexy for rectal prolapse. Tech Coloproctol 2006;10:318–22.

166. Douard R, Frileux P, Brunel M, et al. Functional results after the Orr-Loygue transabdominal rectopexy for complete rectal prolapse. Dis Colon Rectum 2003;46:1089–96.
167. Marchal F, Bresler L, Ayav A, et al. Long-term results of Delorme's procedure and Orr-Loygue rectopexy to treat complete rectal prolapse. Dis Colon Rectum 2005;48:1785–90.
168. Collinson R, Boons P, Van Duijvendijk P, et al. Laparoscopic anterior rectopexy improves both obstructed defecation and faecal incontinence in patients with rectal intussusception. Gut 2007;56:A50.
169. Cristaldi M, Collinson R, Boons P, et al. Laparoscopic anterior rectopexy: a new approach that still cures rectal prolapse, but also improves preoperative constipation without inducing new-onset constipation. Dis Colon Rectum 2007;50:721.

Constipation and Pelvic Outlet Obstruction

Traci L. Hedrick, MD*, Charles M. Friel, MD

KEYWORDS

- Constipation • Slow transit constipation • Pelvic outlet obstruction
- Obstructed defecation • Manometry • Defecography

KEY POINTS

- The diagnosis of constipation is confirmed using the Rome III criteria.
- In addition to history and physical, it is prudent to obtain a colonoscopy in patients with new onset constipation. Further testing may be deferred until a trial of lifestyle modifications and medical therapy fails.
- Surgery is reserved for select patients with colonic inertia that fail medical management and have no evidence of globalized intestinal dysmotility.
- The first-line treatment for patients with pelvic dyssynergy is biofeedback.
- Rectoceles are present in up to 81% of asymptomatic women.
- Large rectoceles that require digital splinting may benefit from repair.
- A stoma may benefit select patients that fail other treatment modalities for constipation.

 A video of defecography for rectocele diagnosis accompanies this article at http://www.gastro.theclinics.com

INTRODUCTION

Constipation is one of the most common medical complaints among Americans, affecting up to 25% of the population.[1] The cause of constipation is oftentimes multidisciplinary, including dietary habits, genetics, psychosocial issues, medications, medical illness, and primary diseases of the colon and rectum. A clear understanding of the available diagnostic modalities and management strategies is imperative for health care providers from any discipline who will undoubtedly treat patients with constipation.

DEFINITION

The complaint of constipation is quite subjective, making it difficult to reliably define. A team of international experts published diagnostic criteria (Rome III) based on the

Department of Surgery, University of Virginia, PO Box 800709, Charlottesville, VA 22908, USA
* Corresponding author.
E-mail address: th8q@virginia.edu

Gastroenterol Clin N Am 42 (2013) 863–876
http://dx.doi.org/10.1016/j.gtc.2013.09.004
0889-8553/13/$ – see front matter © 2013 Elsevier Inc. All rights reserved.

presence of the criteria listed in **Box 1** for at least 3 months with onset of symptoms 6 months before diagnosis.[2]

CAUSE AND PATHOLOGY

Constipation can result from numerous conditions and medications. Perhaps the most common contributing factor to constipation is dietary. The western diet consists primarily of processed grains and, as such, is devoid of adequate amounts of fiber. Fiber intake correlates with stool bulk, which is important for colonic distension, stimulation of normal peristalsis, and efficient propulsion of stools. Furthermore, medical illnesses ranging from diabetes and hypothyroidism to neurologic illness, psychiatric disease, rheumatologic conditions, and anything leading to immobilization contributes to constipation. Finally, numerous medications lead to constipation, ranging from antihypertensives to antidepressants, iron supplements, and opioids. Mechanical causes of constipation must also be carefully considered including colon stricture, malignancy, and endometriosis. Idiopathic chronic constipation can be divided into 3 subtypes.

CONSTIPATION SUBTYPES

1. Motility disorders (11% of patients): May be isolated to the colon (colonic inertia) but can affect the entire bowel in up to 20% of patients with colonic inertia; often associated with constipation since childhood and laxative dependence
2. Irritable bowel syndrome (71% of patients): Frequently associated with abdominal pain that is relieved by defecation and irregular bowel habits; a diagnosis of exclusion
3. Pelvic outlet obstruction (13%–50%): Also known as obstructed defecation syndrome, anismus, and pelvic dyssynergy; characterized by sensation of incomplete evacuation, prolonged straining, and need for digital manipulation.[3,4]

INITIAL EVALUATION
History and Physical

The factors listed in **Box 2** should be taken as part of a full history during evaluation of the patient with constipation. Although the physical examination is oftentimes

---

Box 1
Rome III criteria for the diagnosis of constipation

- Must include at least 2 of the following
  - Fewer than 3 stools per week
  - Hard stools in at least 25% of defecations
  - Manual maneuvers to facilitate at least 25% of defecations (eg, support of pelvic floor or digital stimulation)
  - Straining during at least 25% of defecations
  - Sensation of incomplete evacuation for at least 25% of defecations
  - Sensation of anorectal blockage for at least 25% of defecations
- Loose stools rarely present without the use of laxatives
- Insufficient criteria for irritable bowel syndrome

Symptoms must be present for at least 3 months with onset of symptoms 6 months before diagnosis.

Box 2
Important components of the history and physical examination in patients with constipation

History

- Stool size, frequency, consistency
- Characterize evacuation
- Age of onset
- Diet and exercise habits
- Medical and surgical history
- Medications
- Psychiatric illness, sexual abuse
- Other pelvic floor symptoms (eg, urinary dysfunction, prolapse)

Physical examination

- Abdominal examination: distension, palpation of mass/hardened stool
- Pelvic floor evaluation: vaginal, perineal, and rectal examination to evaluate for rectocele, full-thickness rectal prolapse, bulging of perineum

---

unremarkable, it does remain an important part of the evaluation. Abdominal examination may reveal distension and a palpable mass as the result of hardened stool in extreme cases. Close inspection of the pelvic floor is also important. With the patient in the left lateral decubitus position or the prone jackknife position on a Ritter table, a rectal examination should be performed to evaluate for fecal impaction, tenderness, or masses. The patient should then be asked to strain. The examiner should look for bulging into the vaginal introitus indicating a rectocele, full-thickness rectal prolapse, or bulging of the perineum below the ischial tuberosities, which indicates perineal descent syndrome. Finally, the puborectalis muscle should be palpated with the examiner's finger in the anal canal by hooking the examining finger posteriorly over the coccyx and asking the patient to strain. Under normal conditions the anal canal should relax. However, in patients with anismus or dyssynergia, there can be an inability to relax or paradoxic puborectalis contraction when the patient strains. The sensitivity and specificity of such examination was found to be 75% and 87%, respectively, in one study.[5]

Testing

It is prudent to obtain a colonoscopy in patients with constipation to rule out an underlying malignancy. In addition, a complete blood cell count, thyroid-stimulating hormone, and chemistry panel should be obtained in patients with acute onset constipation or signs and symptoms worrisome for malignancy. Further testing may be deferred until a trial of lifestyle modifications including fiber supplementation, hydration, and exercise along with the use of laxatives fails to resolve the patient's symptoms (**Fig. 1**). Commonly used testing methods are described in **Table 1**.

TREATMENT
Medical Treatment

Medical treatment begins with avoidance of constipating medications, increasing fiber intake to 20 to 25 g per day with adequate hydration, and regular exercise. A

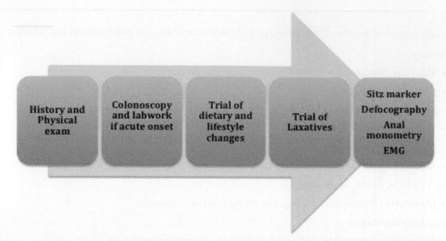

Fig. 1. Algorithm for evaluating patients with constipation. Further testing may be deferred until a trial of lifestyle modifications, fiber therapy, and laxatives fails to resolve the patient's symptoms.

full discussion of the medical treatment of constipation is beyond the scope of this article. However, psyllium, stool softeners, and stimulant and osmotic laxatives are commonly used in the treatment of constipation. Osmotic laxatives such as polyethylene glycol and lactulose seem to be the most effective in the treatment of constipation based on the literature.[6] Other agents include lubiprostone, misoprostol, and colchicine, which have been used in patients with severe constipation with limited success.

Colonic Inertia

Most patients are women and complaints may include bloating, obstipation, and abdominal pain. Patients with colonic inertia have typically suffered with constipation since childhood, although it is not uncommon for women to present after pelvic surgery or childbirth. The diagnosis is confirmed with a sitz marker study; however, pelvic outlet obstruction should also be ruled out.

Surgical options

Surgical options for colonic inertia include total abdominal colectomy with ileorectal anastomosis, subtotal colectomy with ileosigmoid anastomosis, subtotal colectomy with cecorectal anastomosis, and segmental colectomy. The goal with all these procedures is to remove enough colon to relieve the constipation without inadvertently leaving the patient with disabling diarrhea and incontinence. As such, segmental colectomy and subtotal colectomy are appealing. There are no prospective studies comparing these methodologies, only small case series. Lundin and colleagues[7] demonstrated that 23 of 28 patients undergoing segmental colectomy were pleased with their outcome. Similarly, Marchesi and colleagues[8] demonstrated good functional results with open and laparoscopic subtotal colectomy with cecorectal anastmososis. Niether of these procedures is widely performed, however, due to the risk of recurrent or persistent constipation and the difficulty in identifying appropriate patients based on diagnostic testing. In addition, there have been reports of restorative proctocolectomy in the setting of chronic constipation. However, this should only be considered in a highly select and motivated patient population and long-term functional results are lacking.[9]

Table 1
Commonly tests used in the evaluation of constipation and pelvic outlet obstruction

Test	Description	Evaluates	Normal	Abnormal
Manometry	Uses pressure transducers to measure anal canal pressures and rectoanal inhibitory reflex (RIR)	Rectal sensation and compliance, reflexive relaxation of internal anal sphincter	Sphincter relaxes with straining, pressure in anal canal decreases RIR, rectal distension results in relaxation of internal anal sphincter	• Dyssynergy, pressure increases with straining • Presence of RIR excludes Hirshsprung
Colon transit study	Patient ingests capsule of 24 radiopaque markers, radiograph on consecutive days	Colonic motility	80% of markers passed out or to rectum by day 5	• Slow transit, if 5 or more do not reach rectum by day 5 • Pelvic outlet, markers congregate in rectosigmoid
Defecography	150 mL of barium paste inserted into rectum and anal canal; patient then asked to evacuate paste on specially designed radiograph table/commode	Pelvic floor relaxation—anorectal angle (ARA), perineal descent, and puborectalis length	Resting ARA: 70–140°	• Dyssynergy, less than 15° change in ARA angle and less than 1 cm descent of perineum during evacuation • Perineal descent syndrome, greater than 3 cm descent during evacuation • Presence of rectocele, enterocele, or sigmoidocele
Balloon expulsion	50 mL water-filled balloon placed in rectum and evacuated	Functional ability	Pass the balloon	Failure to pass balloon suggests dyssynergy or anismus
Dynamic MRI	Various protocols described, not standardized	Pelvic floor anatomy	Similar to defecography	Similar to defecography
Electromyography	Electrodes placed in anal sphincter and electrical activity of puborectalis evaluated during evacuation	Puborectalis	Puborectalis relaxes during straining with decreased electrical activity	Dyssynergy, increased electrical activity during straining

Currently, total abdominal colectomy with ileorectal anastomosis (either open or laparoscopic) is the most widely performed procedure for colonic inertia and has demonstrated adequate long-term results.[10] Any surgical procedure must be performed in a highly selective population:

- Severe medically refractory constipation
- No evidence of secondary or structural causes for constipation
- Slow transit on colonic motility study (ie, sitz marker test)
- Normal gastric and small bowel motility (whole gut transit scintigraphy, gastric emptying study, or small bowel follow through)
- Ability to relax pelvic floor musculature
- Understands surgical risks and long-term expectations

The patients should be fully evaluated to exclude secondary causes such as hypothyroidism. Colonoscopy should be performed to rule out a structural abnormality. Patients should also be evaluated with whole gut transit scintigraphy, a gastric emptying study, or small bowel follow through to assess for the presence of a diffuse gastrointestinal dysmotility disorder, which can accompany colonic inertia in 30% of patients.[3] Total colectomy is generally not beneficial in patients with globalized dysmotility. A validated constipation score should be obtained to help categorize the type of incontinence and to monitor progress after therapy.[11]

Defecography should be performed to evaluate for the presence of pelvic outlet obstruction, which can affect up to 20% of patients with colonic inertia and complicates management. Increasingly, more surgeons offer total colectomy after preoperative biofeedback with demonstration of pelvic floor relaxation. Previously, the results of colectomy in the setting of colonic inertia and combined pelvic outlet disorder were disappointing.[12] However, more recent reports indicate similar patient satisfaction scores on follow-up surveys administered to patients with and without obstructed defecation syndrome (ODS) following colectomy for slow transit constipation.[13,14]

Finally, the patients should obviously be counseled extensively about the surgical risks of the operation but also must be given realistic expectations. Although total colectomy is highly effective at improving the daily number of bowel movements in patients with colonic inertia, the effect on the patient's overall quality of life isless well defined.[15]

PELVIC OUTLET OBSTRUCTION

Pelvic outlet obstruction is a broad term that refers to a patient's perceived inability to empty the rectum normally. There are many additional terms (rectal outlet obstruction, evacuatory dysfunction, ODS) used throughout the literature to describe the same constellations of findings. The term obstructed defecation or ODS seems to be the most current commonly applied term and is used throughout this article. ODS may or may not be associated with constipation because many patients have both normal consistency and number of bowel movements daily. Pelvic outlet obstruction may be classified as demonstrated in **Box 3**.

Symptoms include the following:
- Rectal pain
- Feeling of incomplete evacuation
- Need for digitation or perineal massage to evacuate
- Dependency on enemas
- Prolonged straining
- Fecal incontinence

Box 3
Classification scheme in patients with pelvic outlet obstruction

1. Functional outlet obstruction
   a. Short-segment Hirschsprung disease
   b. Anismus (pelvic floor dyssynergia)
   c. Neuropathy: spinal cord lesion, multiple sclerosis
2. Mechanical outlet obstruction
   a. Internal intussusception
   b. Enterocele
   c. Sigmoidocele
   d. Rectocele
   e. Rectal prolapse

FUNCTIONAL OUTLET OBSTRUCTION
Short-segment Hirshsprung

Short-segment Hirshsprung is a disorder characterized by the lack of ganglion cells within the myenteric plexus of the rectum. Occasionally, patients may not be diagnosed with Hirschsprung disease until adulthood. In this setting, the patients have generally struggled with constipation their entire life and the aganglionic segement is short. The presence of a rectoanal inhibitory reflex on anal manometry excludes the diagnosis. If the reflex is absent, a full-thickness rectal biopsy is necessary to confirm the diagnosis. Surgical treatment consists of a transanal rectal myectomy to excise a portion of the internal anal sphincter in cases of short segment aganglionosis. Resection of the aganglionic segment with coloanal anastomosis is reserved for patients with refractory symptoms or longer segment aganglionosis.

Pelvic Dyssynergy

Pelvic dyssynergy (anismus, spastic pelvic floor syndrome, paradoxic puborectalis) results from failure of the puborectalis sling to relax during defecation, resulting in obstructed defecation. Diagnosis is based on anal manometry demonstrating increased electrical activity of the puborectalis during straining and defecography demonstrating less than 15° of change in the anorectal angle and less than 1 cm of perineal descent during evacuation. The first-line treatment of pelvic dyssynergy is biofeedback. Other treatment modalities that have been described for patients refractory to biofeedback are injection of botulinum toxin into the puborectalis muscle as well as sacral nerve stimulation (SNS).

Biofeedback
Biofeedback is a commonly used treatment modality that is particularly effective in the treatment of pelvic dyssynergy. It is a behavioral approach that uses anorectal manometers to reflect patient responses during attempted expulsion of the apparatus. It relies on the dedication and a quality therapeutic relationship between the therapist and patient to achieve maximal results. Unfortunately, criteria for patient selection and practice protocols are not well defined. Therefore, it is not widely available and often times not covered by insurance. **Table 2** summarizes 3 randomized controlled trials, which demonstrate significant patient reported and physiologic improvement with

Table 2
Randomized controlled trials evaluating the use of biofeedback in patients with obstructed defecation

Author/Year	Indication	Patients	Control/Treatment	Findings
Roa et al,[35] 2007	Chronic constipation and dyssynergic defecation	77	Biofeedback vs sham feedback vs diet/exercise/laxatives	Biofeedback improved constipation and global bowel satisfaction over sham and standard therapy
Chiarioni et al,[36] 2006	Pelvic floor dyssynergia	109	Biofeedback vs polyethylene glycol plus weekly counseling sessions	Biofeedback improved greater reductions in straining, sensation of incomplete evacuation, and use of enemas and electromyography
Heymen et al,[37] 2007	Pelvic floor dyssynergia	84	Biofeedback vs diazepam vs placebo	Biofeedback superior to diazepam and placebo in relief of symptoms and electromyography

biofeedback over standard therapy in patients with pelvic dyssynergy. It has minimal efficacy in the treatment of slow transit constipation.[16]

Botulinum toxin
Injection of botulinum toxin (60–100 U) in the puborectalis and external anal sphincter has shown promise in the treatment of patients with isolated pelvic dyssynergy.[17–19] However, repeated injections may be necessary and this practice has not become widespread as of yet.

SNS
SNS can be performed by surgically inserting electrodes into the S3 foramen and stimulation of these nerves with a low-amplitude electrical stimulation. It is currently used for the treatment of both urinary and fecal incontinence. Over the last decade there have been several small studies using SNS for constipation.[20] Most of these studies have been in patients with slow transit constipation but some also have been in patients with obstructive defecation. In most of these studies there has been some improvement in both the frequency and the degree of straining. However, the numbers of patients are still quite small and, while the results show some promise, no definitive conclusions can be reached about the true efficacy of SNS at this time.

MECHANICAL OUTLET OBSTRUCTION
Internal Intussusception

Rectal intussusception was previously thought to represent the precursor to full-thickness rectal prolapse and a principal cause of ODS. However, intussusception is found incidentally on defecography in one-third of women[21,22] and only 2% of patients with internal intussusception progress to full-thickness rectal prolapse.[23,24] The mainstay of treatment of the patient with internal intussusception is biofeedback. Intussusception and full-thickness rectal prolapse is discussed in detail in an article elsewhere in this issue.

Enterocele/Sigmoidocele

Enteroceles and sigmoidoceles occur as the result of herniation of the peritoneum through the uterosacral ligaments at the vaginal apex leading to separation of the rectovaginal septum. This herniation may contain small bowel (enterocele) or sigmoid colon (sigmoidocele) and may impede defecation leading to pelvic discomfort and perineal pressure with straining. They can be categorized as 1st, 2nd, and 3rd degree; in general, 1st and 2nd degree sigmoidoceles are treated without surgery. Sigmoidectomy is occasionally warranted to some 3rd degree sigmoidoceles. In extreme cases, an enterocele may ulcerate the vaginal mucosa, leading to evisceration. The diagnosis is confirmed on defecography, with triple contrast in the small intestine and vagina in addition to the usual barium paste in the rectum. Although not universally symptomatic, an enterocele or sigmoidocele that impairs rectal emptying on defecography likely contributes to the patient's symptoms.

Surgical options are available for a clinically significant enterocele or sigmoidocele. However, patients should be carefully counseled that outcomes vary. Surgical options include a sacrculpopexy with or without mesh or resection rectopexy in the setting of a concomitant rectal prolapse with constipation. Perineal approaches are also available. The key to the surgical approach is obliteration of the peritoneal defect with approximation of the peritoneum of the anterior rectal wall, posterior bladder, and vagina. This approach is often referred to as the Moskowitz repair.

Rectocele

A rectocele is the result of a hernia within the rectovaginal septum causing the rectum to bulge into the posterior wall of the vagina. Rectocele is commonly found in patients with ODS. The diagnosis is typically made on physical examination (**Fig. 2**) and defecography (Video 1). However, rectoceles are present in up to 81% of asymptomatic women.[21,22] A study looking at 239 patients presenting with ODS found that the presence of a rectocele did not correlate with the severity of ODS-type symptoms or pelvic dyssynergy, suggesting that rectoceles may be the result, as opposed to the cause, of ODS.[25] Rectoceles less than 2 cm are unlikely to cause symptoms and generally do not require surgical repair. Large rectoceles that require digital splinting of the vagina or perineum to empty (as demonstrated in the attached Video 1) are likely of clinical significance and may benefit from repair. Rectoceles are

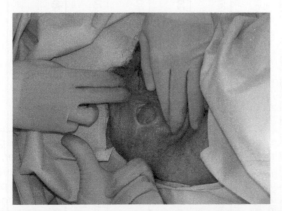

Fig. 2. This figure demonstrates the presence of a rectocele evident on physical examination as a palpable weakness through the anterior wall of the rectum.

Table 3
Studies regarding Stapled Transanal Rectal Resection (STARR) for obstructive defecation syndrome

Authors/Year	Country	Study Years	n	Study Type	Conclusions
Jayne et al,[28] 2009	UK Germany Italy	2006–2008	2838	Nonrandomized prospective multicenter audit	Improvement in obstructive defecation symptoms, symptom severity, and incontinence. Morbidity "acceptable"
Titu et al,[29] 2009	UK	2001–2007	230	Case series	Improved incontinence, obstructive symptoms. Major complications in 7%, including 2 colostomies. Urgency quite common, but improves with time
Goede et al,[30] 2011	UK	2001–2010	344	Case series	Improvement in obstructive symptoms and fecal incontinence, Fecal urgency 72% at 2 mo, 11% at 12 mo, 0% at 48 mo. Patient satisfaction 90%
Stuto et al,[31] 2011	Italy	2006–2009	2171	Nonrandomized prospective multicenter audit	Improvement in obstructive defecation symptoms, symptom severity, and incontinence. Morbidity "acceptable"
Bock et al,[32] 2013	Switzerland	2007–2010	70	Case series	Improvement in obstructive defecation symptoms and symptom severity. No improvement of incontinence. Results deteriorated over 4-y follow-up Fecal urgency resolved over time

generally repaired via a perineal or transvaginal approach. The basic premise of the operation is to re-create the rectovaginal septum using native tissue or biologic mesh.

Stapled Transanal Rectal Resection Procedure

Over the last decade a novel approach to obstructive defecation in the setting of rectal intussusception and/or rectocele has been developed. Following the successful implementation of transanal stapling for hemorrhoids, a similar concept was introduced for the treatment of obstructive defecation.[26] In this procedure 2 fires of the stapler are used. The first effectively resects the anterior rectal wall, removing some of the redundancy often associated with this disorder. Similarly a second fire of the stapler resects the posterior wall. A more recent variation on this technique uses a contour stapler and has been described as the Transtar procedure.[27] Conceptually, the resulting rectal resection removes the redundancy of the distal rectum allowing for a less "obstructed" pathway to defecation.

Most of the reports in the literature regarding the stapled transanal rectal resection procedure procedure are from Europe and many show encouraging results with improvement in obstructive defecation scores, fecal incontinence, and quality of life (Table 3).[28–34] Despite this, concerns about serious complications and the long-term implications of staples in the distal rectum have deterred rapid acceptance of this procedure in the United States.[33,34] There have been reports of rectal pain, rectal pressure, incontinence, pelvic sepsis, and rectovaginal fistulae, to name a few. Unfortunately, the literature is hard to interpret, partly due to the diverse patient population and also to the lack of prospective, randomized studies. Therefore, patients referred for this procedure need to be carefully selected and informed of both the benefits and the potential risks. To maximize the benefits and minimize potential complications, this procedure should clearly only be performed by experts in the field specifically trained to do this procedure.

Stomas

Another consideration in patients with severe constipation or disabling pelvic floor dysfunction is a stoma. If other treatment modalities fail, a functional colostomy or ileostomy can significantly improve the quality of life in a select group of patients. Patients with significant pelvic floor dysfunction can be treated with a colostomy, whereas the patient with colonic inertia will likely require an ileostomy. Either can be accomplished laparoscopically and are generally very well tolerated even in the poorest of operative candidates. It is incredibly helpful for the patients to meet with an enterostomal therapist preoperatively for extensive education and expectation management.

SUMMARY

The treatment of constipation and ODS is complex and requires a multidisciplinary approach. Careful evaluation is paramount to identify the cause of the symptoms correctly and formulate a treatment strategy. The mainstays of treatment of patients with constipation are dietary and lifestyle alterations with laxatives if necessary. Physiologic, radiographic, and endoscopic testing benefit the patient that remains symptomatic after conservative measures fail. Frequently there are associated pelvic floor abnormalities, which often respond to biofeedback and less commonly surgery. Extensive counseling and education are keys to patient satisfaction in outlining expected goals of therapy.

SUPPLEMENTARY DATA

A video related to this article can be found at http://dx.doi.org/10.1016/j.gtc.2013. 09.004.

REFERENCES

1. Koloski NA, Jones M, Wai R, et al. Impact of persistent constipation on health-related quality of life and mortality in older community-dwelling women. Am J Gastroenterol 2013;108(7):1152–8.
2. Drossman DA. Rome III: the new criteria [review]. Chin J Dig Dis 2006;7(4):181–5.
3. Vrees MD, Weiss EG. The evaluation of constipation. Clin Colon Rectal Surg 2005;18(2):65–75.
4. Rao SS. Dyssynergic defecation [review]. Gastroenterol Clin North Am 2001; 30(1):97–114.
5. Tantiphlachiva K, Rao P, Attaluri A, et al. Digital rectal examination is a useful tool for identifying patients with dyssynergia. Clin Gastroenterol Hepatol 2010;8(11): 955–60 [Evaluation Studies Research Support, N.I.H., Extramural Research Support, Non-U.S. Gov't].
6. Ramkumar D, Rao SS. Efficacy and safety of traditional medical therapies for chronic constipation: systematic review. Am J Gastroenterol 2005;100(4): 936–71 [Comparative Study Meta-Analysis Review].
7. Lundin E, Karlbom U, Pahlman L, et al. Outcome of segmental colonic resection for slow-transit constipation. Br J Surg 2002;89(10):1270–4 [Research Support, Non-U.S. Gov't].
8. Marchesi F, Percalli L, Pinna F, et al. Laparoscopic subtotal colectomy with anti-peristaltic cecorectal anastomosis: a new step in the treatment of slow-transit constipation. Surg Endosc 2012;26(6):1528–33 [Evaluation Studies].
9. Asipu D, Jaffray B. Treatment of severe childhood constipation with restorative proctocolectomy. Arch Dis Child 2010;95(11):867–70 [Case Reports].
10. Pikarsky AJ, Singh JJ, Weiss EG, et al. Long-term follow-up of patients undergoing colectomy for colonic inertia. Dis Colon Rectum 2001;44(2):179–83 [Research Support, Non-U.S. Gov't].
11. Agachan F, Chen T, Pfeifer J, et al. A constipation scoring system to simplify evaluation and management of constipated patients. Dis Colon Rectum 1996;39(6): 681–5.
12. Bernini A, Madoff RD, Lowry AC, et al. Should patients with combined colonic inertia and nonrelaxing pelvic floor undergo subtotal colectomy? Dis Colon Rectum 1998;41(11):1363–6.
13. Hassan I, Pemberton JH, Young-Fadok TM, et al. Ileorectal anastomosis for slow transit constipation: long-term functional and quality of life results. J Gastrointest Surg 2006;10(10):1330–6 [discussion: 1336–1337].
14. Reshef A, Alves-Ferreira P, Zutshi M, et al. Colectomy for slow transit constipation: effective for patients with coexistent obstructed defecation. Int J Colorectal Dis 2013;28(6):841–7.
15. Knowles CH, Scott M, Lunniss PJ. Outcome of colectomy for slow transit constipation. Ann Surg 1999;230(5):627–38 [Research Support, Non-U.S. Gov't Review].
16. Chiarioni G, Salandini L, Whitehead WE. Biofeedback benefits only patients with outlet dysfunction, not patients with isolated slow transit constipation. Gastroenterology 2005;129(1):86–97 [Clinical Trial Research Support, N.I.H., Extramural Research Support, U.S. Gov't, P.H.S.].

17. Hompes R, Harmston C, Wijffels N, et al. Excellent response rate of anismus to botulinum toxin if rectal prolapse misdiagnosed as anismus ('pseudoanismus') is excluded. Colorectal Dis 2012;14(2):224–30.

18. Maria G, Cadeddu F, Brandara F, et al. Experience with type A botulinum toxin for treatment of outlet-type constipation. Am J Gastroenterol 2006;101(11):2570–5.

19. Farid M, El Monem HA, Omar W, et al. Comparative study between biofeedback retraining and botulinum neurotoxin in the treatment of anismus patients. Int J Colorectal Dis 2009;24(1):115–20 [Randomized Controlled Trial].

20. Thomas GP, Dudding TC, Rahbour G, et al. Sacral nerve stimulation for constipation [review]. Br J Surg 2013;100(2):174–81.

21. Dvorkin LS, Gladman MA, Epstein J, et al. Rectal intussusception in symptomatic patients is different from that in asymptomatic volunteers. Br J Surg 2005;92(7):866–72.

22. Shorvon PJ, McHugh S, Diamant NE, et al. Defecography in normal volunteers: results and implications. Gut 1989;30(12):1737–49 [Research Support, Non-U.S. Gov't].

23. Ellis CN, Essani R. Treatment of obstructed defecation. Clin Colon Rectal Surg 2012;25(1):24–33.

24. Mellgren A, Schultz I, Johansson C, et al. Internal rectal intussusception seldom develops into total rectal prolapse. Dis Colon Rectum 1997;40(7):817–20 [Research Support, Non-U.S. Gov't].

25. Hicks CW, Wakamatsu M, Pulliam S, et al. Are rectoceles the cause or the result of obstructed defecation syndrome (ODS)? A prospective anorectal physiology study. Colorectal Dis 2013;15(8):993–9.

26. Corman ML, Carriero A, Hager T, et al. Consensus conference on the stapled transanal rectal resection (STARR) for disordered defaecation. Colorectal Dis 2006;8(2):98–101 [Consensus Development Conference Practice Guideline Research Support, Non-U.S. Gov't].

27. Isbert C, Reibetanz J, Jayne DG, et al. Comparative study of Contour Transtar and STARR procedure for the treatment of obstructed defecation syndrome (ODS)–feasibility, morbidity and early functional results. Colorectal Dis 2010; 12(9):901–8 [Comparative Study].

28. Jayne DG, Schwandner O, Stuto A. Stapled transanal rectal resection for obstructed defecation syndrome: one-year results of the European STARR Registry. Dis Colon Rectum 2009;52(7):1205–12 [discussion: 12–4], [Multicenter Study Research Support, Non-U.S. Gov't].

29. Titu LV, Riyad K, Carter H, et al. Stapled transanal rectal resection for obstructed defecation: a cautionary tale. Dis Colon Rectum 2009;52(10):1716–22.

30. Goede AC, Glancy D, Carter H, et al. Medium-term results of stapled transanal rectal resection (STARR) for obstructed defecation and symptomatic rectal-anal intussusception. Colorectal Dis 2011;13(9):1052–7.

31. Stuto A, Renzi A, Carriero A, et al. Stapled trans-anal rectal resection (STARR) in the surgical treatment of the obstructed defecation syndrome: results of STARR Italian Registry. Surg Innov 2011;18(3):248–53 [Research Support, Non-U.S. Gov't].

32. Bock S, Wolff K, Marti L, et al. Long-term outcome after transanal rectal resection in patients with obstructed defecation syndrome. Dis Colon Rectum 2013;56(2): 246–52.

33. Pescatori M, Gagliardi G. Postoperative complications after procedure for prolapsed hemorrhoids (PPH) and stapled transanal rectal resection (STARR) procedures [review]. Tech Coloproctol 2008;12(1):7–19.

34. Naldini G. Serious unconventional complications of surgery with stapler for haemorrhoidal prolapse and obstructed defaecation because of rectocoele and rectal intussusception. Colorectal Dis 2011;13(3):323–7.

35. Rao SS, Seaton K, Miller M, et al. Randomized controlled trial of biofeedback, sham feedback, and standard therapy for dyssynergic defecation. Clin Gastroenterol Hepatol 2007;5:331–8.
36. Chiarioni G, Whitehead WE, Pezza V, et al. Biofeedback is superior to laxatives for normal transit constipation due to pelvic floor dyssynergia. Gastroenterology 2006;130:657–64.
37. Heymen S, Scarlett Y, Jones K, et al. Randomized, controlled trail shows biofeedback to be superior to alternative treatments for patients with pelvic floor dyssynergia-typr constipation. Dis Colon Rectum 2007;50(4):428–41.

Sexually Transmitted and Anorectal Infectious Diseases

Molly M. Cone, MD[a], Charles B. Whitlow, MD[b],*

KEYWORDS

- Anorectal • Sexually transmitted disease • Infection

KEY POINTS

- Patients with acute proctitis who have recently practiced anal receptive intercourse and who have anorectal exudates on examination or polymorphonuclear leukocytes detected on Gram stain should be treated with a 1-time intramuscular dose of ceftriaxone 250 mg and doxycycline 100 mg orally twice a day for 7 days while awaiting laboratory results.
- Patients with painful perianal ulcers or rectal mucosal ulcers should be presumptively treated for herpes simplex virus (HSV) and lymphogranuloma venereum chlamydia until diagnosis is established.
- The classic anoscopic examination for gonorrhea includes thick purulent discharge that is expressed from the anal crypts with pressure on the anus.
- *Chlamydia* serovars D through K are those responsible for urethritis, cervicitis/pelvic inflammatory disease, neonatal disease, and can cause proctitis. Serovars L1, L2, and L3 can cause lymphogranuloma venereum.
- Syphilis typically presents with sores that appear at the location where it entered the body. Extragenital or anal chancres (in contrast with genital lesions) are generally painful and resolve after 3 to 6 weeks whether treated or not. Lymphadenopathy may be present.
- HSV proctitis is suggested by the presence of severe anorectal pain; sacral parasthesias; diffuse ulceration of the distal rectal mucosa; and, at times, difficulty urinating.
- The sexually transmitted diseases discussed are generally treated the same in a human immunodeficiency virus–positive patient. The US Centers for Disease Control and Prevention recommends close follow-up of lesions and symptoms because the risk of recurrent or persistent disease may be higher.
- Acquired immunodeficiency syndrome ulcers are generally higher in the anal canal with a broad base and ulceration that may involve the muscle. Severe pain is common.
- Anogenital warts, or condyloma accuminata, are caused by human papillomavirus (HPV) 6 or 11 in 90% of cases.
- Ninety-five percent of anal cancers are linked to HPV.

The authors have no disclosures.
[a] Department of Colon and Rectal Surgery, Vanderbilt University Medical Center, Nashville, TN, USA; [b] Department of Colon and Rectal Surgery, Ochsner Clinic Foundation, 1514 Jefferson Highway, New Orleans, LA 70121, USA
* Corresponding author.
E-mail address: cwhitlow@ochsner.org

Gastroenterol Clin N Am 42 (2013) 877–892
http://dx.doi.org/10.1016/j.gtc.2013.09.003
0889-8553/13/$ – see front matter © 2013 Elsevier Inc. All rights reserved.

SEXUALLY TRANSMITTED AND INFECTIOUS DISEASES OF THE ANUS AND RECTUM
General Presentation and Initial Management

Anal or perianal ulcers and proctitis are the most common manifestations of anorectal sexually transmitted infections that bring a patient to the attention of a colon and rectal surgeon. Principles based on prevalence of disease can aid in the work-up and treatment. In the United States, most young, sexually active patients with anal or anal canal ulcers have herpes simplex virus (HSV). Although syphilis is another consideration, the incidence is less common. Even more infrequent are chancroid and donovanosis ulcerations. Diagnosis based on a patients history and physical examination can be inaccurate, thus it is recommended by the US Centers for Disease Control and Prevention (CDC) that all patients who have anal or perianal ulcers be evaluated with serologic tests for syphilis and a diagnostic evaluation for herpes either by culture or polymerase chain reaction (PCR). Human immunodeficiency virus (HIV) testing should be performed on all patients with anal or perianal ulcers who are not already known to be infected. Proctitis from sexually transmitted infections occurs predominantly among those involved in anal receptive intercourse. This inflammation of the rectum can be associated with rectal discharge, pain, and tenesmus. The most common sexually transmitted pathogens involved are *Neisseria gonorrhoeae*, *Chlamydia trachomatis*, *Treponema pallidum*, and HSV. Proctitis from HSV can be especially severe in patients with HIV.

Because results from testing can take more than 48 hours, it is often necessary to begin empiric treatment. Patients with acute proctitis who have recently practiced anal receptive intercourse and who have demonstrable anorectal exudates on examination or polymorphonuclear leukocytes on Gram stain should be treated with a 1-time intramuscular (IM) dose of ceftriaxone 250 mg and doxycycline 100 mg orally twice a day for 7 days while awaiting laboratory results. For patients with painful perianal ulcers or rectal mucosal ulcers, presumptive treatment of HSV and lymphogranuloma venereum (LGV) chlamydia should be initiated.[1]

Reporting

To assist local health authorities in partner notification, assess morbidity trends, and help with appropriate allocation of resources, timely reporting of STDs is necessary. In every state, the following cases should be reported: syphilis, gonorrhea, chlamydia, chancroid, HIV, and acquired immunodeficiency syndrome (AIDS). Requirements for reporting other STDs vary by state.

Prevention

The most reliable way to avoid transmission of STDs is to abstain from oral, vaginal, and anal sex or to be in a long-term, mutually monogamous relationship with an uninfected partner. For persons who are being treated for an STD, counseling that encourages abstinence from sexual intercourse until completion of the course of medication is crucial.[1]

Barriers, such as male latex condoms, are highly effective in preventing the sexual transmission of HIV when used correctly.[2] Condoms can also reduce the risk for other STDs, including chlamydia, gonorrhea, and trichomoniasis.[3,4] Although data are more limited, consistent and correct use of latex condoms also reduces the risk for genital herpes, syphilis, and chancroid when the infected area or site of potential exposure is covered.[5,6] Condoms lubricated with spermicides are no more effective than other lubricated condoms in protecting against the transmission of HIV and other STDs.[7] Furthermore, spermicides containing nonoxynol-9 can damage the cells lining the rectum, which may provide a portal of entry for HIV and other sexually transmissible diseases. Therefore, it should not be used as a microbicide or lubricant during anal intercourse by men who have sex with men (MSM) or by women.[1]

MOST COMMON PATHOGENS AND TREATMENTS
Gonorrhea

Over the past few years, reported cases of gonococcal disease have increased in both men and women across all ethnic groups and in all regions of the United States.[8] The CDC states that in 2011 there were 321,849 cases reported in the United States, which is a 4% increase since 2010. Rates among women continue to be higher than those among men, and the age group most frequently affected is 15 to 44 years.

Anorectal gonococcal disease is most common among MSM and women. Transmission is typically by oral-anal or anoreceptive intercourse, although women may also develop anorectal infection by spread from cervical or urethral gonorrhea because they frequently harbor disease in both areas.[9]

Although most women and approximately half of men with anorectal gonorrhea are asymptomatic,[10] patients may experience tenesmus, anorectal pain, constipation, or mucopurulent discharge.[11] To differentiate this from different causes of proctitis, work-up should include a history involving sexual practices, external anal examination, and anoscopy. In general, findings are nonspecific, including erythema and friable mucosa. The classic anoscopic examination for gonorrhea includes thick purulent discharge that is expressed from the anal crypts with pressure on the anus.[12] If anorectal exudate is detected or if a Gram stain of the anorectal secretions shows polymorphonuclear leukocytes, the CDC recommends initiation of treatment with ceftriaxone and doxycycline while awaiting final culture results.[1]

Infection with N gonorrhoeae can Facilitate HIV Transmission with more than a 3-Fold Increase in HIV Transmission Among MSM

Testing for N gonorrhoeae has historically been performed with culture,[13,14] which has the advantage of identification of the bacteria as well as analyzing antibiotic sensitivities. The culture should be taken by a cotton swab inserted 3 to 4 cm into the rectal vault. This swab is then placed on agar, most commonly Thayer-Martin, because it prevents the overgrowth of other endogenous flora. The specimen must then be transported and stored in a CO_2-rich environment. The sensitivity of culture for anorectal gonorrhea is poorly reported and ranges from 27% to 85%.[15]

Newer tests with promise are classified as nucleic acid amplification tests (NAATs). The transcription-mediated amplification shows greater sensitivity (100%) compared with culture (66.7%–71%) and similar specificity (>95% vs 99% for culture).[16,17] This test does not require the careful handling required for culture and can detect gonorrhea and chlamydia simultaneously. In less than 48 hours it can give results, but it is more expensive and cannot provide information on antibiotic susceptibility. There are currently no FDA-approved commercial tests for nongenital testing, but there are 19 states and 12 commercial laboratories that are Clinical Laboratory Improvement Amendments (CLIA) certified and listed in conjunction with the CDC who have standardized methods of testing with good results.[18] In high-risk populations, specifically MSM, the CDC recommends that men who have had receptive anal intercourse during the preceding year be tested for rectal infection with N gonorrhoeae and C trachomatis and states that an NAAT of a rectal swab is the preferred approach.[1]

N gonorrhoeae has shown the ability to develop antimicrobial resistance. In the late 1990s and 2000s fluoroquinolone resistance became widespread leaving cephalosporins as the only recommended antibiotic class for first-line treatment. More recently the minimum concentration of cefixime used to treat gonorrhea has increased, suggesting that its efficacy may be decreasing. For this reason, the CDC's recommendations for treatment were updated to no longer recommend cefixime. They now include combination therapy with ceftriaxone 250 mg IM and either azithromycin 1 g orally as a single dose, or doxycycline 100 mg orally twice daily for 7 days.[19] This treatment regimen ensures the treatment of both gonorrhea and chlamydia because they are frequent concomitant pathogens. Treatment does not differ in HIV-positive patients.

Chlamydia

With an estimated 2.86 million infections occurring annually in the United States, chlamydia is the most frequently reported bacterial sexually transmitted infection. Chlamydia is most prevalent among sexually active young persons aged 14 to 24 years and non-Hispanic black people.[20] Rectal chlamydia is also common among MSM, with a positivity rate in a screening population of 3% to 10.5%.[21,22]

There are multiple distinct variations within the species of C trachomatis. Grouped into serovars, D through K are those responsible for urethritis, cervicitis/PID, and neonatal disease, and they can also cause proctitis. Chlamydia can infect the rectum in both men and women, either through receptive anal sex or via spread from the cervix and vagina in women with chlamydia. Although rectal chlamydia is often asymptomatic, similar to gonorrhea it can cause symptoms of proctitis including rectal pain, discharge, or bleeding.[20] The incubation period for Chlamydia is 5 to 14 days.[12]

Testing for Chlamydia should be performed if suspicion arises based on history and examination. Findings for symptomatic proctitis from serovars D to K are similar to gonorrhea, including friable mucosa and mucus discharge. Annual rectal screening has only been shown to be advantageous in MSM who are sexually active. MSM who have multiple or anonymous partners should be screened every 3 to 6 months.[1]

Obtaining a diagnosis for rectal chlamydia can be challenging. Culture is limited to research and reference laboratories because of the technical expertise and expense required. Serology can support the diagnosis, but is not standardized, performed infrequently, and requires a high level of expertise to interpret. There is also a paucity of data for men with rectal infections, which may affect the test's performance. Antigen detection by swab has generally shown good sensitivity and specificity for urogenital chlamydia; however, for rectal swab, the limited data suggest a sensitivity of less than 50%.[23] Several studies have shown that NAATs on rectal specimens are more sensitive than culture in detecting rectal chlamydia and still have high specificity. In particular, the use of a transcription-mediated amplification method seems to show consistently strong results.[24,25] Although uniformly validated rectal NAAT is not available, as stated before, some laboratories in the United States have met testing validation requirements under the CLIA regulations and perform NAATs on rectal specimens.

Treatment of Chlamydia proctitis serovars D to K (non-LGV) includes either azithromycin 1 g orally once, or doxycycline 100 mg orally twice a day for 7 days. Either regimen has a greater than 97% efficacy of eradicating the bacteria after 1 week.[26] Abstaining from sex for 1 week after initiation of treatment decreases transmission, and treatment of partners decreases reinfection.[12]

LGV

LGV disease is also caused by the species C trachomatis; however, the serovars are most commonly L1, L2, or L3. The most common clinical manifestation overall is unilateral tender inguinal or femoral lymphadenopathy. Among those with rectal exposure via anal receptive sex, LGV can result in proctocolitis causing mucoid or bloody rectal discharge, fevers, anal pain, or tenesmus. It is an invasive, systemic infection and can lead to colorectal fistulas and strictures if not treated early. Examination may reveal inguinal lymphadenopathy, genital ulcers, or rectal ulcers. Diagnosis is generally based on clinical suspicion and can be verified by NAAT. PCR-based genotyping can also be used to differentiate LGV from non-LGV chlamydia, but, in the absence of specific LGV diagnostic testing, those with a clinical syndrome suspicious for LGV should be treated. Treatment includes doxycycline 100 mg orally twice daily for 21 days. An alternative regimen is erythromycin base 500 mg orally 4 times a day for 21 days. Although treatment cures the infection, there may be resultant scarring from the tissue's reaction to the infection.[1]

Syphilis

Syphilis, caused by *T pallidum*, is a systemic disease that has been divided into a series of overlapping stages. Each year, the CDC estimates that approximately 55,000 people in the United States present with new syphilis infections. Of those diagnosed in 2011 (the most recent year with available statistics), 30% were in the earliest and most infectious stage of syphilis. Seventy-two percent of cases of primary and secondary syphilis were diagnosed in MSM.[27] Transmission occurs by direct contact with an infectious lesion. The early lesions are very infectious, with an estimated transmission rate of one-third of patients exposed.[28]

On average, it takes a week for symptoms to appear after infection, but it can take as long as 90 days. Initially 1 or multiple sores appear at the location where syphilis entered the body. Extragenital or anal chancres are generally painful and resolve after 3 to 6 weeks whether treated or not. Lymphadenopathy may be present.[27] Weeks to a few months later, approximately one-quarter of untreated patients develop secondary syphilis, manifested as a systemic illness including rash, fevers, malaise, and diffuse lymphadenopathy. Secondary syphilis may also include mucous membrane lesions of the anus and rectum and proctitis. Condyloma lata, or large, raised, gray or white lesions may also develop in areas including the groin.[29] Untreated, a patient goes into a latent stage without signs or symptoms. Fifteen percent of these patients develop late-stage syphilis, which can occur 10 to 30 years after the initial infection, and can develop paralysis, dementia, damage to multiple organs, and resultant death.

Syphilis is linked to HIV infection because the presence of open sores makes it easier to transmit and acquire. If exposed when syphilis sores are present, the risk of acquiring HIV is 2 to 5 times higher than if uninfected with syphilis.[27]

In the past, diagnosis of syphilis was by visualization of the spirochete via darkfield microscopy; however, this is technologically difficult. Venereal disease research laboratory (VDRL) and rapid plasma reagin (RPR) (nontreponemal tests) are often used for screening because they are simple and inexpensive. They are not as specific for syphilis and, if reactive, the patient should undergo a treponemal test to confirm the diagnosis. Treponemal tests include fluorescent treponemal antibody absorption tests (FTA-ABS) and other immunoassays that detect antibodies that are specific for syphilis.[27]

Syphilis generally responds well to curative treatment in its early stages. A single IM dose of 2.4 million units of benzathine penicillin G cures a person who has had syphilis for less than a year. For those with syphilis for longer than a year, additional doses are needed.[30] For patients allergic to penicillin, the data are limited, but in nonpregnant patients doxycycline 100 mg orally twice daily for 14 days or tetracycline 500 mg 4 times daily for 14 days are acceptable alternatives. All patients with syphilis should undergo testing for HIV. For follow-up, clinical and serologic evaluation should occur at 6 and 12 months after treatment. Those with symptoms that persist or recur, or those with a nontreponemal titer that is 4 times baseline, should be considered treatment failures or to be reinfected. Repeat testing for HIV and treatment with benzathine penicillin G for 3 doses once a week is the treatment.[1] Sexual partners should be deemed at risk and testing with presumptive treatment should be considered.

Donovanosis (Granuloma Inguinale)

Klebsiella granulomatis (formally known as *Calymmatobacterium granulomatis*) is an intracellular bacterium that can cause ulcerative disease of the genitalia and anus. Although uncommon in the United States, it is endemic in some tropical and developing areas of the world. It manifests most commonly with genital ulcerative lesions, but they may also occur on the anus. The lesions are described as beefy red because of their vascularization, and bleed easily.[1] Sclerotic lesions can develop on the anus and cause stenosis.[12] Regional lymphadenopathy or subcutaneous granulomas (pseudobuboes) may also occur.

Testing for donovanosis is difficult because the organism is difficult to culture. Diagnosis requires visualization of dark-staining Donovan bodies on biopsy. Healing generally proceeds inward from the ulcer margins and prolonged therapy is usually necessary to permit reepithelialization of the ulcers. Even after apparently effective therapy, relapse can occur 6 to 18 months later. Recommended regimen by the CDC includes doxycycline 100 mg orally twice a day for at least 3 weeks and until all lesions have completely healed. Alternatives consist of azithromycin, ciprofloxacin, erythromycin, or trimethoprim-sulfamethoxazole. If improvement is not evident within the first few days of therapy, the addition of an aminoglycoside such as gentamicin should be considered.[1]

Chancroid

Haemophilus ducreyi is the causative organism behind the ulcerating STD known as chancroid. It has become more and more infrequently reported in the United States, with only 24 cases in 2010 occurring in 9 states. Although this likely reflects a decline in incidence, it is also a difficult bacterium to culture, so it may be underdiagnosed. It is most common in parts of the Caribbean and Africa.[1,31] The transmission is through breaks in the skin during sexual contacts. Hours to days after exposure, a person may develop a tender papule with erythema that goes on to develop into a pustule then an ulceration. In general, these are painful and, although most common on the genitalia, can occur in the perianal region.[12]

As mentioned earlier, the test for chancroid is difficult and involves identifying *H ducreyi*. Gram stain may show gram-negative rods in small groups with a sensitivity of 40% to 60%.[12] A special culture media, not widely available, is needed to attempt culture. With this, the sensitivity is still less than 80%.[32] There are a few laboratories that offer PCR testing, but this is not widely available either.

For this reason, a probable diagnosis followed by treatment should be made based on the following criteria: presence of one or more painful genital ulcers; no evidence of *T pallidum* infection; regional lymphadenopathy that is typical of chancroid; and ulcer exudate that is negative for HSV.

Treatment is with azithromycin 1 g orally, ceftriaxone 250 mg IM once, ciprofloxacin 100 mg orally twice a day for 3 days, or erythromycin base 500 mg orally twice a day for 3 days. Successful treatment cures the infection, prevents transmission, and resolves the symptoms. In advanced cases, scarring can result. The patient should be reexamined in 3 to 7 days to ensure improvement.[1]

HSV

Two types of HSV have been identified as causing genital herpes, HSV-1 and HSV-2. Herpes is a chronic, lifelong viral infection. HSV-2 is thought to cause most cases of recurrent genital herpes, but an increasing proportion of anogenital herpetic infections have been attributed to HSV-1.[1] The CDC estimates that 776,000 people in the United States each year develop new herpes infections. One in 6 people aged 14 to 49 years have genital HSV-2 infection.[33] Transmission is via anal, vaginal, or oral sex. The virus can be released from skin that does not appear to have a lesion.

Most people with HSV are asymptomatic or mistake the lesions for another skin condition. It is estimated that 81% of infected individuals are unaware of their diagnosis,[34] which increases the rate of transmission because the infector is ignorant of the disease. Incubation period ranges from 2 to 12 days after exposure. Clinical manifestations include one or more vesicles on or near the anus, genitals, or mouth (**Fig. 1**). These vesicles break and leave painful ulcers that may take several weeks to heal. The first outbreak is often associated with a longer duration of the lesions and may involve systemic symptoms such as fever, lymphadenopathy, or body aches. Recurrences are typically shorter in duration and less severe. The number of outbreaks tends to decrease over time and is less frequent among those with HSV-1 than for those with HSV-2.[33] Acute HSV infection can also manifest as proctitis. HSV proctitis is suggested by the presence of severe anorectal pain, sacral parasthesias, diffuse ulceration of the distal rectal mucosa, and at times difficulty urinating.[35] Nearly half of patients with HSV proctitis also get tender inguinal lymphadenopathy. It is acquired by anorectal intercourse and in homosexual men is second only to gonorrhea as a cause of proctitis.[12]

There are several diagnostic tests available. The current reference standard is viral culture with collection of a sample from the sore, then, once viral growth is seen, specific cell staining to differentiate HSV-1 and HSV-2. PCR can also test for viral DNA or RNA and is more accurate and rapid than culture, with rates of detection more than 4:1 favoring the PCR.[36] Serologic tests are also available to detect antibodies to the herpes virus. Several enzyme-linked immunosorbent assay tests are FDA approved and available commercially to detect HSV-1, but the tests to detect HSV-2 have more frequent false-positives.[37] For the symptomatic patient, testing with both a direct test (ie, culture or PCR) and an indirect test (ie, serum) can help determine whether the infection is new. In a new infection, a patient has a positive culture or PCR with a negative serologic test. The serum is positive with recurrent disease.[33]

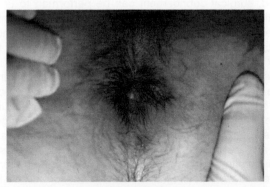

Fig. 1. Perianal HSV.

There is no cure for herpes. Antiviral medications have been shown in genital herpes to prevent or shorten outbreaks while taking the medication. Daily suppressive therapy can also reduce the likelihood of transmission between partners. Treatment of anorectal herpes is mostly supportive, including oral pain medication and warm soaks. Oral acyclovir was shown to decrease the duration of viral shedding in herpes proctitis if given as 400 mg 5 times a day for 10 days. There was a trend toward decreased symptoms but it was not statistically significant.[38] Ulcerative perianal lesions can be treated similarly to genital lesions with acyclovir 400 mg orally 3 times a day for 7 to 10 days for the first clinical episode. For recurrent disease, acyclovir 400 mg orally 3 times a day for 5 days can be given and, for suppression, treatment consists of acyclovir 400 mg orally twice a day. Suppressive therapy does not eliminate the possibility of viral shedding or latent infection. Antiviral alternatives include famciclovir or valacyclovir.[1]

When counseling patients with HSV it is important to stress that abstinence is recommended when lesions are present, that people may be infective even when asymptomatic, and to explain the nature of the virus with its latent and recurrent phases.[12]

HIV

The number of people living with HIV has continued to increase over the past decade because of advances in treatment. The CDC estimates that 1,148,200 people in the United States are HIV positive, including more than 200,000 people who are unaware of their infection. Despite education efforts, the pace of new infections persists at a rate of 50,000 per year. The estimated number of people diagnosed with AIDS in the United States in 2011 was 32,052, with an estimated total of 487,692 people living with an AIDS diagnosis.[39]

It has been suggested that up to 34% of HIV-positive patients develop anorectal problems requiring medical attention. Common symptoms include pain, lumps/warts, bleeding, discharge, or pruritis.[40] Most often they present with a disease common to the general population, including benign anorectal disease and sexually transmitted infections. In one study of 677 HIV-positive patients who presented with an anorectal complaint (most with early stage HIV), more than 60% had at least one additional sexually transmitted disease (STD).[41] The management of infectious anorectal conditions in the HIV-positive patient is frequently similar to those without HIV. The CDC recommends closer follow-up of lesions and symptoms because the risk of recurrent or persistent disease may be higher.

In an HIV-positive patient with an anal fissure, the fissure must be distinguished from an AIDS-related anal ulcer or an STD. AIDS ulcers are generally higher in the anal canal with a broad base and ulceration that may involve the muscle. Severe pain is common. If this is suspected, surgical debridement can be performed to unroof and remove necrotic debris, allow for biopsy, and appropriate testing for potentially treatable or contributing causes of ulceration, including malignancy, HSV, chancroid, syphilis, or tuberculosis. Injection of steroids into the lesion provides relief from the pain in most patients, but may not affect healing.[12]

AIDS has also been shown to affect healing from treatment of noninfectious anorectal disease. These patients may have failed or significantly delayed wound healing. This poor healing has been associated with a decreased CD4 count and leukocyte count.[12,42] In general for noninfectious anorectal disease, late-stage (AIDS) patients are managed conservatively (similarly to patients with Crohn disease) with goals of draining infection and improving symptoms. For example, patients with abscesses are treated with antibiotics and small incision followed by catheter drainage; those with fistulas are treated with draining setons; thrombosed external hemorrhoids that produce severe pain and are not improving in the typical time frame can be excised;

symptomatic internal hemorrhoids should be banded or excised in these patients as a last resort (maximal medical treatment of the hemorrhoids and any underlying diarrhea or constipation should be the initial treatment). However, despite the best medical treatment, some patients continue to have severe symptoms that markedly affect their quality of life. Symptomatic improvement may be accomplished in these patients even if a persistent perianal wound remains. Early stage patients (HIV positive) are treated with standard operative procedures appropriate to their anorectal disorder.

Human Papillomavirus

The most common STD in the United States is human papillomavirus (HPV), a DNA papovavirus that can infect the genital, oropharyngeal, or anal area. Most HPV infections are asymptomatic or unrecognized. There are more than 100 types of HPV with more than 40 that can infect the anogenital area. The high-risk, or oncogenic, HPV types are 16 and 18, which are the cause of cervical cancer and are associated with other anogenital cancers in men and women, as well as a portion of oropharyngeal cancers. Low-risk, or nononcogenic HPV, types 6 and 11, are the cause of anogenital warts. Persistence of infection with the oncogenic HPV types is the strongest risk factor for developing dysplasia and cancers. Spread of the disease is by sexual contact with infected individuals that may or may not have gross lesions.[12] The perianal area can be infected by proximity without a history of anal receptive intercourse. It is estimated that greater than 50% of sexually active persons become infected in their lifetimes.[1]

Anogenital warts, or condyloma accuminata, are caused by HPV-6 or HPV-11 in 90% of cases. Symptoms may include bleeding, presence of a lump/wart, or pruritus. On examination the lesions have been described as cauliflowerlike, gray or fleshy pink growths externally. Within the anal canal, they tend to be distal to the dentate line and appear as small papules.[12] Diagnosis is generally made by inspection, but can be confirmed by biopsy. In general, biopsy should be considered if the lesion is atypical, the patient is immunosuppressed, the diagnosis is uncertain, the lesions do not respond to therapy, or the warts are fixed or ulcerated.[1]

Treatment involves removal or destruction of all obvious disease for relief of symptoms. Wart size, number, location, patient preference, cost, side effects, patient preference, and provider experience should influence treatment choice. Presence of immunosuppression and compliance with therapy must also be considered.[43] One treatment method is excision or destruction, which can be done with excision, fulguration, or cryotherapy for small lesions in the office. Larger lesions likely require sedation or general anesthesia. Electrodessication is fulguration with the electrocautery until the lesion becomes gray/white followed by abrading the tissue with gauze and repeating until the condyloma is removed. To decrease morbidity, this may need to be done in 2 or more sessions. Clearance rates for condyloma are estimated to be 60% to 90%, with recurrence in up to 30% of patients.[44,45] Eradication of the visible condylomas does not eliminate HPV infectivity. Also, the presence of anal condyloma has been shown to be associated with higher rates of anal cancer.[46,47] Although this may be more reflective of sexual practices and risk than a causal relationship, it should be considered.

Other treatments include topical agents such as imiquimod or podofilox. Imiquimod increases local production of cytokines modifying the local immune response. In patients treated with imiquimod only, complete response or complete clearance occurs in 40% to 50% of cases.[48,49] It is applied 3 nights per week to the perianal area, left on for 6 to 8 hours, and then should be washed off. Treatment may take up to 16 weeks, and, although no systemic side effects are expected, local skin irritation can occur.

There are also data to support use of imiquimod following destruction of lesions to decrease recurrence of condyloma.[50]

Podofilox, the purified component in the plant resin podophyllin, is inexpensive, safe, and easy to use. It is an antimitotic drug that destroys the wart and is applied twice a day for 3 days followed by 4 days of no therapy. This routine can be repeated up to 4 times. Local irritation may develop.[43] Clearance rates have been reported from 28% to 74%.[51,52]

Polyphenon E 15% ointment, a proprietary extract of green tea approved by the FDA in 2006 for use with external genital and perianal warts, has been shown to clear anal condylomas compared with placebo. A thin layer of ointment is applied 3 times daily until resolution of the warts is achieved but for no more than 16 weeks. Clearance of up to 51% of patients with a significant improvement compared with placebo has been reported.[53] Small lesions within the anal canal can be treated topically with tri-chloroacetic acid.[12]

Patients infected with HIV are more likely to develop genital warts and to have more persistent disease because of the decreased cell-mediated immunity. The treatment modalities are the same for HIV-positive patients but patients may not respond as well, requiring more frequent treatments. Cancer arising in or resembling a condyloma may occur more frequently so confirmation of diagnosis with biopsy is often warranted.[1]

In 2006, a vaccine for HPV was licensed for use in the United States. At first it was indicated for women aged 9 to 26 years, but this was expanded in 2009 to include men aged 9 to 26 years. The vaccine protects against HPV types 6, 11, 16, and 18; the types that are typically associated with condylomas and anogenital cancers. It is rec-ommended that women who have received the vaccine should continue routine cer-vical cancer screening because 30% of cervical cancers are caused by HPV types other than 16 or 18.[8] Based on this, the assumption that some degree of risk remains for anal cancer is reasonable.

Ninety-five percent of anal cancers are linked to HPV. In 2013, it is estimated that 7060 people in the United States will be diagnosed with anal cancer and 880 will die from it.[54] Although still poorly understood, it is thought that anal cancer may prog-ress along the same pathway as many cancers, including cervical, with precursor le-sions known as anal intraepithelial neoplasia. For this reason, anal cytology has been suggested as a screening tool for detecting patients with dysplasia. Similar to a cer-vical Pap smear, an anal Pap smear involves introduction of a cotton tip applicator in the anal canal for sampling of cells. When tested against high-resolution anoscopy with biopsy, anal Pap smear had a 70% sensitivity and a positive predictive value of 97% for abnormal cells.[55] Although the usefulness of this test is still being evaluated, it is thought that, in some high-risk populations such as MSM or HIV-positive patients, early detection of cellular abnormalities and treatment may lead to an eventual decline in anal cancer, similar to that seen with cervical cancer after introduction of the cervical Pap smear. At present, there is no routine screening test for HPV recommended by the CDC.

High-resolution anoscopy (HRA) with targeted surgical treatment of high-grade squamous intraepithelial lesions (AIN) has been shown in select studies to be a ther-apeutic option for those with a large area of cellular abnormality or with low-volume disease that is not suitable for office therapy (**Figs. 2** and **3**). Over 10 years, a 1.2% rate of progression to cancer was reported in a high-risk population treated with HRA-guided therapy, suggesting that control of AIN is effective at decreasing the risk of cancer.[56] Thus, evaluation and treatment of a patient with an abnormal anal Pap smear using HRA could potentially decrease the possibility of cancer. Research in this area is ongoing.

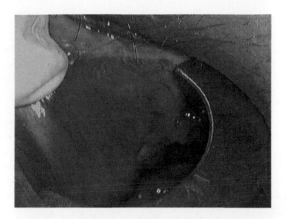

Fig. 2. HRA.

Giant Condyloma (Buschke-Löewenstein)

Associated with HPV types 6 and 11, giant condylomas are large, cauliflower like lesions on the perineum or penis that are histologically unique among condylomas. They show marked papillomatosis, thickened rete ridges, acanthosis, and increased mitotic activity.[12] Although often benign, the giant condyloma can infiltrate the surrounding tissues, behaving in a malignant fashion. They are thought to lie on the continuum between benign condylomata acuminate and squamous cell carcinoma, and may harbor foci of in situ or invasive squamous cell cancer.[57]

Treatment is with wide local excision with a margin greater than 1 cm. The wounds are then treated with skin grafts, tissue flaps, or left to heal by secondary intent (**Figs. 4–6**). For lesions with unattainable resection margins or poor surgical candidates, chemoradiation has been reported as an option.[57]

Molluscum Contagiosum

Caused by a poxvirus, molluscum is a benign superficial skin disease characterized by small pearly papules with a central depression. The lesions average 2 to 5 mm and are usually painless but can be tender or pruritic. It is generally a self-limited condition and resolves spontaneously in 6 to 12 months, but can take years. Immunocompromised hosts may have a more severe form of the disease with increased number and

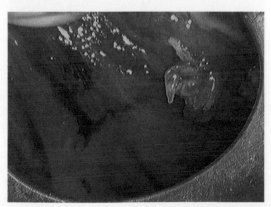

Fig. 3. HRA with Lugol solution.

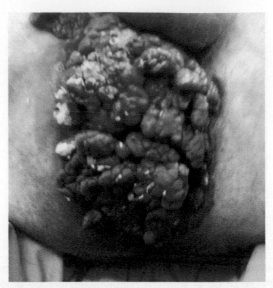

Fig. 4. Perianal giant condyloma.

size of lesions. Diagnosis is generally clinical but, in HIV-positive or AIDS-infected patients, a biopsy may be necessary to rule out other conditions such as malignancy or fungal infection. Biopsy reveals eosinophilic inclusions (molluscum bodies) in the epidermis.[12] Although molluscum is largely self-limited in an immunocompetent host, issues including desire to prevent transmission may prompt treatment. Lesions can be removed with eradication methods including cryotherapy, electrodessication, or curettage. Lesions can also be treated with topical compounds including podophyllotoxin and imiquimod, although neither is FDA approved for this indication.[58,59]

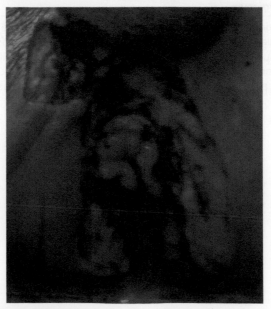

Fig. 5. Resection of perianal giant condyloma.

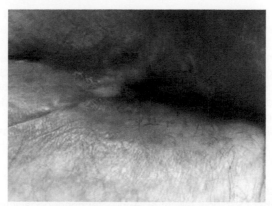

Fig. 6. Healing by secondary intent after resection of perianal giant condyloma.

SUMMARY

Syndromic treatment of sexually transmitted anorectal infections includes treatment of proctitis or ulcerations. Proctitis is treated with antibiotics targeting gonorrhea and chlamydia unless other organisms are suspected. In the United States, perianal ulcerations are most commonly from HSV infection and therefore are treated with antivirals and measures to relieve local discomfort. Diagnostic testing for STDs of the anorectum depends on the likely organisms involved and local resources. Current treatment recommendations from the CDC for bacterial STDs should be reviewed periodically because antibiotic resistance for some organisms continues to increase.

Anal condylomas are treated with topical agents, excision/destruction, or a combination of the two. In homosexual HIV-positive men, anal HPV infection is associated with a marked increased risk for developing anal cancer. Strategies for decreasing this risk may include close surveillance, anal Pap smears, and HRA.

In addition to an increased risk of anal cancer, HIV patients frequently experience anorectal complaints. The treatment of these complaints is determined by the severity of the HIV disease and the symptoms. In some instances more aggressive treatment may be warranted to give adequate symptomatic relief, despite risking a chronic wound problem.

Patient counseling about causes and prevention of STDs is an integral part of minimizing the spread of these diseases. In addition, surgeons who treat these patients should be aware of the reporting requirements for these diseases in the states in which they practice.

REFERENCES

1. Workowski KA, Berman S. Sexually transmitted diseases treatment guidelines, 2010. MMWR Recomm Rep 2010;59(RR-12):1–110.
2. Weller S, Davis K. Condom effectiveness in reducing heterosexual HIV transmission. Cochrane Database Syst Rev 2002;(1):CD003255.
3. Holmes KK, Levine R, Weaver M. Effectiveness of condoms in preventing sexually transmitted infections. Bull World Health Organ 2004;82(6):454–61.
4. Ness RB, Randall H, Richter HE, et al. Condom use and the risk of recurrent pelvic inflammatory disease, chronic pelvic pain, or infertility following an episode of pelvic inflammatory disease. Am J Public Health 2004;94(8):1327–9.

5. Wald A, Langenberg AG, Krantz E, et al. The relationship between condom use and herpes simplex virus acquisition. Ann Intern Med 2005;143(10): 707–13.

6. Martin ET, Krantz E, Gottlieb SL, et al. A pooled analysis of the effect of condoms in preventing HSV-2 acquisition. Arch Intern Med 2009;169(13):1233–40.

7. Male latex condoms and sexually transmitted diseases. Centers For Disease Control And Prevention. Available at: www.cdc.gov/condomeffectiveness/latex.htm. Accessed May 11, 2013.

8. 2011 Sexually transmitted disease surveillance. Center for Disease Control and Prevention. Available at: http://www.cdc.gov/std/stats11/gonorrhea.htm. Accessed May 11, 2013.

9. Hook EW III, Handsfield HH. Gonococcal infection in the adult. Sexually transmitted diseases. New York: McGraw-Hill; 1999.

10. Klein EJ, Fisher LS, Chow AW, et al. Anorectal gonococcal infection. Ann Intern Med 1977;86(3):340–6.

11. Sherrard J, Barlow D. Gonorrhoea in men: clinical and diagnostic aspects. Genitourin Med 1996;72(6):422–6.

12. Whitlow C, Gottesman L, Bernstein MA. Sexually transmitted diseases. In: Beck DE, editor. The ASCRS textbook of colon and rectal surgery. New York: Springer; 2011. p. 295–307.

13. Laga M, Manoka A, Kivuvu M, et al. Non-ulcerative sexually transmitted diseases as risk factors for HIV-1 transmission in women: results from a cohort study. AIDS 1993;7(1):95–102.

14. Craib KJ, Meddings DR, Strathdee SA, et al. Rectal gonorrhoea as an independent risk factor for HIV infection in a cohort of homosexual men. Genitourin Med 1995;71(3):150–4.

15. Schink JC, Keith LG. Problems in the culture diagnosis of gonorrhea. J Reprod Med 1985;30(Suppl 3):244–9.

16. Bachmann LH, Johnson RE, Cheng H, et al. Nucleic acid amplification tests for diagnosis of Neisseria gonorrhoeae and Chlamydia trachomatis rectal infections. J Clin Microbiol 2010;48(5):1827–32.

17. Schachter J, Moncada J, Liska S, et al. Nucleic acid amplification tests in the diagnosis of chlamydial and gonococcal infections of the oropharynx and rectum in men who have sex with men. Sex Transm Dis 2008;35(7):637–42.

18. CLIA verified labs for non-genital CT and GC NAATS. Available at: http://nnptc.org/resources/phlabs-html/. Accessed May 12, 2013.

19. Centers for Disease Control and Prevention (CDC). Update to CDC's sexually transmitted diseases treatment guidelines, 2010: oral cephalosporins no longer a recommended treatment for gonococcal infections. MMWR Morb Mortal Wkly Rep 2012;61(31):590–4.

20. Chlamydia-CDC fact sheet. Available at: http://www.cdc.gov/std/chlamydia/STDFact-chlamydia-detailed.htm#_ENREF_6. Accessed May 11, 2013.

21. Marcus JL, Bernstein KT, Stephens SC, et al. Sentinel surveillance of rectal chlamydia and gonorrhea among males–San Francisco, 2005-2008. Sex Transm Dis 2010;37(1):59–61.

22. Pinsky L, Chiarilli DB, Klausner JD, et al. Rates of asymptomatic nonurethral gonorrhea and chlamydia in a population of university men who have sex with men. J Am Coll Health 2010;60(6):481–4.

23. Tay YK, Goh CL, Chan R, et al. Evaluation of enzyme immunoassay for the detection of anogenital infections caused by Chlamydia trachomatis. Singapore Med J 1995;36(2):173–5.

24. Cosentino LA, Campbell T, Jett A, et al. Use of nucleic acid amplification testing for diagnosis of anorectal sexually transmitted infections. J Clin Microbiol 2010; 50(6):2005–8.
25. Geisler WM. Diagnosis and management of uncomplicated Chlamydia trachomatis infections in adolescents and adults: summary of evidence reviewed for the 2010 Centers for Disease Control and Prevention sexually transmitted diseases treatment guidelines. Clin Infect Dis 2010;53(Suppl 3):S92–8.
26. Lau CY, Qureshi AK. Azithromycin versus doxycycline for genital chlamydial infections: a meta-analysis of randomized clinical trials. Sex Transm Dis 2002; 29(9):497–502.
27. Syphilis-CDC fact sheet. Available at: http://www.cdc.gov/std/syphilis/STDFact-Syphilis.htm. Accessed May 18, 2013.
28. Hook EW 3rd, Marra CM. Acquired syphilis in adults. N Engl J Med 1992; 326(16):1060–9.
29. Gjestland T. The Oslo study of untreated syphilis; an epidemiologic investigation of the natural course of the syphilitic infection based upon a re-study of the Boeck-Bruusgaard material. Acta Derm Venereol Suppl (Stockh) 1955; 35(Suppl 34):3–368 Annex I-LVI.
30. Syphilis treatment and care. Available at: http://www.cdc.gov/std/syphilis/treatment.htm. Accessed May 18, 2013.
31. 2010 Sexually transmitted diseases surveillance. Available at: http://www.cdc.gov/std/stats10/other.htm#foot1. Accessed May 18, 2013.
32. Lockett AE, Dance DA, Mabey DC, et al. Serum-free media for isolation of Haemophilus ducreyi. Lancet 1991;338(8762):326.
33. Genital herpes-CDC fact sheet. Available at: http://www.cdc.gov/std/herpes/stdfact-herpes.htm. Accessed May 19, 2013.
34. Schillinger JA, McKinney CM, Garg R, et al. Seroprevalence of herpes simplex virus type 2 and characteristics associated with undiagnosed infection: New York City, 2004. Sex Transm Dis 2008;35(6):599–606.
35. Goodell SE, Quinn TC, Mkrtichian E, et al. Herpes simplex virus proctitis in homosexual men. Clinical, sigmoidoscopic, and histopathological features. N Engl J Med 1983;308(15):868–71.
36. Wald A, Huang ML, Carrell D, et al. Polymerase chain reaction for detection of herpes simplex virus (HSV) DNA on mucosal surfaces: comparison with HSV isolation in cell culture. J Infect Dis 2003;188(9):1345–51.
37. Mark HD, Nanda JP, Roberts J, et al. Performance of focus ELISA tests for HSV-1 and HSV-2 antibodies among university students with no history of genital herpes. Sex Transm Dis 2007;34(9):681–5.
38. Rompalo AM, Mertz GJ, Davis LG, et al. Oral acyclovir for treatment of first-episode herpes simplex virus proctitis. JAMA 1988;259(19):2879–81.
39. HIV in the United States: at a glance. Available at: http://www.cdc.gov/hiv/statistics/basics/ataglance.html. Accessed May 18, 2013.
40. Yuhan R, Orsay C, DelPino A, et al. Anorectal disease in HIV-infected patients. Dis Colon Rectum 1998;41(11):1367–70.
41. Beck DE, Jaso RG, Zajac RA. Proctologic management of the HIV-positive patient. South Med J 1990;83(8):900–3.
42. Morandi E, Merlini D, Salvaggio A, et al. Prospective study of healing time after hemorrhoidectomy: influence of HIV infection, acquired immunodeficiency syndrome, and anal wound infection. Dis Colon Rectum 1999;42(9):1140–4.
43. Genital warts. Available at: http://www.cdc.gov/std/treatment/2010/genital-warts.htm. Accessed May 19, 2013.

44. Wiley DJ, Douglas J, Beutner K, et al. External genital warts: diagnosis, treatment, and prevention. Clin Infect Dis 2002;35(Suppl 2):S210–24.

45. Jensen SL. Comparison of podophyllin application with simple surgical excision in clearance and recurrence of perianal condylomata acuminata. Lancet 1985; 2(8465):1146–8.

46. McCloskey JC, Metcalf C, French MA, et al. The frequency of high-grade intraepithelial neoplasia in anal/perianal warts is higher than previously recognized. Int J STD AIDS 2007;18(8):538–42.

47. Holly EA, Whittemore AS, Aston DA, et al. Anal cancer incidence: genital warts, anal fissure or fistula, hemorrhoids, and smoking. J Natl Cancer Inst 1989; 81(22):1726–31.

48. Beutner KR, Spruance SL, Hougham AJ, et al. Treatment of genital warts with an immune-response modifier (imiquimod). J Am Acad Dermatol 1998;38(2 Pt 1): 230–9.

49. Beutner KR, Tyring SK, Trofatter KF Jr, et al. Imiquimod, a patient-applied immune-response modifier for treatment of external genital warts. Antimicrob Agents Chemother 1998;42(4):789–94.

50. Hoyme UB, Hagedorn M, Schindler AE, et al. Effect of adjuvant imiquimod 5% cream on sustained clearance of anogenital warts following laser treatment. Infect Dis Obstet Gynecol 2002;10(2):79–88.

51. Greenberg MD, Rutledge LH, Reid R, et al. A double-blind, randomized trial of 0.5% podofilox and placebo for the treatment of genital warts in women. Obstet Gynecol 1991;77(5):735–9.

52. Lafuma A, Monsonego J, Moyal-Barracco M, et al. A model-based comparison of cost effectiveness of imiquimod versus podophyllotoxin for the treatment of external anogenital warts in France. Ann Dermatol Venereol 2003;130(8–9 Pt 1):731–6 [in French].

53. Stockfleth E, Beti H, Orasan R, et al. Topical polyphenon E in the treatment of external genital and perianal warts: a randomized controlled trial. Br J Dermatol 2008;158(6):1329–38.

54. National Cancer Institute: anal cancer. Available at: http://www.cancer.gov/cancertopics/types/anal/. Accessed May 23, 2013.

55. Nathan M, Singh N, Garrett N, et al. Performance of anal cytology in a clinical setting when measured against histology and high-resolution anoscopy findings. AIDS 2010;24(3):373–9.

56. Pineda CE, Berry JM, Jay N, et al. High-resolution anoscopy targeted surgical destruction of anal high-grade squamous intraepithelial lesions: a ten-year experience. Dis Colon Rectum 2008;51(6):829–35 [discussion: 835–7].

57. Tytherleigh MG, Birtle AJ, Cohen CE, et al. Combined surgery and chemoradiation as a treatment for the Buschke-Lowenstein tumour. Surgeon 2006;4(6): 378–83.

58. Syed TA, Lundin S, Ahmad SA. Topical 0.3% and 0.5% podophyllotoxin cream for self-treatment of condylomata acuminata in women. A placebo-controlled, double-blind study. Dermatology 1994;189(2):142–5.

59. Theos AU, Cummins R, Silverberg NB, et al. Effectiveness of imiquimod cream 5% for treating childhood molluscum contagiosum in a double-blind, randomized pilot trial. Cutis 2004;74(2):134–8, 141–2.

Anal Squamous Intraepithelial Neoplasia

Pablo A. Bejarano, MD[a], Marylise Boutros, MD[b],
Mariana Berho, MD[a],*

KEYWORDS

- Anal carcinoma • Dysplasia • Anal intraepithelial neoplasia • Human papilloma virus

KEY POINTS

- AIN can be managed by close observation, topical treatments, photodynamic therapy and surgery.
- Surgical approaches for AIN include anal mapping with wide local excision with or without flaps, or more limited removal using targeted destruction with high-resolution anoscopy.

INTRODUCTION

Although anal squamous cell carcinoma (SCC) remains an uncommon malignancy its occurrence has been steadily rising in the United States. Previous to the AIDS epidemic the incidence reported was of 0.7 per 100,000 individuals[1]; subsequently the rate rose to approximately 2 per 100,000.[2] Extensive research conducted during the last decades has shown that this disease is more closely related to genital rather than to gastrointestinal malignancies. Historically women have been more frequently affected by these tumors than males; however, newer studies have revealed similar rates between the two genders. It has been postulated that the higher proportion of anal SCC is linked to an increased number of lifetime sexual partners for both men and women, changing sexual practices including both women and men engaging in anoreceptive intercourse, and an increased number of men having sex with men (MSM).[3,4] Similarly to colonic malignancies in which invasive adenocarcinoma evolves from premalignant lesions (adenoma-carcinoma sequence),[5] anal SCC progress through a continuum of preinvasive lesions known as anal intraepithelial neoplasia (AIN). Timely diagnosis of AIN is therefore of paramount importance to lower the incidence of invasive carcinoma, which frequently carries a very poor prognosis. Diagnosis, follow-up, and treatment of AIN is complex and not standardized, which may be partly related to poor communication of biopsy and cytology findings between

[a] RT Institute of Pathology and Laboratory Medicine, Cleveland Clinic Florida, 2950 Cleveland Clinic Boulevard, Weston, FL 33331, USA; [b] Department of Surgery, McGill University, Jewish General Hospital, Montreal, QC, Canada
* Corresponding author.
E-mail address: mberho@ccf.org

Gastroenterol Clin N Am 42 (2013) 893–912
http://dx.doi.org/10.1016/j.gtc.2013.09.005

pathologists and clinicians as a result of a disparate and confusing terminology used to classify these lesions. This article focuses on general aspects of epidemiology and on clarifying the current terminology of intraepithelial squamous dysplasia, its relationship with human papilloma virus (HPV) infection, and the current methods used to diagnose and treat this condition.

HISTORICAL PERSPECTIVE

Although premalignant and malignant lesions of the anus and perianal region had long been described, it was not until 1962 when Turell recognized that anal skin and anal canal SCC were histologically and biologically distinct lesions.[6] Turell realized that perianal tumors often displayed keratinization when examined histologically and were associated with a favorable clinical course; SCC of the anal canal, however, usually exhibited poor histologic differentiation and often metastasized to inguinal and pelvic lymph node metastasis. Subsequently, a possible etiologic relationship between HPV, anal warts, and in situ and invasive SCC was not proposed until 1971 by Oriel and Whimster[7] who used electron microscopy for the identification of HPV particles on these lesions.

Fenger and Nielsen[8] described dysplasia for the first time in 1981. The same authors in a relatively small (19 patients) but revealing study linked anal and uterine cervix neoplasia and proposed adoption of a similar terminology to the already existing cervical intraepithelial neoplasia (CIN) as anal canal intraepithelial neoplasia I–III.[1]

More recently extensive research has provided conclusive evidence between the association of HPV and AIN and the link between certain HPV types and the likelihood of developing high-grade squamous dysplasia and invasive carcinoma[9,10] The rise of the AIDS epidemic has further advanced the understanding of the risk factors associated with the development of this disease and its natural history and those clinicopathologic factors that influence clinical progression.[11,12]

EPIDEMIOLOGY AND INCIDENCE

The exact incidence of AIN is difficult to estimate. Impaired cellular-mediated immunity, as found in patients with AIDS and organ transplant recipients, is a strong risk factor for low- and high-grade AIN.[13–15] The relationship between HPV-driven disease and the host immune defense mechanisms is complex and numerous factors besides an adequate CD4 count play a role in the natural progression of the infection.[16]

The iatrogenic immunosuppression that follows organ transplantation has been shown to increase the incidence of high-grade dysplasia and anal cancer 10- to 100-fold compared with the general population, especially in women, who are affected twice as often as men.[17] Most of these data have been compiled from patients receiving drugs that typically elicit a profound dysfunction of the cellular arm of the immune system (calcinurin inhibitors, azathioprin). Current studies are being conducted to assess the impact of newer medications that exert a more selective immunomodulation and may therefore be associated with lower risk of developing high-grade AIN and anal cancer.[18]

The frequency of anal cancer and AIN is significantly increased in men and women infected with HIV independent of the route by which the virus was acquired. It is, however, especially prevalent in MSM, who are 20 times more likely to develop this disease than heterosexuals.[19] HIV-positive MSM carry the highest incidence of HPV-related disease including high-grade AIN and invasive SCC. In a meta-analysis conducted in Australia the pooled prevalence of high-grade AIN and invasive SCC was 29.1% and 21.5% and 45.9 per 100,000 and 5.1 per 100,000 in HIV-positive

MSM versus HIV-negative MSM, respectively. Furthermore, the detection of HPV-16 and -18 was much higher in HIV-positive MSM than in HIV-negative MSM.[4] HIV-infected women have a nearly sevenfold increased risk of anal cancer compared with the general population.[20]

There is a clear but not fully characterized relationship between these two sexually transmitted viruses, HIV and HPV. It has been shown that HPV infection is more likely to persist in HIV-positive patients and to evolve in a more aggressive clinical fashion possibly related to the inadequate cellular immunity, which is critical in the clearance of viral organisms.[21] Infection with multiple types of HPV is also more commonly noted in HIV-positive patients.[22] It has also been shown that HPV infection itself increases the risk of acquiring HIV. In a study conducted in the United States, a cohort of 1409 MSM with HPV disease had a significantly higher chance of HIV seroconversion than in HPV-negative individuals (hazard ratio, 3.5; 95% confidence interval, 1.2–10.6).[23]

PREDICTIVE FACTORS FOR PROGRESSION TO HIGH-GRADE AIN AND INVASIVE CARCINOMA

There are no solid data on the rate of progression regarding low- to high-grade AIN and invasive carcinoma. Two studies with a follow-up of almost two decades have revealed that overall 5% of high-grade AIN evolves into invasive carcinoma.[14,24] In a study of HIV-positive and HIV-negative MSM, Palefsky and coworkers[14] found a rate of progression from low- to high-grade AIN in 62% and 36% of patients, respectively. These findings were similar to another study of 41 HIV-positive MSM in whom normal epithellum or low-grade AIN evolved into high-grade AIN over a 17-month period.[24]

The presence of high-risk viral phenotypes, multiple HPV-type infections, low levels of CD4 lymphocytes, and smoking have all been suggested as factors that accelerate progression to high-grade AIN and invasive carcinoma.[14,22]

The use of highly active antiretroviral therapy in patients with HIV has dramatically decreased the incidence of most defining AIDS cancers. However, the incidence of high-grade AIN and anal cancer have not been affected by the introduction of highly active antiretroviral therapy. The explanation for this observation remains unknown.[25,26]

The natural history of AIN progression in HIV-negative heterosexual men and women is much less understood and solid data addressing this issue are lacking. In a large ongoing study in 431 women with follow-up at the 4-month interval, it was shown that 50% had incidental anal HPV, which was sequentially acquired after cervical infection. Interestingly, in 87% of these patients the infection resolved within 1 year, which is much shorter than the approximately 2-year duration typically reported for elimination of cervical HPV.[27]

HPV AND ITS ROLE IN AIN AND INVASIVE SCC

The similarities between anal and cervical preinvasive and invasive squamous lesions can be partly explained by the anatomic and histologic resemblances between these two organs. That is, both have a transformation zone composed of a squamous-columnar epithelial junction in which the columnar epithelium of the lower rectum commonly undergoes squamous metaplasia.[28] Most AIN and invasive carcinoma arise within this area. There is compelling scientific evidence that HPV is the cause of premalignant and malignant squamous tumors of the lower anogenital tract including uterine, cervix, vagina, vulva, anus, perianal skin, and scrotum. Numerous molecular virology studies performed in cell lines and in human tissue have demonstrated the capability of HPV to induce transformation from nonneoplastic epithelium to AIN1 to AIN 3 and finally invasive carcinoma.[10,29]

Human papilloma are small double-stranded DNA viruses with an exquisite predilection for squamous epithelium. Currently, more than 130 HPV types have been characterized and within the different types some viruses show specific tropism for either cutaneous or mucosal tissue.[11,15,30] Anogenital infection is usually linked to a group of 30 to 40 types that can be divided into those predominantly associated with indolent, self-limited disease, including condylomas, AIN1, and, CIN1 (subtypes 6, 11, 42, 43, and 44) and those most commonly isolated from high-grade lesions and invasive carcinomas (subtypes 6, 18, 31, 33, 35, 39, 45, 50, 51, 55, 56, 58, 59, and 68).[16,31] Understanding the differences in the potential to induce malignant transformation among the different types of HPV has been instrumental in guiding follow-up and treatment in affected men and women. Furthermore, in 2008, Harald zur Hausen was awarded the Nobel Prize for his discovery of the role HPV types 16 and 18 play in the development of cervical cancer. The association between high-risk HPV types and cervical cancer is robust with very strong odds ratios for HPV 16 and 18 and tight confidence limits.[31]

HPV prevalence in high- and low-grade AIN has been reported at 91% and 88%, respectively.[32,33] HPV types 16 and 18 are the most commonly identified in high-grade dysplasia and invasive SCC (72% and 69%, respectively).[33] Contrary to low-risk HPV types that remain in the host cells as a plasmid, high-risk types become integrated into the keratynocyte leading to overexpression of oncogenes and inhibition of tumor-suppressor genes and DNA aneuploidy. This state of genetic chaos allows the progression from low- to high-grade dysplasia and invasive carcinoma.[34]

THE EVOLUTION OF THE NOMENCLATURE AND GRADING

Historically, grading of the dysplastic changes within the anal canal squamous mucosa was based in great part on the subjective opinion of the examining pathologist and classified into three categories: (1) mild, (2) moderate, or (3) severe. These three categories were then renamed AIN1, 2, and 3 extrapolating the data that existed on the uterine cervix (CIN1, 2, and 3) and its association with HPV.[1] This approach was supported by the fact that the uterine cervix and the anal canal have common embryologic pathways. Studies on cervical lesions highlighted that CIN1 and 3 had the lowest interobserver variability among pathologists, but CIN2 lacked consistency among observers.[35,36] This poor reproducibility was also demonstrated for the anal region,[37] and thus the term AIN2 or moderate dysplasia was interpreted by clinicians as equivocal for the possibility of a preneoplastic lesion. This uncertainty made it difficult among clinicians to decide on a specific therapy. It became evident that this intermediate category lacked biologic correlation because it merely combined a low-grade lesion with a premalignant disease, which cannot be accurately distinguished on hematoxylin and eosin stained sections. This observation explained the poor reproducibility among observers. Further complicating the issue, cases formerly diagnosed as moderate dysplasia (grade 2) turned out to be severe dysplasia on follow-up.[6,38]

Another point of potential confusion is that the American Joint Committee on Cancer promoted the term squamous intraepithelial lesion (SIL) either as low or high grade, whereas the World Health Organization still recommended the use of AIN terminology low- and high-grade categories. SIL and CIN therefore described the same types of lesions and could be interchangeable.

With advancements made in the biology of HPV the grading was modified to reflect the behavior of the HPV infection and its effects on the anal squamous mucosa,[38] and the term squamous intraepithelial lesion was introduced with a two-tier grading system: low grade corresponding to AIN1 and high grade to AIN2 and AIN3.

The pathology community recognized the need to standardize the nomenclature related to this topic to avoid potential serious misunderstandings in the communication of pathology results. There was a clear need to unify the concepts of SIL and AIN, and to modify the grading system in a way that it would better guide treatment. The proposal is to abandon dysplasia grade 2 not only to follow the route established by the Bethesda grading for cytology, but more importantly to apply the knowledge propelled by several advances in molecular pathology that shed light into the natural history of HPV infection and further strengthened the concept of a two-tiered grading system for squamous dysplasia.

It is now known that HPV infection can take two behavior routes: either that of a transient infection in which the virus replicates in an active but self-limited manner; or in the form of a persistent carrier state, which is associated with the development of carcinoma. In this regard, the grading of AIN can then be classified into two-tier, low-grade SIL (LSIL), which reflects a transient, self-limited infection, and high-grade SIL (HSIL), which is associated with chronic and long-standing infection. Expression of biomarkers by immunohistochemistry, such as p16, is in keeping with this two-tier grading system wherein the HSIL cases stain strongly and consistently and the LSIL stain negative. This immunoprofile further supports the two- versus a three-tier system. Immunohistochemical stain for p16 is an excellent tool to discriminate between an indolent lesion (transient infection) and one associated with carcinoma (persistent infection).[39–41]

The two-tier system of LSIL and HSIL is similar to that for other genital areas including the cervix, vagina, vulva, perianus, and penis. Ideally, a uniform, reproducible, and standardized histologic evaluation would be applied to all these sites to reduce diagnostic variability among pathologists and thus facilitate accuracy for research purposes. Based on this premise and with the goal of obtaining unity in the definitions of dysplasia, in 2012 the College of American Pathologists and the American Society for Colposcopy and Cervical Pathology through the work of approximately 60 physicians from various specialties who are experts in anogenital disease sponsored standardization of the terminology for HPV-related lesions affecting the epithelium of the anal canal. The recommendation of using a two-grade system was also endorsed by numerous other professional societies and government agencies. This support gave the current nomenclature an "official" connotation: LSIL and HSIL (**Figs. 1** and **2**).[28]

PATHOLOGY OF AIN

Anal intraepithelial HPV-associated squamous lesions are classified as LSIL and HSIL. The gross appearance of AIN is polymorphic because the lesions may present as plaques, papules, eczema, or papilloma-like areas. The presence of induration or ulceration may be seen when the lesion is an invasive carcinoma.

Microscopically, the changes are limited to the epithelium where there is increased cellularity accompanied by nucleomegaly, pleomorphism, increased nuclear to cytoplasmic ratio, irregular nuclear contours, and denser chromatin. In LSIL the changes predominately effect the lower third of the full epithelial thickness, with maturation starting at the middle third, leaving the upper third close to normal. Although mitosis may be observed, abnormal mitotic figures and marked nuclear atypia are not characteristic of LSIL. With the presence of HPV cytopathic changes, such as koilocytosis, multinucleation, nuclear irregularity, and perinuclear clearing of the cytoplasm, may

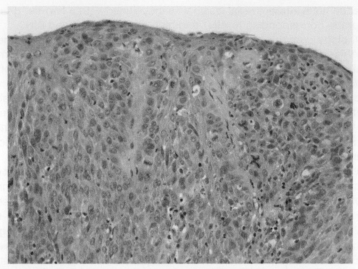

Fig. 1. HSIL showing full-thickness atypia with lack of maturation and the presence of nuclear pleomorphism throughout with abnormal mitotic figures.

be present, but these features do not correspond to HSIL. The mere presence of HPV cytopathic changes, such as koilocytosis, in the absence of high-grade lesion should be classified as a LSIL.

For HSIL, in addition to the findings of LSIL, there is lack of maturation in the upper two-thirds of the epithelium. Mitotic figures, typical or abnormal, are also present in the middle or the upper third of the epithelium. Abnormal mitosis and marked nuclear atypia are not characteristic of an LSIL, but may be present in a sample with maturation starting at the middle third and upward creating diagnostic uncertainty. In this situation a strong positive stain for p16 facilitates diagnosis of HSIL.[39]

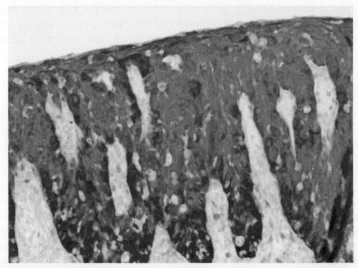

Fig. 2. Immunohistochemical stain for p16 showing strong reactivity in a case of HSIL.

Another cause for diagnostic uncertainty arises when the sample is distorted, particularly as a result of the cauterization effect on tissues. In this situation, the distortion makes evaluation of the dysplastic lesion difficult to distinguish between low- and high-grade lesions. Immunostaining for p16 may be helpful in this situation. **Figs. 3** and **4** show HSIL, which involves the transition zone and extends into the proximal colonic mucosa.

Another difficult scenario is when, in an otherwise low-grade lesion or the presence of condyloma, there are focal areas that raise the possibility of a proximal high-grade lesion as seen in **Figs. 5** and **6**. Immunostaining for p16 is helpful to exclude the presence of HSIL. As seen in the photomicrograph negative p16 not only distinguishes tangentially cut basal cells from HSIL, but it helps to separate LSIL, immature squamous metaplasia, atrophy, and regenerative/reactive changes. The staining in these lesions is either absent or only focal. True diagnostic stain for HSIL should be diffuse and strong in the nuclei alone or in both nuclei and cytoplasm.

ANAL CYTOLOGY

In populations at high risk, there is a need for a screening method to help reduce morbidity and mortality by detecting precursor lesions for invasive SCC similar to that established for cervical carcinoma. Before the implementation of cervical screening, the incidence of SCC of the cervix in the United States was 35 to 40 cases per 100,000, which then decreased to 8 per 100,000 after implementation of screening. The incidence of anal carcinoma ranges from 42 to 137 cases per 100,000 person-years in the HIV-positive population,[42,43] presenting an argument that implementing screening cytology may impact the incidence of anal carcinoma.

Anal cytology is not commonly used in daily practice, and it is still unknown if its use as a screening method will reduce mortality from SCC. Several studies have reported data in support of and against its implementation as a screening tool. Although anal

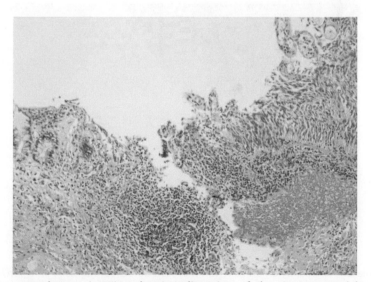

Fig. 3. Squamocolumnar junction showing distortion of the tissues caused by cautery. Although the possibility of HSIL may be considered with uncertainty, immunostain for p16 supports the view that this is HSIL because there is strong staining. Moreover, it demonstrates that the dysplastic cells are using the colonic glandular mucosa to spread.

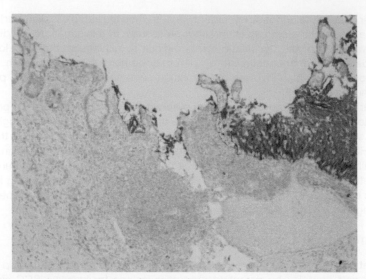

Fig. 4. Squamocolumnar junction showing distortion of the tissues caused by cautery. Although the possibility of HSIL may be considered with uncertainty, immunostain for p16 supports the view that this is HSIL because there is strong staining. Moreover, it demonstrates that the dysplastic cells are using the colonic glandular mucosa to spread.

cytology has a high degree of sensitivity (ranging from 80% to 93% ability to detect abnormalities), its specificity drops considerably when compared with biopsy and many cases are upgraded on the biopsy tissue. The diagnosis of atypical squamous cells of undetermined significance in anal cytology has been changed to HSIL in up

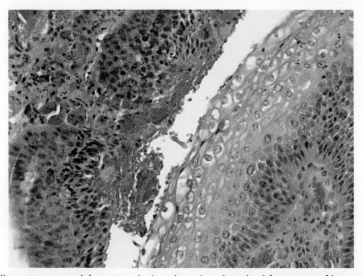

Fig. 5. Adjacent to a condylomatous lesion there is a detached fragment of hyperchromatic cells admixed with blood. This fragment may represent HSIL or a tangentially cut basal layer of squamous mucosa with reactive changes. As expected the stain for p16 is negative in the condyloma part, but it is likewise negative in the detached cells supporting the absence of HSIL.

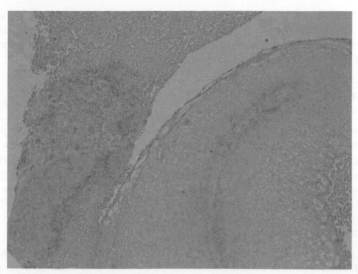

Fig. 6. Adjacent to a condylomatous lesion there is a detached fragment of hyperchromatic cells admixed with blood. This fragment may represent HSIL or a tangentially cut basal layer of squamous mucosa with reactive changes. As expected the stain for p16 is negative in the condyloma part, but it is likewise negative in the detached cells supporting the absence of HSIL.

to 46% to 67% of cases and from LSIL on cytology to HSIL on biopsy specimens in up to 56% of cases. Although anal cytology seems to be a good screening tool, it is not accurate at determining the severity of anal SIL. Therefore, there is agreement that any cytologic abnormality needs to be followed up by anoscopy and biopsy to determine the true nature of the abnormality.[44–49]

Depending on the method used for the sample collection the cytologist may be faced with difficulties in interpreting the findings. Conventional smears may contain abundant cellular debris, fecal material, and higher numbers of keratinized or anucleated epithelial cells associated with parakeratosis, and even parasites[50] risking uncertain evaluation. Conversely, hand liquid-based cytology renders a cleaner background facilitating the detection and identification of atypical cells. For the individual obtaining the swab it is important to make sure that the transitional zone is sampled for accuracy. Likewise, the yield of a certain interpretation is dependent on the cellularity of the specimen; the more epithelial cells present the higher the likelihood of an accurate diagnosis.[51]

Another compounding factor is that, although cytologists may be very familiar with the analysis of cervical smears, they may lack experience in anal cytology. Currently, there is a lack of standardized terminology specifically for evaluation of anal cytology. The existing nomenclature has been extrapolated from the Bethesda system used for cervical samples. Nonetheless, in certain studies involving designated examiners there has been moderate-to-good agreement among cytopathologists who are evaluating anal cytology samples from HIV-positive MSM.[52,53] Similar to that observed for biopsy tissues, the use of p16 immunohistochemical staining and the use of high-risk HPV DNA testing increases the probability of detecting high-grade lesions.[52,54]

TREATMENT OF AIN

The optimal management of AIN remains controversial because of the subclinical nature of the condition, the unclear natural history of the disease, and the multiple possible treatment strategies ranging from expectant management to excisions requiring flap reconstruction. In the last two decades, advances in histopathologic classification and prospective evaluation of diagnostic and treatment methods have advanced the understanding of this disease and its treatment.

IDENTIFICATION
Clinical Identification

AIN is often asymptomatic and the diagnosis is either an incidental histologic finding when perianal lesions, such as hemorrhoids, are excised or when high-risk patients are screened.[55–57] Although rare, patients may report pruritis and/or bleeding, and may have clinical findings, such as raised, scaly, white, erythematous, pigmented, or fissured perianal lesions; these should be biopsied (**Fig. 7**). The appearance of an ulcerated lesion may herald invasion and should be investigated promptly.[55,56]

Identification by Screening

Because of the numerous similarities in disease processes, the methods for AIN screening arose from the experience acquired in managing CIN. Screening procedures for AIN include anal cytology and high-resolution anoscopy (HRA) with biopsies.[55,56]

Anal Papanicolaou smear cytology consists of rotating a cytology brush in the anal canal to sample cells.[56] The goal of anal cytology is to identify high-risk individuals with dysplasia who would benefit from more intensive screening by HRA. The sensitivity and specificity of anal cytology compared with biopsy-proved dysplasia range from 47% to 93% and from 16% to 92%, respectively.[56,57] In a large prospective study, the sensitivity of anal cytology in biopsy-proved anal dysplasia was 69% in

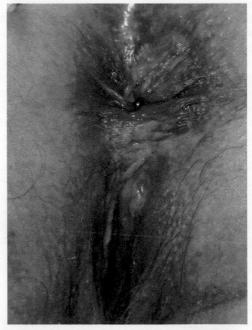

Fig. 7. Perianal and perivulvar high-grade intraepithelial neoplasia.

HIV-positive and 47% in HIV-negative men at their first visit, rising to 81% and 50%, respectively, when all surgical visits were included.[55,58] In another study, the sensitivity of abnormal cytology to detect high-grade anal neoplasia was 87% in HIV-positive men, and 55% in HIV-negative MSM.[59] Anal cytology may be a useful screening tool for detection of AIN; however, it does not delineate the exact site and extent of disease.[55]

HRA is colposcopy of the anus after application of 3% acetic acid to differentiate normal from abnormal tissue.[56,59] After application of acetic acid, tissues harboring dysplasia become white. These tissues are then examined for changes associated with HSIL including vascular signs, such as punctation and mosaicism (**Fig. 8**), and epithelial patterns, such as honeycombing and hyperpigmentation.[60,61] LSIL also becomes whitened with the application of acetic acid; however, these lesions are generally raised and have warty vessels.[57] After a full evaluation with acetic acid, areas of diagnostic uncertainty can be examined with the application of Lugol iodine. The nonkeratinized mucosa involved with dysplasia turns yellow because of the absence of glycogen, whereas normal anal mucosa turns dark brown.[60] Identified areas for HSIL involvement by HRA are destroyed (discussed in the next section), and suspicious areas are biopsied for evaluation and subsequent treatment. In a study of 263 women, HRA correctly predicted normal epithelium in 90% and HSIL in 75% of histologically proved biopsies; however, HRA missed biopsy-proved LSIL in 50% of cases.[55] In another study comparing HRA characteristics with histopathology of 385 anal lesions in 121 HIV-positive and 31 HIV-negative MSM, the positive predictive value of HRA in HSIL was 49%.[61]

NONOPERATIVE TREATMENT
Expectant Management

Because of the unknown natural history of dysplasia, some advocate a strategy of watchful waiting reserving interventions only for clinically identified, palpable lesions. This approach requires a physical examination every 4 to 6 months.[56] In several studies of HIV-positive patients with HSIL who were managed with observation and surgical intervention only for palpable lesions, 11% to 16% of patients progressed

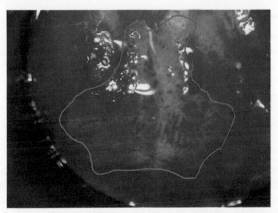

Fig. 8. Acetowhite lesion with punctation, mosaicism, and ringed glands with AIN 3 histology. (*From* Berry JM, Palefsky JM, Jay N, et al. Performance characteristics of anal cytology and human papillomavirus testing in patients with high-resolution anoscopy-guided biopsy of high-grade anal intraepithelial neoplasia. Dis Colon Rectum 2009;52:241; with permission.)

to anal cancer with 1 to 7 years.[34,62,63] One study reported progression from LSIL to HSIL in 62% and 36% of HIV-positive and HIV-negative patients, respectively.[14] Thus, expectant management may be better suited for select lower-risk patients, such as HIV-negative patients with LSIL, in whom lower rates of disease progression have been found.

In addition, because of the high prevalence of concomitant CIN, it is recommended that all females with AIN undergo a complete gynecologic evaluation.[56]

Topical Treatments

Topical 5% imiquimod cream, an immunomodulator, has been shown to be effective for AIN in cohort studies and case series.[56] It is typically applied three times per week for 16 weeks. Repeat courses can be used. In a recent meta-analysis, a complete response was achieved in almost half of patients (predominantly high-risk HIV-positive MSM), with additional partial response in 34% at a mean follow-up of 11 to 39 months.[56,64] Side effects include burning, irritation, erosions, and infection, which may adversely affect patient compliance.[56] Some authors suggest that topical immunomodulators may be best used to treat LSIL and anal warts, and as adjuncts to targeted therapy for HSIL.[65] As with other treatments for AIN, recurrence and metachronous lesions are still problematic and surveillance is essential. Although these results are encouraging, long-term data on rates of recurrence and progression to anal cancer are still needed.

Topical 5-fluorouracil (5-FU) has been described for use in AIN for 25 years.[56] Topical 5-FU is applied for 9 to 16 weeks, although recurrence may be minimized with longer use.[56] Initial clinical response rates are reported as high as 90%; however, recurrence may occur in up to 50%.[56] In a recent prospective study, 5-FU was applied twice weekly for 16 weeks to HRA-identified AIN lesions in 46 HIV-positive MSM. Thirty-nine percent achieved complete clearance of AIN, 17% had a partial response, and 37% did not respond. One patient progressed from low- to high-grade AIN. At 6-months follow-up, 50% of complete responders had recurred. Most patients experienced side-effects during therapy, but only two patients discontinued treatment. The authors suggested that pretreatment with topical 5-FU might facilitate subsequent ablative therapy.[66]

Photodynamic Therapy

Photodynamic therapy uses an oral or intravenous photosensitizer that is taken up by the affected tissues of the anal canal followed by activation of the sensitizer with a specific light wavelength that selectively destroys the dysplastic cells.[55,57] Several small case series have demonstrated the safety and feasibility of photodynamic therapy for the treatment of AIN, resulting in significant downstaging (HSIL to LSIL) and remission in short-term follow-up, and only mild discomfort.[55,57] To date, there are no large prospective studies using this treatment method.

Vaccination

Vaccination against HPV-16 and -18 may be considered in high-risk patients including HIV-positive patients and MSM to prevent the development of malignancy.[56] It has been shown to be safe and feasible.[55,56] Trials of the various HPV-16 and -18 vaccines have shown nearly 100% efficacy against high-grade lesions of the cervix, vulva, and vagina in uninfected women younger than 26 years of age and the quadrivalent vaccine that includes HPV-6, -11, -16, and -18 has shown efficacy against anogenital disease.[67] A recent double-blind randomized trial assessed quadrivalent HPV vaccination in 602 healthy MSM, 16 to 26 years of age, who either received quadrivalent

HPV vaccination or placebo. Efficacy of the HPV vaccine against AIN associated with HPV-6, -11, -16, or -18 was 50.3% in the intention-to-treat group and 77.5% in the per-protocol efficacy group. The rate of HSIL related to infection with HPV-6, -11, -16, or -18 was reduced by 54.2% in the intention-to-treat group and by 74.9% in the per-protocol efficacy group. The corresponding risks of persistent anal infection with HPV-6, -11, -16, or -18 were reduced by 59.4% and 94.9%, respectively. No vaccine-related serious adverse events occurred.[68] Thus, vaccination seems promising; however, the exact vaccine composition, timing of administration, and overall indications continue to be investigated.[56]

OPERATIVE TREATMENT

A variety of approaches to destroy and excise AIN have been used to eradicate disease and prevent progression to anal SCC.

Wide Local Excision

Traditionally, AIN was managed with wide local excision (WLE), which implies removal of all involved anoderm and perianal skin; in women, this may require excision of part of the labia, vulva, and vagina.[69] The extent of resection can be determined using one or a combination of three methods: (1) macroscopically negative margins; (2) preoperative mapping using punch biopsies under local anesthetic to sample the anal canal, including the dentate line, anal verge, and perianal skin (2 cm from the anal verge) at the four major and four minor points of the compass (24 biopsy specimens total), and any abnormal-appearing skin not in the routine biopsy positions[70]; and (3) intraoperative frozen section analysis until microscopically negative margins are obtained. Marchesa and colleagues[71] compared the incidence of local recurrence for high-grade perianal dysplasia managed with WLE based on a macroscopically negative margin and WLE based on preoperative punch biopsy mapping with intraoperative frozen sections ensuring 1-cm microscopic negative margins. They reported a local recurrence of 53.3% for the former compared with 23.1% for the latter. However, all patients who developed local recurrence after either method of WLE underwent repeat local excision without further recurrence or progression to invasive carcinoma within a median follow-up of 104 months. Following WLE, smaller defects can be closed primarily or allowed to heal by secondary intention, whereas larger defects may require split-thickness skin grafts, subcutaneous flaps, or myocutaneous flaps.[69,72,73] Furthermore, for bilateral and extensive WLE, constipating regimens[74] and temporary diversion may be required until perineal healing is achieved. Unfortunately, despite these aggressive procedures with significant potential morbidity (anal stenosis and fecal incontinence), the recurrence rates continue to be high (9%–63%).[55,56,60] The authors and the editors prefer a two-staged operation after punch biopsy, as shown in **Fig. 9**, and as defined previously, permanent section histopathologic specimen analysis is undertaken. The definitive operation includes WLE based on these results. Frozen section analysis is not recommended because of its relative inaccuracy and the additional intraoperative time required to perform it.

Targeted Destruction

Alternatively, targeted destruction of HSIL after HRA identification can be performed using electrocautery, infrared coagulator (IRC) ablation, or cryotherapy. These techniques have the potential to destroy lesions harboring AIN without the morbidity associated with WLE (**Fig. 10**).[56] However, regardless of the tissue destruction technique used, recurrence rates following HRA-based treatments are high, especially in HIV-positive patients and those with multifocal disease.[57]

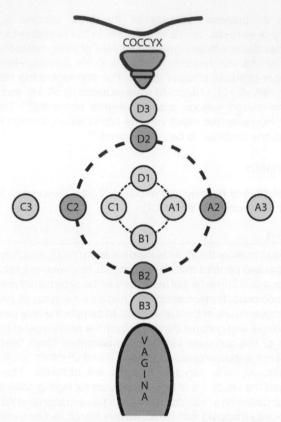

Fig. 9. Preoperative mapping procedure for wide local excision of high-grade dysplasia. (*Modified from* Beck DE, Fazio VW, Jagelman DG, et al. Perianal Bowen's disease. Dis Colon Rectum 1988;31:422; with permission.)

Chang and colleagues[75] prospectively assessed electrocautery ablation of HRA-detected lesions in 37 males and reported a 79% and 0% recurrence rate in HIV-positive and HIV-negative patients, respectively, for a mean follow-up of more than 2 years. However, with repeated HRA examinations, biopsies, and destruction, no patients developed anal cancer. More than 50% of patients reported uncontrolled pain for a mean of 3 weeks after the procedure; however, no patients developed incontinence, stenosis, postoperative infection, or significant bleeding after surgical treatment.[75] In a subsequent report using HRA-targeted electrocautery destruction in HIV-negative patients, all LSIL were cured and 45% of patients with HSIL recurred and were retreated.[60]

Targeted destruction of HRA-identified lesions can be performed using an IRC as an office-based procedure. Goldstone and colleagues[76] report promising results for office-based IRC ablation of HRA-identified HSIL-confirmed lesions in 96 MSM with more than 4 years follow-up. In HIV-negative and HIV-positive MSM, the probability of curing an individual lesion after the first ablation was 80% and 67%, respectively. However, the recurrence rate of HSIL was 62% and 91% in HIV-negative and HIV-positive MSM, respectively, mainly because of metachronous lesions (52% and 82%, respectively). With close surveillance and repeated treatment, 82% of HIV-positive and 90% of HIV-negative patients were HSIL-free at their last follow-up visit. Importantly, no patients developed anal carcinoma, and the only complication was

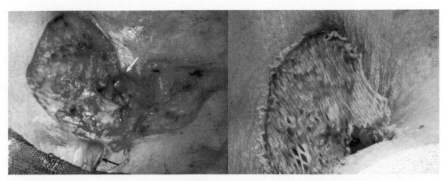

Fig. 10. Wide local excision for HSIL requiring split-thickness skin graft flap reconstruction (*white arrow*, anal canal; *black arrow*, vagina).

pain controlled with mild narcotics. Similarly, Pineda and colleagues[57] reported 10 years' experience with operating room ablation and additional office-based IRC for HRA-identified lesions in 246 HIV-positive patients with HSIL (80% were large-volume, nearly circumferential disease). They report that with routine surveillance and multiple procedures (most secondary procedures were office-based IRC), 78% were free of HSIL at last follow-up visit and only 1.2% progressed to anal carcinoma.[57] These encouraging results demonstrate that treatment of high-risk lesions produces lower progression to cancer than expectant management.[77,78] HRA-targeted destruction has several advantages: improved visualization allowing for better detection of previously unseen disease and the ability to spare normal tissue, thus reducing complications.[65] However, HRA-targeted therapy requires routine and intensive follow-up because of the high recurrence rate of AIN, especially among high-risk patients.[56,65]

SURVEILLANCE

Once established in the anal epithelium, AIN rarely regresses in HIV-positive individuals.[55,56] In these high-risk patients, progression to HSIL may be as high as 50% within 2 years, and the lifetime risk of progression to invasive cancer may be as high as 10% to 50%.[56] The natural history of untreated AIN in immunocompetent patients seems more indolent; however, it remains uncertain. The American Society of Colon and Rectal Surgeons recommends that patients with AIN be monitored with surveillance examinations at 3- to 6-month intervals as long as dysplasia is present.[56] The guidelines stress the importance of close follow-up particularly for HIV-positive patients, those with a history of other HPV-related genital malignancies, solid organ transplant patients, or MSM.[56] Although close follow-up is recommended for patients with AIN, much debate exists regarding the optimal and most cost-effective surveillance strategy. To date, there is a paucity of randomized or prospective cohort studies that demonstrate improved survival and long-term disease-free status for any specific surveillance strategy.

REFERENCES

1. Fenger C, Nielsen VT. Intraepithelial neoplasia of the anal canal. The appearance and relation to genital neoplasia. Acta Pathol Microbiol Immunol Scand A 1986;94:343–9.

2. Siegel R, Naishadham D, Jemal A. Cancer statistics. CA Cancer J Clin 2012;62: 10–29.
3. Palefsky JM. Human papillomavirus infection and anogenital neoplasia in human immunodeficiency virus positive men and women. J Natl Cancer Inst 1998;23:15–20.
4. Machalek D, Poynten M, Fengyi J, et al. Anal human papillomavirus infection and associated neoplastic lesions in men who have sex with men: a systematic review and metanalysis. Lancet Oncol 2012;13:487–500.
5. Cho KR, Vogelstein B. Genetic alterations in the adenoma–carcinoma sequence. Cancer 1992;70:1727–31.
6. Turell R. Epidermoid squamous cell cancer of perianus and anal canal. Surg Clin North Am 1962;42:1235–41.
7. Oriel J, Whimster I. Carcinoma in situ associated with virus-containing anal warts. Br J Dermatol 1971;84:71–5.
8. Fenger C, Nielsen VT. Dysplastic changes in the anal canal epithelium in minor surgical specimens. Acta Pathol Microbiol Immunol Scand A 1981;89:463–5.
9. Darragh T, Winkler B. Anal cancer and cervical cancer screening; key differences. Cancer 2011;119:5–19.
10. Frisch M, Glimelius B, van den Brule AJ, et al. Sexually transmitted infection as a cause of anal cancer. N Engl J Med 1997;337:1350–8.
11. Zbar AP, Fenger C, Efron J, et al. The pathology and molecular biology of anal intraepithelial neoplasia: comparison with cervical and vulvar intraepithelial carcinoma. Int J Colorectal Dis 2002;17:203–15.
12. Stanley M. Genital human papillomavirus infections: current and prospective therapies. J Natl Cancer Inst Monogr 2003;31:117–24.
13. Ogunbiyi O, Scholefiel J, Raftery A, et al. Prevalence of anal human papillomavirus infection and anal intraepithelial neoplasia in renal allograft recipients. Br J Surg 1994;81:365–7.
14. Palefsky J, Holly EA, Hogeboom CJ, et al. Virologic, immunologic and clinical parameters in the incidence and progression of anal squamous intraepithelial lesions in HIV-positive and HIV-negative homosexual men. J Acquir Immune Defic Syndr Hum Retrovirol 1998;17:314–9.
15. Friedman HB, Saah AJ, Sherman ME, et al. Human papillomavirus and anal squamous intraepithelial lesions and human immunodeficiency virus in a cohort of gay men. J Infect Dis 1998;178:45–52.
16. Moscicki AB, Schiffman M, Kjaer S, et al. Updating the natural history of HPV and anogenital cancer. Vaccine 2006;24(Suppl 3):S3/42–51.
17. Adami J, Gabel H, Lindelof B, et al. Cancer risk following organ transplantation: a nationwide cohort study in Sweden. Br J Cancer 2003;89:1221–7.
18. Mathew T, Kreis H, Friend P. Two year incidence of malignancy in sirolimus treated renal transplant patients: results from five multicenter studies. Clin Transplant 2004;18:446–9.
19. Daling JR, Madeleine MM, Johnson LG, et al. Human papilloma virus, smoking and sexual practices in the etiology of anal cancer. Cancer 2004;101:270–80.
20. Shiels MS, Cole SR, Kirk GD, et al. A metanalysis of the incidence of non-AIDS cancers in HIV infected individuals. J Acquir Immune Defic Syndr 2009;52: 611–22.
21. Lacey CJ. Therapy for genital human papillomavirus-related disease. J Clin Virol 2005;32:S82–90.
22. De Pokomandy A, Rouleau D, Ghattas G, et al. Highly active antiretroviral therapy for progression and progression to high grade anal intraepithelial neoplasia

in men who have sex with men and are infected with human immunodeficiency virus. Clin Infect Dis 2011;52:1174–81.

23. Chin-Hong PV, Husnik M, Cranston RD, et al. Anal human papillomavirus infection is associated with HIV acquisition in men who have sex with men. AIDS 2009;23(9):1135–42.

24. Lacey HB, Wilson GE, Tilston P, et al. A study of anal intraepithelial neoplasia in HIV positive homosexual men. Sex Transm Infect 1999;75:172–7.

25. Bower M, Powles T, Newsom D, et al. HIV associated anal cancer: has highly active antiretroviral therapy reduced the incidence or improved the outcome. J Acquir Immune Defic Syndr 2004;37:1563–5.

26. Powles T, Robinson D, Stebbing J, et al. Highly active antiretroviral therapy and the incidence of non-AIDS defining cancers in people with HIV infection. J Clin Oncol 2009;27:884–90.

27. Shvetsov YB, Hernandez BY, McDuffie K, et al. Duration and clearance of anal human papilloma infection among women: the Hawaii HPV cohort study. J Infect Dis 2010;201:1331–9.

28. Darragh TM, Colgan JT, Cox JT, et al. The lower anogenital squamous terminology standardization project for HPV-associated lesions: background and consensus recommendations from the College of American Pathologists and the American Society for Colposcopy and Cervical Pathology. J Low Genit Tract Dis 2012;16:205–42.

29. Zaki SR, Judd R, Coffiel LM, et al. Human papillomavirus and anal carcinoma. Retrospective analysis by in situ hybridization and the polymerase chain reaction. Am J Pathol 1992;140:1345–55.

30. Stanley M. Pathology and epidemiology of HPV infection in females. Gynecol Oncol 2010;110:S5–10.

31. Munoz N, Bosch FX, de Sanjosé S, et al. Risk factors for cervical intraepithelial neoplasia grade III/carcinoma in situ in Spain and Colombia. Cancer Epidemiol Biomarkers Prev 1993;2:423–31.

32. Hoots BE, Palefsky JM, Pimenta JS. Human papillomavirus type distribution in anal cancer and anal intraepithelial lesions. Int J Cancer 2009;124:2375–83.

33. Gohy L, Gorska I, de Podomanky A, et al. Genotyping of human papillomavirus in anal biopsies and anal swabs collected from HIV-seropositive men with anal dysplasia. J Acquir Immune Defic Syndr 2008;49:32–9.

34. Watson AJ, Smith BB, Whitehead MR, et al. Malignant progression of anal intra epithelial neoplasia. ANZ J Surg 2006;76:715–7.

35. Stoler MH, Vichnin MD, Ferenczy A, et al. The accuracy of colposcopic biopsy: analysis from the placebo arm of the Gardasil clinical trials. Int J Cancer 2011; 128:1354–62.

36. Castle PE, Stoler MH, Solomon D, et al. The relationship of community biopsy-diagnosed cervical intraepithelial neoplasia grade 2 to the quality control pathology-reviewed diagnoses: an ALTS report. Am J Clin Pathol 2007;127: 805–15.

37. Carter PS, Sheffield JP, Shepherd N, et al. Interobserver variation in the reporting of the histopathological grading of anal intraepithelial neoplasia. J Clin Pathol 1994;47:1032–4.

38. Northfelt DW, Swift PS, Palefsky JM. Anal neoplasia. Pathogenesis, diagnosis, and management. Hematol Oncol Clin North Am 1996;10:1177–87.

39. Walts AE, Lechago J, Gose S. P16 and Ki67 immunostaining is a useful adjunct in the assessment of biopsies for HPV-associated anal intraepithelial neoplasia. Am J Surg Pathol 2006;30:795–801.

40. Bala R, Pinsky BA, Beck AH, et al. p16 is superior to ProEx C in identifying high-grade squamous intraepithelial lesions (HSIL) of the anal canal. Am J Surg Pathol 2013;37:659–68.
41. Pirog EC, Quint KD, Yantiss RK. P16/CDKN2A and Ki-67 enhance the detection of anal intraepithelial neoplasia and condyloma and correlate with human papillomavirus detection by polymerase chain reaction. Am J Surg Pathol 2010;34: 1449–55.
42. Piketty C, Selinger-Leneman H, Grabar S, et al. Marked increase in the incidence of invasive anal cancer among HIV infected patients despite treatment with combination antiretroviral therapy. AIDS 2008;22:1203–11.
43. Chaturvedi AK, Madeleine MM, Biggar RJ, et al. Risk of human papillomavirus-associated cancers among persons with AIDS. J Natl Cancer Inst 2009;101: 1120–30.
44. Betancourt EM, Wahbah NN, Been LC, et al. Anal cytology as a predictor of anal intraepithelial neoplasia in HIV-positive men and women. Diagn Cytopathol 2013;41:697–702.
45. Jimenez JB, Frieyro-Elicegui M, Padilla-España L, et al. Anal intraepithelial neoplasia in a sexually transmitted diseases outpatient clinic: correlation with cytological screening. J Eur Acad Dermatol Venereol 2013. [Epub ahead of print].
46. Mathews WC, Sitapati A, Caperna JC, et al. Measurement characteristics of anal cytology, histopathology, and high-resolution anoscopic visual impression in an anal dysplasia screening program. J Acquir Immune Defic Syndr 2004;37: 1610–5.
47. Panther LA, Wagner K, Proper J, et al. High resolution ansoscopy findings for men who have sex with men: inaccuracy of anal cytology as a predictor of histologic high-grade anal intraepithelial neoplasia and the impact of IHI serostatus. Clin Infect Dis 2004;38:1490–2.
48. Nahas CS, da Silva Filho EV, Segurado AA, et al. Screening anal dysplasia in HIV-infected patients: is there an agreement between anal pap smear and high-resolution anoscopy-guided biopsy? Dis Colon Rectum 2009;52: 1854–63.
49. Weis SE, Vecino I, Pgoda JM, et al. Prevalence of anal intraepithelial neoplasia defined by anal cytology screening and high-resolution anoscopy in a primary care population of HIV-infected men and women. Dis Colon Rectum 2011;54: 433–41.
50. Darragh TM. Anal cytology. In: Wilbur DC, Henry MR, editors. College of American Pathologists practical guide to gynecologic cytopathology: morphology, management and molecular methods. Northfied (IL): CAP Press; 2008. p. 177–81.
51. Arain S, Walts AE, Thomas P, et al. The anal pap smear: cytomorphology of squamous intraepithelial lesions. Cytojournal 2005;2:4.
52. Darragh TM, Tokugawa D, Castle PE, et al. Interrater agreement of anal cytology. Cancer 2013;121:72–8.
53. Lytwyn A, Salit IE, Raboud J, et al. Interobserver agreement in the interpretation of anal intraepithelial neoplasia. Cancer 2005;103:1447–56.
54. Etienney I, Vuong S, Si-Mohamed A, et al. Value of cytologic papanicolaou smears and polymerase chain reaction screening for human papillomavirus DNA in detecting anal intraepithelial neoplasia. Cancer 2012;118:6031–8.
55. Abbasakoor F, Boulos PB. Anal intraepithelial neoplasia. Br J Surg 2005;92: 277–90.

56. Steele SR, Varma MG, Melton GB, et al, on behalf of the Standards Practice Task Force of the American Society of Colon and Rectal Surgeons. Practice parameters for anal squamous neoplasms. Dis Colon Rectum 2012;55:735–49.
57. Pineda CE, Berry JM, Jay N, et al. High-resolution anoscopy targeted surgical destruction of anal high-grade squamous intraepithelial lesions: a ten-year experience. Dis Colon Rectum 2008;51:829–35.
58. Palefsky JM, Holly EA, Hogeboom CJ, et al. Anal cytology as a screening tool for anal squamous intraepithelial lesions. J Acquir Immune Defic Syndr 1997;14: 415–22.
59. Berry JM, Palefsky JM, Jay N, et al. Performance characteristics of anal cytology and human papillomavirus testing in patients with high-resolution anoscopy-guided biopsy of high-grade anal intraepithelial neoplasia. Dis Colon Rectum 2009;52:239–47.
60. Pineda CE, Berry JM, Jay N, et al. High resolution anoscopy in the planned staged treatment of anal squamous intraepithelial lesions in HIV-negative patients. J Gastrointest Surg 2007;11:1410–6.
61. Jay N, Berry JM, Hogeboom CJ, et al. Colposcopic appearance of anal squamous intraepithelial lesions: relationship to histopathology. Dis Colon Rectum 1997;40(8):919–28.
62. Devaraj B, Cosman BC. Expectant management of anal squamous dysplasia in patients with HIV. Dis Colon Rectum 2006;49:36–40.
63. Sobhani I, Walker F, Roudot-Thorval F, et al. Anal carcinoma: incidence and effect of cumulative infections. AIDS 2004;18:1561–9.
64. Mahto M, Nathan M, O'Mahony C. More than a decade on: review of the use of imiquimod in lower anogenital intraepithelial neoplasia. Int J STD AIDS 2010;21: 8–16.
65. Pineda CE, Welton ML. Controversies in the management of anal high-grade squamous intraepithelial lesions. Minerva Chir 2008;63:389–99.
66. Richel O, Wieland U, de Vries HJ, et al. Topical 5-fluorouracil treatment of anal intraepithelial neoplasia in human immunodeficiency virus-positive men. Br J Dermatol 2010;163(6):1301–7.
67. Franceschi S, De Vuyst H. Human papillomavirus vaccines and anal carcinoma. Curr Opin HIV AIDS 2009;4(1):57–63.
68. Palefsky JM, Giuliano AR, Goldstone S, et al. HPV vaccine against anal HPV infection and anal intraepithelial neoplasia. N Engl J Med 2011;365(17): 1576–85.
69. Cleary RK, Schaldenbrand JD, Fowler JJ, et al. Perianal Bowen's disease and anal intraepithelial neoplasia: review of the literature. Dis Colon Rectum 1999; 42:945–51.
70. Strauss RJ, Fazio VW. Bowen's disease of the anal and perianal area: a report and analysis of twelve cases. Am J Surg 1979;137:231–4.
71. Marchesa P, Fazio VW, Oliart S, et al. Perianal Bowen's disease: a clinicopathologic study of 47 patients. Dis Colon Rectum 1997;40:1286–93.
72. Margenthaler JA, Dietz DW, Mutch MG, et al. Outcomes, risk of other malignancies, and need for formal mapping procedures in patients with perianal Bowen's disease. Dis Colon Rectum 2004;47:1655–61.
73. Wietfeldt ED, Thiele J. Malignancies of the anal margin and perianal skin. Clin Colon Rectal Surg 2009;22:127–35.
74. Reynolds VH, Madden JJ, Franklin JD, et al. Preservation of anal function after total excision of the anal mucosa for Bowen's disease. Ann Surg 1984;199: 563–8.

75. Chang GJ, Berry JM, Jay N, et al. Surgical treatment of high-grade anal squamous intraepithelial lesions: a prospective study. Dis Colon Rectum 2002;45: 453–8.
76. Goldstone RN, Goldstone AB, Russ J, et al. Long-term follow-up of infrared coagulator ablation of anal high-grade dysplasia in men who have sex with men. Dis Colon Rectum 2011;54:1284–92.
77. Goldstone SE. Invited commentary: high-resolution anoscopy targeted surgical destruction of anal high-grade squamous intraepithelial lesions: a ten-year experience. Dis Colon Rectum 2008;51:835–6.
78. Beck DE, Fazio VW, Jagelman DG, et al. Perianal Bowen's disease. Dis Colon Rectum 1988;31:419–22.

Management of Radiation Proctitis

Ankit Sarin, MD, MHA[a], Bashar Safar, MBBS, MRCS[b],*

KEYWORDS

- Radiation proctitis • Radiation colitis • Sucralfate • Short-chain fatty acids
- Hyperbaric oxygen • Formalin • Endoscopic laser therapy
- Argon plasma coagulation

KEY POINTS

- Radiation proctitis is a common complication of radiation therapy but most instances of proctitis are self-limited and respond to medical management.
- Rates of both acute and chronic proctitis have been decreasing with improved radiation therapy techniques that allow the targeted delivery of higher doses of radiation.
- The paucity of well-controlled, blinded, randomized studies makes it impossible to fully assess the comparative efficacy of the different endoscopic and medical therapies for chronic radiation proctitis. Despite this limitation, endoscopic therapies, particularly argon plasma coagulation (APC), seem to be the most effective in managing well-defined bleeding from radiation proctitis.
- Although focal ablative tools such as lasers, contact probes, and APC may be helpful when bleeding occurs from a limited number of identifiable ectatic vessels, a larger field of arteriovenous malformations or oozing may be more difficult to control.
- Methods allowing a broader field of treatment, such as formalin instillation or the newer methods of radiofrequency ablation (RFA) and cryotherapy, may theoretically be advantageous in this setting. In particular, the unexpected finding of neosquamous epithelialization with RFA may have further advantages in preventing recurrent symptoms and needs to be further evaluated in larger randomized trials.

INTRODUCTION

Radiation therapy is commonly used as part of the multidisciplinary treatment strategies of pelvic malignancies of gynecologic, urologic, and anorectal origin with well-established benefits. Radiation proctitis following pelvic radiation therapy can range from a dose-limiting side effect in its acute stage to major morbidity affecting health-related quality of life in its chronic stage. Many series have suggested an

Disclaimers: None.
Sources of Support: None.
[a] Division of Colon and Rectal Surgery, University of California-San Francisco, San Francisco, CA, USA; [b] Department of Surgery, Ravitch Division, The Johns Hopkins Hospital, Blalock 618, Baltimore, MD, USA
* Corresponding author.
E-mail address: bsafar1@jhmi.edu

incidence of 5% or less after pelvic radiation, but a review of published controlled trials of adjuvant therapies suggests that 30% might be more realistic (**Fig. 1**).[1] There are also data to suggest that the proportion of patients who seek help for subsequent symptoms represent only a fraction of affected patients.[2]

Patients with prostate, cervical, and anal cancers are the most commonly affected, although the epidemiology of radiation proctitis is difficult to characterize because of the range of cancers for which pelvic radiation therapy is used, and the diversity of dosing regimens and modes of therapy. Predisposing factors that may be associated with increased risk of late complications of radiation include preexisting comorbid conditions, tumor stage, total radiation dosage, the volume treated, dose distribution, and concurrent therapies.[3] Most radiation oncologists now rely on advanced techniques, such as the use of three-dimensional treatment planning software, to target maximal dose to the intended organ while minimizing exposure to the rectum. Despite this, in a randomized control trial on dose escalation using three-dimensional treatment planning and conformal radiotherapy among patients with prostate cancer, a third of patients had more than 25% of their rectal volume exposed to radiation therapy. This exposure resulted in a doubling of the 5-year risk for development of late radiation proctitis (37% vs 13% among patients with <25% of rectal volume exposed).[4]

No standard guidelines exist for diagnosis and management of radiation proctitis. This article reviews the definitions, staging, and clinical features of radiation proctitis, and then summarizes the different modalities currently available for the treatment of acute and chronic radiation proctitis.

DEFINITIONS

Acute radiation proctitis refers to radiation-induced injury during the time of radiation therapy and for a short period (up to 6 months) after completion, usually defined as 6 months. Nearly all patients develop at least transient symptoms consistent with this acute process.

Chronic radiation proctitis can continue from the acute phase or begin after a variable latent period (typically at least 90 days). Most patients develop symptoms at a median of 8 to 12 months after completion of radiotherapy.[5]

HISTOLOGIC AND CLINICAL FEATURES OF ACUTE VERSUS CHRONIC RADIATION PROCTITIS

In the acute phase of radiation proctitis, extensive mucosal inflammation, eosinophilic infiltration of the submucosa, crypt atrophy, and crypt abscesses are observed on

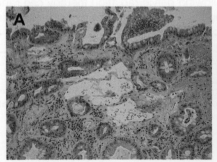
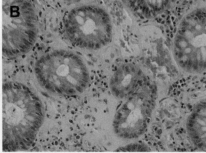

Fig. 1. Radiation proctitis. (*A*) Magnification ×20. (*B*) Magnification ×40. (*Courtesy of* Ilke Nalbantoglu, MD, Department of Pathology, Washington University, St Louis, MO.)

histology. This damage causes symptoms such as diarrhea, mucus discharge, cramping, bloating, tenesmus, anal pain or incontinence, and minor rectal bleeding. Of these symptoms, the most common is diarrhea, which affects from 50% to 75% of patients.[6]

Chronic damage is characterized by obliterative enteritis with ulceration and fibrous induration of the gut.[7] The cardinal sign of chronic radiation proctitis that distinguishes it from acute radiation proctitis is the presence of small-vessel vasculopathy.[8] Clinical manifestations of chronic radiation damage are characterized by rectal urgency, incontinence, pain, bleeding, mucous discharge, and strictures. Rectal fistula or perforation can, rarely, occur.

CLASSIFICATION

Most studies grade late rectal adverse events using the Radiation Therapy Oncology Group scoring criteria, shown in **Table 1**.[9] The objective of a more specific rectal toxicity profile is to help physicians and patients make more informed management decisions after radiation therapy.

DIAGNOSIS

In most patients, the diagnosis can be confirmed by colonoscopy or sigmoidoscopy. Mucosal features consistent with radiation injury include pallor with friability, and telangiectasias.[10] Although mucosal biopsies are not diagnostic, they can help to exclude other causes of proctitis such as infection or inflammatory bowel disease. Rectal biopsy to evaluate rectal bleeding because of radiation proctitis seems to be an important factor in the development of rectal fistulas.[11] For this reason, rectal biopsies should be performed judiciously depending on the clinical indication as well as the dose and fractionation of previous pelvic radiation therapy. If required, they should be directed at the posterior and lateral walls to avoid the irradiated areas in patients with prior prostate therapy.[12]

PREVENTION

The main approach to the prevention of radiation proctitis is the use of newer conformal radiation therapy techniques. These advances include intensity-modulated radiation

Table 1
Modified Radiation Therapy Oncology Group rectal toxicity scale

Grade 1	Mild and self-limiting	Minimal, infrequent bleeding or clear mucus discharge, rectal discomfort not requiring analgesics, loose stools not requiring medications
Grade 2	Managed conservatively, lifestyle (performance status) not affected	Intermittent rectal bleeding not requiring regular use of pads, erythema of rectal lining on proctoscopy, diarrhea requiring medications
Grade 3	Severe, alters patient lifestyle	Rectal bleeding requiring regular use of pads and minor surgical intervention, rectal pain requiring narcotics, rectal ulceration
Grade 4	Life threatening and disabling	Bowel obstruction, fistula formation, bleeding requiring hospitalization, surgical intervention required

therapy and intensity-guided radiation therapy, and minimize the dose of radiation to the rectum while maximizing dose to the tumor.

Amifostine is a prodrug that is metabolized to a thiol metabolite that is thought to scavenge reactive oxygen species. When administered intravenously, it has shown some promise in small trials with short follow-up in preventing symptoms of acute proctitis as well as decreasing the severity of chronic proctitis symptoms.[13–15] Sucralfate has also been evaluated for prophylaxis against acute radiation injury. However, placebo-controlled phase III trials have detected no benefit from either topical or oral sucralfate.[16,17]

TREATMENT

Potential therapy for chronic radiation proctitis includes 3 broad categories (**Table 2**)[18]:

(1) Medical: enemas, oral agents, topical applications, and oxygen therapy.

(2) Endoscopic: argon plasma coagulation (APC), laser, cryotherapy, and electrocoagulation.

Table 2 Potential therapy for chronic radiation proctitis			
	Type of Therapy	**Proposed Mechanism**	**Role**
Medical therapies	Butyrate	Nutrient for healing colonocytes	Used primarily in acute radiation proctitis
	5-Aminosalicylic acid derivatives	Antiinflammatory	As first-line therapy in chronic radiation proctitis with mixed results
	Sucralfate	Prevents microvascular injury	
	Metronidazole	Antiinflammatory	
	Short-chain fatty acid	Nutrient for healing colonocytes	
	Vitamin A	Antiinflammatory	
	Topical formalin	Chemical cauterization	
	Hyperbaric oxygen	Promotes healing	Not widely available but shows some efficacy
Endoscopic therapies	Dilatation		For radiation-related strictures
	Heater and bipolar cautery	Thermoelectric cauterization	More effective than medical therapies, especially in controlling rectal bleeding, but not widely available; APC is preferred to laser coagulation or cryotherapy
	Nd:YAG, KTP laser	Noncontact electrocoagulation	
	Cryotherapy	Thermal cauterization	
	Argon plasma coagulation	Noncontact electrocoagulation	
	Radiofrequency ablation	Noncontact electrocoagulation	
Surgical therapies	Diverting ostomy	Diversion of fecal stream	High risk of postoperative morbidity; reserved for severe rectal strictures and rectal fistulas
	Reconstruction with flaps	Vascularized tissue mobilized	
	Proctectomy	Removal of damaged tissue	

Abbreviations: APC, argon plasma coagulation; KTP, potassium titanyl phosphate; laser Nd:YAG, neodymium/yttrium aluminum garnet argon.

(3) Surgical: there have been no large controlled trials evaluating the different treatments for radiation proctitis, and management strategies are derived primarily from institutional experience, case reports, and small clinical trials.

MEDICAL THERAPIES
Butyrate

Butyrate is used primarily in acute radiation proctitis, for which it has shown some benefit in hastening recovery,[19,20] and other treatments have not been shown to be efficacious. Butyrate is the main short-chain fatty acid (SCFA) used by colonocytes for nutrition and this is attributed to its protective effect during recovery from radiation trauma.

Amino Salicylic Acid Derivatives

Antiinflammatory agents in this group, such as sulfasalazine and mesalazine, have been reported to have a role in the management of radiation proctitis.[21] The antiinflammatory actions of 5-aminosalicylic acid (5-ASA) occur through a variety of mechanisms, most notably via a reduction of prostaglandin production.[22,23] At first, it was thought that 5-ASA was an effective medical agent for the treatment of chronic radiation proctitis.[22] However, several small trials of 5-ASA for radiation proctitis have produced mixed results. Some produced symptomatic improvement or no clinical changes, whereas others produced worsening of clinical symptoms.[21,24–26] Other antiinflammatory agents that are used in combination with sulfasalazine or 5-ASA include oral or rectal steroids such as prednisone, betamethasone, or hydrocortisone. Steroids have multiple mechanisms of action that produce antiinflammatory effects, which range from stabilization of lysosomes in neutrophils to prevent degranulation to upregulation of antiinflammatory genes via binding to glucocorticoid receptors.[27] The efficacy of corticosteroids alone has been poorly studied and anecdotal clinical experience with this approach has been disappointing.

Sucralfate

Several reports have suggested that topical sucralfate may improve symptoms of radiation proctitis or proctosigmoiditis.[22,28–31] Sucralfate is a highly sulfated polyanionic disaccharide. Its postulated mechanisms of action include a reduction in the extent of microvascular injury and protection of epithelial surfaces from radiation damage.[32,33]

In a prospective, double-blind trial, 37 patients with proctosigmoiditis were randomly assigned to a 4-week course of oral sulfasalazine (3.0 g/d) plus prednisolone enemas (20 mg twice daily) or sucralfate enemas (2.0 g twice daily).[22] Clinical improvement was noted in both groups at the end of the study. However, the response was better for sucralfate enemas alone, which were also better tolerated.

Another report from the same investigators included 26 patients with moderate to severe radiation proctosigmoiditis who were treated with sucralfate enemas (20 mL of a 10% suspension twice daily) until bleeding stopped or failure of therapy was acknowledged.[28] A good response (decreased number of episodes of bleeding) was observed in 77% of patients by 4 weeks, and 92% by 16 weeks. These results await confirmation in larger controlled trials.

Metronidazole

Metronidazole is a nitroimidazole whose complete mechanism of action is unclear but is thought to be via the reduction of the nitro group in an anaerobic environment.[34] The efficacy of metronidazole was evaluated in study that included 60 patients with rectal bleeding and diarrhea who were randomly assigned to treatment with mesalamine plus betamethasone enemas with or without oral metronidazole.[35] The incidence of rectal bleeding and mucosal ulcers was lower in the metronidazole groups at 1, 3, and 12 months. Diarrhea and edema were also reduced in this group.

SCFA Enemas

SCFAs are the preferred nutrients for colonocytes and also exert a trophic effect on the colonic mucosa by stimulating a physiologic pattern of proliferation and promoting cellular differentiation. Their use may be impaired in chronic radiation proctitis. Radiation-associated mucosal atrophy may interfere with mitochondrial fatty acid oxidation, and supplementation of SCFA in the form of enemas could overcome this deficiency and improve the energy supply to colonocytes. Moreover, the dilatory effect of SCFA on arteriolar walls may also contribute by improving mucosal ischemia. Fatty acid enemas have been effective for treatment of diversion colitis, and some case reports suggest a possible benefit in radiation proctitis.[36] However, no significant improvement in symptoms was found in a placebo-controlled study.[37]

Vitamin A

Oxidative stress is thought to be a major mechanism in the development of chronic radiation proctitis, and agents with antioxidant properties such as vitamins A and C have been used in an attempt to limit tissue damage related to oxidation. In a study by Kennedy and colleagues,[38] which only included 10 patients, the use of vitamins E and C significantly decreased the rate of diarrhea and urgency. Another study was a pilot, placebo-controlled trial involving 18 patients with radiation proctitis.[39] Response (defined as a reduction in 2 or more symptoms by at least 2 points on a validated scale) was observed significantly more often in the group randomized to retinol palmitate (vitamin A). In addition, 5 placebo nonresponders subsequently responded to active treatment during crossover.

Formalin

Rubinstein and colleagues[40] reported the first published successful use of 4% formalin in a patient who had required colostomy and 39 U of blood transfusion. Application directly to the mucosa produces local chemical cauterization, reducing bleeds by sealing the neovascularized telangiectatic spots and ulcers. The success of bleeding control is related to the accurate localization and application of formalin to all the affected points. Several variations in technique have been described. Most commonly, the treatment consists of proctoscopy with direct application with a cotton tip applicator or gauze of 4% or buffered 10% formalin in contact with the hemorrhagic rectal mucosa or of instillation into the rectum of 20 to 100 mL of 3.6% to 4% solution. Direct contact of the formalin with the anoderm should be avoided because it can be irritating to the skin. Endoscopic flushing out of residual formaldehyde with saline is usually recommended. The success in controlling bleeding ranges from 80% to 100% but there is real, albeit small, risk of pelvic sepsis, rectal wall necrosis, or development of rectovaginal fistulae.[41] The risk of late strictures or incontinence is also real and is increased in patients with anal cancer treated with radiation.[42] Given these complications, the use of formalin should be restricted to patients with hemorrhagic proctitis.

Hyperbaric Oxygen

The theoretic benefit of hyperbaric oxygen therapy may be via inhibition of bacterial growth, preservation of marginally perfused tissue, and inhibition of toxin production. Hyperbaric oxygen therapy has an angiogenic effect and has been shown to cause an

8-fold or 9-fold increase in the vascular density of soft tissues compared with air-breathing controls.[43] Several studies have suggested a marginal benefit, although this has never been well defined.[44–47] Assessment of response has tended to be a vague description of the resolution of symptoms instead of a tangible system that can be used for statistical analysis.

ENDOSCOPIC THERAPIES
Endoscopic Dilation

Balloon dilation can be effective in patients with obstructive symptoms from radiation-related strictures who do not respond to stool softeners, provided that the strictured segment is short.[48] The risk of perforation is increased in patients with long or angulated strictures. Such patients may require surgery if obstruction is clinically significant.

Endoscopic Lasers and Cryoablation

The potassium titanyl phosphate (KTP) and neodymium/yttrium aluminum garnet argon (Nd:YAG) lasers have been used to coagulate bleeding ectatic vessels throughout the gastrointestinal tract.[49–53] However, these devices are not widely available.

Nd:YAG laser has a low affinity for hemoglobin and H_2O but is well absorbed by tissue protein, thus making it ideal for deeper vessel coagulation. The potential benefit of this approach was shown in a report in which the Nd:YAG laser was used in 9 patients, of whom 6 required periodic blood transfusion; bleeding was reduced to only occasional spotting in 6 patients, with only 1 continuing to require periodic blood transfusions during follow-up of 24 months.[50] Transmural necrosis, fibrosis, stricture formation, and rectovaginal fistula are some of the complications reported with use of Nd:YAG.

The KTP laser uses the beam from the Nd:YAG laser that is passed through a KTP crystal, reducing the wavelength by half (532 nm).[30] At this wavelength, the energy is absorbed by hemoglobin and the depth of penetration is shallower (1–2 mm) than hat of Nd:YAG, hence the risk of transmucosal damage resulting in necrosis or stricture is less.

In small pilot studies of 7 to 10 patients with radiation proctitis, response to cryoablation spray ablation with a decrease in rectal telangiectasia density and improvement in radiation proctitis symptom severity has been seen.[54,55] One patient suffered cecal perforation caused by gas overdistention. Controlled trials are needed to establish the safety and efficacy of cryoablation for radiation proctitis.

Endoscopic Bipolar and Heater Probe

The advantage of bipolar electrocoagulation and the heater probe compared with laser therapy is that they cause less tissue injury, and permit tangential application of cautery, and that the equipment needed is widely available and inexpensive. The disadvantage is char formation on the tip of the probe, leading to decreased treatment efficiency and requiring repeated cleaning.

These techniques were evaluated in a study involving 21 patients with chronic recurrent hematochezia and anemia caused by radiation-induced injury who were followed for 12 months.[56] Patients were treated with either bipolar coagulation probe or heater probe therapy as needed. Severe bleeding diminished significantly after these treatments compared with the previous 12 months of medical therapy (75% vs 33% and 67% vs 11%, respectively). The decreased rate of bleeding was accompanied by an improvement in the hematocrit in both groups; there were no major complications.

Endoscopic APC

Laser therapy for hemorrhagic chronic radiation proctitis has largely been supplanted by APC, which is less expensive, easier, safer, and more widely available. APC uses high-frequency energy transmitted to tissue by ionized gas. Unlike traditional bipolar devices, the current jumps from the probe to the target lesion, with the arc being broken once the tissue is desiccated. The theoretic advantage is a uniform, more predictable, and limited depth of coagulation (0.5–3 mm),[34] which minimizes the risks of perforation, stenosis, and fistulization. APC has been used to treat a wide spectrum of bleeding lesions in the gastrointestinal tract and has been shown to be effective in controlling bleeding caused by radiation proctitis, although it may require multiple sessions (usually at 4-week intervals).[57–59] Some patients may experience postprocedure rectal pain and cramps, but major complications are rare. Special care is required to avoid spraying too close to the dentate line. In addition, APC may control bleeding even after other treatment methods have failed.[60,61]

Endoscopic Radiofrequency Ablation

Zhou and colleagues[62] reported successful use of endoscopic radiofrequency ablation (RFA) in treating 3 patients with lower gastrointestinal bleeding from chronic radiation proctitis, including 2 who failed other therapies. In all cases, the procedure was well tolerated and hemostasis was effectively achieved after 1 or 2 sessions. Reepithelialization by neosquamous mucosa was observed over areas of prior hemorrhage with no stricturing or ulceration during follow-up of up to 19 months.

Several benefits of RFA have been found compared with other endoscopic treatments for radiation proctitis. The tightly spaced bipolar array of the RFA catheter limits the radiofrequency energy penetration, restricting the RFA treatment to the superficial mucosa, thereby avoiding deep tissue injury in ischemic mucosa and the resulting ulceration and stricturing. RFA also allows broader areas of tissue to be treated simultaneously compared with the point-by-point approach required with heater or bipolar probes. The energy delivered to the surface is consistent and reproducible, thus reducing operator dependence and overtreatment, which may lead to perforations or ulcerations. In addition, the unexpected finding of squamous reepithelialization seen after RFA results in the lack of stricturing and ulceration that is often seen after other thermal ablative procedures.[63]

SURGICAL THERAPIES

Surgery should be reserved for patients who have intractable symptoms such as strictures, pain, or bleeding, because it may be technically demanding because of adhesions and other radiation damage in the pelvis. Fewer than 10% of patients eventually require surgery,[64] which is usually for intractable bleeding, perforation, strictures, and fistulas.

Fecal Diversion

Diverting the fecal stream with a colostomy or ileostomy decreases symptoms of pain, tenesmus, drainage, and infection, and can also improve symptoms related to incontinence and stricture. It has a limited effect on bleeding, although at least one study has shown improvement in bleeding as well.[65] In some patients, a complete diversion improves symptoms and their quality of life to the point that they do not require any further intervention[6,64,66,67] even though the underlying problem is not directly addressed. In one review of 48 patients who had been referred for severe refractory radiotherapy complications that had failed initial treatment, surgery was generally required for patients who presented with a fistula, and permanent diversion was more likely in patients with severe radiation enteritis and distal colonic strictures.[68]

Repair/reconstruction

Local excision and reconstruction such as an advancement flap, although technically feasible, are limited by the presence of poorly vascularized tissues and low healing rates.[69] An exception is the treatment of rectourethral or rectovaginal fistula with a pedunculated gracilis or a Martius flap to facilitate healing by introducing well-vascularized healthy tissue, and preliminary or synchronous diversion of stool and of the urinary stream with an ostomy and a catheter, respectively, is required. Although these procedures may be a technical success, they often result in unacceptable long-term morbidity, including complicated scarring, stricture, and incontinence.

Proctectomy/pelvic Exenteration

Complete rectal resection may be the only option in some patients, such as in cases of complicated fistulous disease, especially when accompanied by significant pain and incontinence, or in cases of severe and intractable bleeding, because diversion rarely controls the bleeding completely. Although this is a definitive treatment, it is accompanied by significant morbidity, including exceedingly high rates of anastomotic leaks in cases of reconstruction and high rates of perineal wound complications when reconstruction is not attempted.[6,67] When surgical treatment is needed, most studies have poor outcomes with high complication rates (15%–80%), and mortalities of 3% to 9%.[64,66,67]

SUMMARY

Radiation proctitis is a common complication of radiation therapy but most instances of proctitis are self-limited and respond to medical management. Rates of both acute and chronic proctitis have been decreasing with improved radiation therapy techniques that allow the targeted delivery of higher doses of radiation.

Because of the paucity of well-controlled, blinded, randomized studies, it is not possible to fully assess the comparative efficacy of the different endoscopic and medical therapies for chronic radiation proctitis. Despite this limitation, endoscopic therapies, particularly APC, seem to be the most effective in managing well-defined bleeding from radiation proctitis and may have some impact on other symptoms as well.[70] Although focal ablative tools such as lasers, contact probes, and APC may be helpful when bleeding occurs from limited number of identifiable ectatic vessels, a larger field of arteriovenous malformations or oozing may be more difficult to control. Methods allowing broader fields of treatment, such as formalin instillation, or the newer methods of RFA and cryotherapy may therefore theoretically be advantageous in this setting. In particular, the unexpected finding of neosquamous epithelialization with RFA may have further advantages in preventing recurrent symptoms[63] and needs to be further evaluated in larger randomized trials.

REFERENCES

1. Ooi BS, Tjandra JJ, Green MD. Morbidities of adjuvant chemotherapy and radiotherapy for resectable rectal cancer: an overview. Dis Colon Rectum 1999;42(3): 403–18.
2. Yeoh EK, Horowitz M. Radiation enteritis. Surg Gynecol Obstet 1987;165(4): 373–9.

3. Coia LR, Myerson RJ, Tepper JE. Late effects of radiation therapy on the gastrointestinal tract. Int J Radiat Oncol Biol Phys 1995;31(5):1213–36.

4. Storey MR, Pollack A, Zagars G, et al. Complications from radiotherapy dose escalation in prostate cancer: preliminary results of a randomized trial. Int J Radiat Oncol Biol Phys 2000;48(3):635–42.

5. Eifel PJ, Levenback C, Wharton JT, et al. Time course and incidence of late complications in patients treated with radiation therapy for FIGO stage IB carcinoma of the uterine cervix. Int J Radiat Oncol Biol Phys 1995;32(5): 1289–300.

6. Anseline PF, Lavery IC, Fazio VW, et al. Radiation injury of the rectum: evaluation of surgical treatment. Ann Surg 1981;194(6):716–24.

7. Haboubi NY, Schofield PF, Rowland PL. The light and electron microscopic features of early and late phase radiation-induced proctitis. Am J Gastroenterol 1988;83(10):1140–4.

8. Hasleton PS, Carr N, Schofield PF. Vascular changes in radiation bowel disease. Histopathology 1985;9(5):517–34.

9. Gelblum DY, Potters L. Rectal complications associated with transperineal interstitial brachytherapy for prostate cancer. Int J Radiat Oncol Biol Phys 2000; 48(1):119–24.

10. O'Brien PC, Hamilton CS, Denham JW, et al. Spontaneous improvement in late rectal mucosal changes after radiotherapy for prostate cancer. Int J Radiat Oncol Biol Phys 2004;58(1):75–80.

11. Theodorescu D, Gillenwater JY, Koutrouvelis PG. Prostatourethral-rectal fistula after prostate brachytherapy. Cancer 2000;89(10):2085–91.

12. Do NL, Nagle D, Poylin VY. Radiation proctitis: current strategies in management. Gastroenterol Res Pract 2011;2011:917941.

13. Liu T, Liu Y, He S, et al. Use of radiation with or without WR-2721 in advanced rectal cancer. Cancer 1992;69(11):2820–5.

14. Athanassiou H, Antonadou D, Coliarakis N, et al. Protective effect of amifostine during fractionated radiotherapy in patients with pelvic carcinomas: results of a randomized trial. Int J Radiat Oncol Biol Phys 2003;56(4):1154–60.

15. Keefe DM, Schubert MM, Elting LS, et al. Updated clinical practice guidelines for the prevention and treatment of mucositis. Cancer 2007;109(5):820–31.

16. O'Brien PC, Franklin CI, Poulsen MG, et al. Acute symptoms, not rectally administered sucralfate, predict for late radiation proctitis: longer term follow-up of a phase III trial–Trans-Tasman Radiation Oncology Group. Int J Radiat Oncol Biol Phys 2002;54(2):442–9.

17. Kneebone A, Mameghan H, Bolin T, et al. Effect of oral sucralfate on late rectal injury associated with radiotherapy for prostate cancer: a double-blind, randomized trial. Int J Radiat Oncol Biol Phys 2004;60(4):1088–97.

18. Phan J, Swanson DA, Levy LB, et al. Late rectal complications after prostate brachytherapy for localized prostate cancer: incidence and management. Cancer 2009;115(9):1827–39.

19. Vernia P, Fracasso PL, Casale V, et al. Topical butyrate for acute radiation proctitis: randomised, crossover trial. Lancet 2000;356(9237):1232–5.

20. Hille A, Herrmann MK, Kertesz T, et al. Sodium butyrate enemas in the treatment of acute radiation-induced proctitis in patients with prostate cancer and the impact on late proctitis. A prospective evaluation. Strahlenther Onkol 2008; 184(12):686–92.

21. Baum CA, Biddle WL, Miner PB Jr. Failure of 5-aminosalicylic acid enemas to improve chronic radiation proctitis. Dig Dis Sci 1989;34(5):758–60.

22. Kochhar R, Patel F, Dhar A, et al. Radiation-induced proctosigmoiditis. Prospective, randomized, double-blind controlled trial of oral sulfasalazine plus rectal steroids versus rectal sucralfate. Dig Dis Sci 1991;36(1):103-7.
23. Hong JJ, Park W, Ehrenpreis ED. Review article: current therapeutic options for radiation proctopathy. Aliment Pharmacol Ther 2001;15(9):1253-62.
24. Goldstein F, Khoury J, Thornton JJ. Treatment of chronic radiation enteritis and colitis with salicylazosulfapyridine and systemic corticosteroids. A pilot study. Am J Gastroenterol 1976;65(3):201-8.
25. Ladas SD, Raptis SA. Sucralfate enemas in the treatment of chronic postradiation proctitis. Am J Gastroenterol 1989;84(12):1587-9.
26. Triantafillidis JK, Dadioti P, Nicolakis D, et al. High doses of 5-aminosalicylic acid enemas in chronic radiation proctitis: comparison with betamethasone enemas. Am J Gastroenterol 1990;85(11):1537-8.
27. Schwiebert LM, Beck LA, Stellato C, et al. Glucocorticosteroid inhibition of cytokine production: relevance to antiallergic actions. J Allergy Clin Immunol 1996; 97(1 Pt 2):143-52.
28. Kochhar R, Sriram PV, Sharma SC, et al. Natural history of late radiation proctosigmoiditis treated with topical sucralfate suspension. Dig Dis Sci 1999;44(5): 973-8.
29. Chun M, Kang S, Kil HJ, et al. Rectal bleeding and its management after irradiation for uterine cervical cancer. Int J Radiat Oncol Biol Phys 2004;58(1):98-105.
30. Sasai T, Hiraishi H, Suzuki Y, et al. Treatment of chronic post-radiation proctitis with oral administration of sucralfate. Am J Gastroenterol 1998;93(9):1593-5.
31. Stockdale AD, Biswas A. Long-term control of radiation proctitis following treatment with sucralfate enemas. Br J Surg 1997;84(3):370.
32. Sandor Z, Nagata M, Kusslatscher S, et al. Stimulation of mucosal glutathione and angiogenesis: new mechanisms of gastroprotection and ulcer healing by sucralfate. Scand J Gastroenterol Suppl 1995;210:19-21.
33. Konturek SJ, Brzozowski T, Majka J, et al. Fibroblast growth factor in gastroprotection and ulcer healing: interaction with sucralfate. Gut 1993;34(7):881-7.
34. Freeman CD, Klutman NE, Lamp KC. Metronidazole. A therapeutic review and update. Drugs 1997;54(5):679-708.
35. Cavcic J, Turcić J, Martinac P, et al. Metronidazole in the treatment of chronic radiation proctitis: clinical trial. Croat Med J 2000;41(3):314-8.
36. al-Sabbagh R, Sinicrope FA, Sellin JH, et al. Evaluation of short-chain fatty acid enemas: treatment of radiation proctitis. Am J Gastroenterol 1996;91(9):1814-6.
37. Talley NA, Chen F, King D, et al. Short-chain fatty acids in the treatment of radiation proctitis: a randomized, double-blind, placebo-controlled, cross-over pilot trial. Dis Colon Rectum 1997;40(9):1046-50.
38. Kennedy M, Bruninga K, Mutlu EA, et al. Successful and sustained treatment of chronic radiation proctitis with antioxidant vitamins E and C. Am J Gastroenterol 2001;96(4):1080-4.
39. Ehrenpreis ED, Jani A, Levitsky J, et al. A prospective, randomized, double-blind, placebo-controlled trial of retinol palmitate (vitamin A) for symptomatic chronic radiation proctopathy. Dis Colon Rectum 2005;48(1):1-8.
40. Rubinstein E, Ibsen T, Rasmussen RB, et al. Formalin treatment of radiation-induced hemorrhagic proctitis. Am J Gastroenterol 1986;81(1):44-5.
41. Luna-Perez P, Rodriguez-Ramirez SE. Formalin instillation for refractory radiation-induced hemorrhagic proctitis. J Surg Oncol 2002;80(1):41-4.
42. de Parades V, Etienney I, Bauer P, et al. Formalin application in the treatment of chronic radiation-induced hemorrhagic proctitis-an effective but not risk-free

procedure: a prospective study of 33 patients. Dis Colon Rectum 2005;48(8): 1535–41.

43. Marx RE, Ehler WJ, Tayapongsak P, et al. Relationship of oxygen dose to angiogenesis induction in irradiated tissue. Am J Surg 1990;160(5):519–24.

44. Dall'Era MA, Hampson NB, Hsi RA, et al. Hyperbaric oxygen therapy for radiation induced proctopathy in men treated for prostate cancer. J Urol 2006;176(1):87–90.

45. Clarke RE, Tenorio LM, Hussey JR, et al. Hyperbaric oxygen treatment of chronic refractory radiation proctitis: a randomized and controlled double-blind crossover trial with long-term follow-up. Int J Radiat Oncol Biol Phys 2008;72(1):134–43.

46. Craighead P, Shea-Budgell MA, Nation J, et al. Hyperbaric oxygen therapy for late radiation tissue injury in gynecologic malignancies. Curr Oncol 2011; 18(5):220–7.

47. Bennett MH, Feldmeier J, Hampson N, et al. Hyperbaric oxygen therapy for late radiation tissue injury. Cochrane Database Syst Rev 2005;(3):CD005005.

48. Triadafilopoulos G, Sarkisian M. Dilatation of radiation-induced sigmoid stricture using sequential Savary-Guilliard dilators. A combined radiologic-endoscopic approach. Dis Colon Rectum 1990;33(12):1065–7.

49. Berken CA. Nd:YAG laser therapy for gastrointestinal bleeding due to radiation colitis. Am J Gastroenterol 1985;80(9):730–1.

50. Barbatzas C, Spencer GM, Thorpe SM, et al. Nd:YAG laser treatment for bleeding from radiation proctitis. Endoscopy 1996;28(6):497–500.

51. Viggiano TR, Zighelboim J, Ahlquist DA, et al. Endoscopic Nd:YAG laser coagulation of bleeding from radiation proctopathy. Gastrointest Endosc 1993;39(4): 513–7.

52. Taylor JG, DiSario JA, Buchi KN. Argon laser therapy for hemorrhagic radiation proctitis: long-term results. Gastrointest Endosc 1993;39(5):641–4.

53. Buchi KN, Dixon JA. Argon laser treatment of hemorrhagic radiation proctitis. Gastrointest Endosc 1987;33(1):27–30.

54. Kantsevoy SV, Cruz-Correa MR, Vaughn CA, et al. Endoscopic cryotherapy for the treatment of bleeding mucosal vascular lesions of the GI tract: a pilot study. Gastrointest Endosc 2003;57(3):403–6.

55. Hou JK, Abudayyeh S, Shaib Y. Treatment of chronic radiation proctitis with cryoablation. Gastrointest Endosc 2011;73(2):383–9.

56. Jensen DM, Machicado GA, Cheng S, et al. A randomized prospective study of endoscopic bipolar electrocoagulation and heater probe treatment of chronic rectal bleeding from radiation telangiectasia. Gastrointest Endosc 1997;45(1): 20–5.

57. Fantin AC, Binek J, Suter WR, et al. Argon beam coagulation for treatment of symptomatic radiation-induced proctitis. Gastrointest Endosc 1999;49(4 Pt 1):515–8.

58. Silva RA, Correia AJ, Dias LM, et al. Argon plasma coagulation therapy for hemorrhagic radiation proctosigmoiditis. Gastrointest Endosc 1999;50(2):221–4.

59. Karamanolis G, Triantafyllou K, Tsiamoulos Z, et al. Argon plasma coagulation has a long-lasting therapeutic effect in patients with chronic radiation proctitis. Endoscopy 2009;41(6):529–31.

60. Tjandra JJ, Sengupta S. Argon plasma coagulation is an effective treatment for refractory hemorrhagic radiation proctitis. Dis Colon Rectum 2001;44(12): 1759–65 [discussion: 1771].

61. Taieb S, Rolachon A, Cenni JC, et al. Effective use of argon plasma coagulation in the treatment of severe radiation proctitis. Dis Colon Rectum 2001;44(12): 1766–71.

62. Zhou C, Adler DC, Becker L, et al. Effective treatment of chronic radiation proctitis using radiofrequency ablation. Therap Adv Gastroenterol 2009;2(3):149–56.
63. Rustagi T, Mashimo H. Endoscopic management of chronic radiation proctitis. World J Gastroenterol 2011;17(41):4554–62.
64. Jao SW, Beart RW Jr, Gunderson LL. Surgical treatment of radiation injuries of the colon and rectum. Am J Surg 1986;151(2):272–7.
65. Ayerdi J, Moinuddeen K, Loving A, et al. Diverting loop colostomy for the treatment of refractory gastrointestinal bleeding secondary to radiation proctitis. Mil Med 2001;166(12):1091–3.
66. Pricolo VE, Shellito PC. Surgery for radiation injury to the large intestine. Variables influencing outcome. Dis Colon Rectum 1994;37(7):675–84.
67. Lucarotti ME, Mountford RA, Bartolo DC. Surgical management of intestinal radiation injury. Dis Colon Rectum 1991;34(10):865–9.
68. Turina M, Mulhall AM, Mahid SS, et al. Frequency and surgical management of chronic complications related to pelvic radiation. Arch Surg 2008;143(1):46–52 [discussion: 52].
69. Marks G, Mohiudden M. The surgical management of the radiation-injured intestine. Surg Clin North Am 1983;63(1):81–96.
70. Hanson B, MacDonald R, Shaukat A. Endoscopic and medical therapy for chronic radiation proctopathy: a systematic review. Dis Colon Rectum 2012; 55(10):1081–95.

Index

Note: Page numbers of article titles are in **boldface** type.

A

Abscess, anal, 774–777
Acyclovir, for herpes simplex virus, 884
Advancement flaps
    endorectal, for anal fistula, 782
    for anal stenosis, 748–751
    for radiation proctitis, 921
    mucosal, for anal fissure, 744–745
Altmeir procedure, for rectal prolapse, 845–847
Amifostine, for radiation proctitis prevention, 916
Amino salicylic acid derivatives, for radiation proctitis, 917
Anal abscess, 774–777
Anal enrichment procedure, for rectal prolapse, 845–847
Anal fissure, 729–745
    acute, 732
    anatomy of, 729–730
    chronic, 732
    epidemiology of, 730
    etiology of, 731
    examination of, 731–732
    physiology of, 729–730
    primary, 730
    symptoms of, 731
    treatment of, 732–745
Anal hygiene, 808–809
Anal sphincters
    anatomy of, 704–705
    artificial, for fecal incontinence, 826–828
    hypertonicity of, anal fissures in, 731
    injury of, incontinence in, 816–817
    physiology of, 709–710
    spasm of, anal fissures in, 731
Anal verge, anatomy of, 703–704
Anismus (pelvic dyssynergy), 869–870
Anogenital warts, 885–886
Anorectal disorders
    abscesses and fistulas, **773–784**
    anatomy of, **701–712,** 773–774
    constipation, 731, **863–876**
    embryology and, 701–702
    fecal incontinence. *See* Fecal continence and incontinence.
    fissures, **729–758**

Gastroenterol Clin N Am 42 (2013) 927–939
http://dx.doi.org/10.1016/S0889-8553(13)00124-6
0889-8553/13/$ – see front matter © 2013 Elsevier Inc. All rights reserved.

gastro.theclinics.com

Anorectal (*continued*)
    hemorrhoids, **759–772**
    imaging for, **701–712**
    intussusception, **837–861**
    pelvic outlet obstruction, **863–876**
    pelvic pain syndrome and, **785–800**
    prolapse, **837–861**
    pruritus ani, **801–813**
    radiation proctitis, **913–925**
    squamous intraepithelial neoplasia, 806–807, **893–912**
    stenosis, **729–758**
    testing for, 715–726
Anorectal physiology, **713–728**
Anoscopy
    for hemorrhoids, 761
    for squamous intraepithelial neoplasia, 886, 902–903
Antegrade continence enema, for fecal incontinence, 830–831
Anterior sling rectopexy, for rectal prolapse, 847–849
Antidepressants, for chronic pelvic pain, 794
Argon plasma coagulation, for radiation proctitis, 920
Artificial bowel sphincter, for fecal incontinence, 826–828
Atopic dermatitis, 803–804
Azithromyin, for chancroid, 882

B

Balloon expulsion test, 716, 721, 867
Beahrs classification, of rectal prolapse, 841
Benzathine penicillin G, for syphilis, 881–882
Berwick's solution, for pruritus ani, 808
Biofeedback
    for fecal incontinence, 821
    for pelvic dyssynergy, 869–870
    for rectal prolapse, 844
Biopsy, for radiation proctitis, 915
Bipolar electrocoagulation, for radiation proctitis, 919
Bleeding, in anal fissure, 731
Botulinum toxin
    for anal fissure, 740–743
    for pelvic dyssynergy, 870
Bowen disease, 806–807
Bulking agents, for fecal incontinence, 823–824
Buschke-Löwenstein lesion, 887
Butyrate, for radiation proctitis, 917

C

Calcium channel blockers, for anal fissure, 737–740
Calcium dobesilate, for hemorrhoids, 764
Cancer, pruritus ani in, 806–807
Candidiasis, pruritus ani in, 805–806

Ceftriaxone
  for chancroid, 882
  for gonorrhea, 880
  for sexually transmitted diseases, 878
Cephalosporins, for gonorrhea, 880
Cerclage, for fecal incontinence, 828–829
Chancres, in syphilis, 881–882
Chancroid, 882
Chemodenervation, for anal fissure, 741
Chlamydia infections, 880–881
Cholestasis, pruritus ani in, 806
Chronic pain syndrome, pelvic, 794
Chronic pelvic pain, **785–800**
  causes of, 788–794
  challenges in, 795
  definition of, 785–786
  epidemiology of, 786
  history of, 786–787
  pain types in, 787
  physical examination in, 787–788
  treatment of, 794–795
Cinedefecography, 709
Ciprofloxacin, for chancroid, 882
Cloaca, embryology of, 702
Clobetasol, for lichen sclerosis, 805
Coagulation, infrared, for hemorrhoids, 766
Coccygodynia, 793
Colectomy, for constipation, 864, 866
Colonic inertia, constipation in, 864, 866
Colonic transit studies, 716, 725–726
  for constipation, 867
  for rectal prolapse, 843
Colonoscopy
  for constipation, 865
  for fecal incontinence, 819–820
  for radiation proctitis, 915
  for rectal prolapse, 842
Colostomy
  for pelvic outlet obstruction, 873
  for radiation proctitis, 920–921
Colposcopy, 903
Condyloma, giant, 887
Condyloma accuminata, 885–886
Condyloma lata, in syphilis, 881–882
Congestion, pelvic, 790
Constipating agents, for fecal incontinence, 820
Constipation, **863–876**
  anal fissures in, 731
  causes of, 864
  definition of, 863–864
  evaluation of, 864–866

Constipation (*continued*)
    incidence of, 863
    pathology of, 864
    pelvic outlet obstruction subtype of, 864, 868–873
    subtypes of, 864
    treatment of, 865–866, 868
Corticosteroids, for pruritus ani, 810
Crohn disease, anal stenosis in, 750
Cryoablation, for radiation proctitis, 919
Cryotherapy
    for hemorrhoids, 766
    for squamous intraepithelial neoplasia, 905–907
Cryptoglandular theory, of anal abscess formation, 774
Culture
    Chlamydia, 880–881
    Haemophilus ducreyi, 882
    herpes simplex virus, 883–884
    Neisseria gonorrhea, 879
Cystitis, interstitial, 791
Cytology, for squamous intraepithelial neoplasia, 899–901

D

Defecation
    for fecal incontinence, 819–820
    pain in, in anal fissure, 731
Defecography, 708–709, 716, 720–721, 867–868
Delorme procedure, for rectal prolapse, 845–847
Dermatitis
    atopic, 803–804
    seborrheic, 804
Devascularization, transanal, for hemorrhoids, 770
Diamond flaps, for anal stenosis, 749
Diet
    anal fissures due to, 731
    constipation due to, 864
    for anal fissure, 732
    for fecal incontinence, 820
    for hemorrhoids, 763
    for pruritus ani, 810
    for rectal prolapse, 844
Digital rectal examination, 716–717
    for chronic pelvic pain, 788
    for constipation, 865
    for fecal incontinence, 818
    for hemorrhoids, 761
    for rectal prolapse, 840
Dilation
    for anal fissure, 744
    for anal stenosis, 745
    for radiation proctitis, 919

Diltiazem, for anal fissure, 737–739
Dimethyl sulfoxide, for interstitial cystitis, 791
Donovanosis, 882
Doppler-guided transanal devascularization, for hemorrhoids, 770
Doxycycline
    for donovanosis, 882
    for lymphogranuloma venereum, 881
    for syphilis, 881–882
Doxycyline
    for gonorrhea, 880
    for sexually transmitted diseases, 878
Drainage, for anal abscesses, 776–777
Drugs, constipation due to, 864

E

Electrocoagulation
    for radiation proctitis, 919
    for squamous intraepithelial neoplasia, 905–907
Electrodessication, for warts, 885
Electromyography, 716, 725
    for constipation, 867
    for fecal incontinence, 819–820
    for rectal prolapse, 844
Endometriosis, 790
Endorectal advancement flaps, for anal fistula, 782
Endorectal ultrasonography, 705–707, 716, 718, 720, 818
Endoscopic therapies, for radiation proctitis, 919–920
Enemas, for fecal incontinence, 820, 830–831
Enteroceles, 871
Enzyme-linked immunosorbent assay, for herpes simplex virus, 883–884
Erythromycin
    for chancroid, 882
    for gonorrhea, 880
    for lymphogranuloma venereum, 881
Excision
    for squamous intraepithelial neoplasia, 905
    of giant condyloma, 887
Excisional hemorrhoidectomy, 767–769
Exteneration, pelvic, for radiation proctitis, 921

F

Famciclovir, for herpes simplex virus, 884
Fat injection, for fecal incontinence, 823–824
Fecal continence and incontinence, **815–836**
    etiology of, 816–817
    evaluation of, 817–820
    in rectal prolapse, 839
    muscles involved in, 704–705
    physiology of, 709–710
    treatment of

Fecal (*continued*)
     medical, 820–821
     surgical, 821–832
Fecal diversion, for radiation proctitis, 920–921
Ferguson (closed) hemorrhoidectomy, 767–768
Fiber
     for anal fissure, 732
     for anal stenosis, 745
     for constipation, 863–864
     for fecal incontinence, 820
     for hemorrhoids, 763
     for rectal prolapse, 844
Fibrin glue, for anal fistula, 781
Fistulas, anal, 774–782
     classification of, 778–779
     diagnosis of, 779
     incidence of, 777
     symptoms of, 779
     treatment of, 779–782
Fistulectomy, for anal fistula, 780
Fistulotomy, for anal fistula, 780
Flavinoids, for hemorrhoids, 764
Fluoroscopy
     for rectal prolapse, 842–843
     in defecography, 708–709, 716, 720–721
5-Fluorouracil, for squamous intraepithelial neoplasia, 904
Formalin, for radiation proctitis, 918
Fryjkman-Goldberg procedure, for rectal prolapse, 850
Fungal infections, pruritus ani in, 805–806

G

Gastrointestinal disorders, chronic pelvic pain in, 791–792
Genital herpes, 883–884
Giant condyloma, 887
Glue, fibrin, for anal fistula, 781
Gluteoplasty, for fecal incontinence, 830
Glyceryl trinitrate, for anal fissure, 733–740
Gonorrhea, 879–880
Goodsall classification, of anal fistulas, 778–779
Graciloplasty, for fecal incontinence, 826
Granuloma inguinale, 882
Gynecologic disorders, chronic pelvic pain in, 790–791

H

Haemophilus ducreyi infections, 882
Heater probe therapy, for radiation proctitis, 919
Hemorrhoid(s), **759–772**
     anatomy of, 760–761
     classification of, 760–763
     history of, 759

physical examination of, 761
physiology of, 760–761
pruritus ani in, 807
treatment of
    nonoperative, 763–766
    operative, 766–770
Hemorrhoidal arteries, anatomy of, 703
Hemorrhoidectomy, anal stenosis after, 745
Herpes simplex virus infections, 883–884
Herpes zoster, pruritus ani in, 806
High-resolution anoscopy, for squamous intraepithelial neoplasia, 886, 902–903
Hirshsprung disease, short-segment, 869
Horseshoe anal abscess, 775–777
House flaps, for anal stenosis, 749
Human immunodeficiency virus infection, 879, 894–895, 904–907
Human immunodeficiency virus infections, 884–885
Human papillomavirus, 885–886, 894–897, 904–905
Hyaluronic acid, for fecal incontinence, 824
Hyperbaric oxygen therapy, for radiation proctitis, 918–919
Hysterectomy, for chronic pelvic pain, 794–795

I

Ileostomy
    for pelvic outlet obstruction, 873
    for radiation proctitis, 920–921
Imiquimod cream
    for squamous intraepithelial neoplasia, 904
    for warts, 885–886
Incontinence. See Fecal continence and incontinence.
Infections, chronic pelvic pain in, 793
Inflammatory diseases, pruritus ani in, 802–805
Infliximab, for anal fistula, 780
Infrared coagulation
    for hemorrhoids, 766
    for squamous intraepithelial neoplasia, 905–907
Interspheric anal abscesses, 775–777
Interstitial cystitis, 791
Intraepithelial neoplasia. See Squamous intraepithelial neoplasia.
Intussusception. See also Rectal prolapse.
    internal, 870
Irritable bowel syndrome
    chronic pelvic pain in, 791–792
    constipation in, 864
Island flaps, for anal stenosis, 749, 751
Isosorbide dinitrate, for anal fissure, 741
Itching (pruritus ani), 801–813

K

Kegel exercises, for rectal prolapse, 844
Klebsiella granulomatis infections, 882

L

Laparoscopy
  for chronic pelvic pain, 794
  for rectal prolapse repair, 851–852
Laser therapy, for radiation proctitis, 919–920
Laxatives, for constipation, 864
Levator syndrome, 793
Lichen planus, 804–805
Lichen sclerosis, 805
Lidocaine, for anal fissure, 739
Lifestyle modifications, for hemorrhoids, 763
LIFT procedure, for anal fistula, 781–782
Ligation, rubber band, for hemorrhoids, 764–766
Lymphatic system, anatomy of, 703
Lymphogranuloma venereum, 880–881

M

Magnetic resonance imaging, 707–708, 716, 722
  for constipation, 867
  for rectal prolapse, 843
Manometry, anal, 716–719
  for constipation, 867
  for fecal incontinence, 818–819
  for rectal prolapse, 843
Mechanical pelvic outlet obstruction, 870–873
Mesalazine, for radiation proctitis, 917
Mesh rectopexy, for rectal prolapse, 847–849
Mesorectum, anatomy of, 703
Metronidazole
  for anal fistula, 780
  for radiation proctitis, 917–918
Milligan-Morgan (open) hemorrhoidectomy, 768
Moskowitz repair, 871
Motility disorders, constipation in, 864
Motor physiology, 709–710
Mucosal advancement flaps, for anal fissure, 744–745
Mucosal sleeve resection, for rectal prolapse, 845–847
Musculoskeletal disorders, chronic pelvic pain in, 792–793
Myectomy, for short-segment Hirshsprung disease, 869

N

NASHA Dx hyaluronic acid, for fecal incontinence, 824
Neisseria gonorrhea infections, 879–880
Neuroablative techniques, for chronic pelvic pain, 794
Nifedipine, for anal fissure, 737, 739–740
Nitrates, for hemorrhoids, 764
Nitric oxide donors, for anal fissure, 732–740
Nonsteroidal anti-inflammatory drugs
  for chronic pelvic pain, 794

for interstitial cystitis, 791
Nucleic acid amplification tests
  for *Chlamydia,* 880–881
  for *Neisseria gonorrhea,* 879

O

Obstructed defecation. *See* Pelvic outlet obstruction.
Orr-Loygue procedure, for rectal prolapse, 850–851
Oxygen therapy, hyperbaric, for radiation proctitis, 918–919

P

Paget disease, 807
Pain, in anal abscesses, 775
Pap smear, for squamous intraepithelial neoplasia, 902–903
Parasitic infections, pruritus ani in, 806
Parks classification, of anal fistulas, 778
Pediculosis, pruritus ani in, 806
Pelvic congestion, 790
Pelvic dyssynergy, 869–870
Pelvic exteneration, for radiation proctitis, 921
Pelvic floor
  defecography of, 708–709
  examination of, for constipation, 865
  muscles of, 705
  prolapse of, 793
  spasms of, 793
Pelvic girdle pain, 792–793
Pelvic nerves, anatomy of, 703–704
Pelvic outlet obstruction, 864, 868–873
  classification of, 868–869
  functional, 869–870
  mechanical, 870–873
Pelvic pain, chronic. *See* Chronic pelvic pain.
Pelvic sepsis, in hemorrhoid ligation, 766
Penicillin(s), for syphilis, 881–882
Pentosan polysulfate sodium, for interstitial cystitis, 791
Perianal abscesses, 774–777
Perianal wink test, 717, 817
Perineal approaches, for rectal prolapse, 845–847
Phlebotonics, for hemorrhoids, 764
Photodynamic therapy, for squamous intraepithelial neoplasia, 904
Physical therapy, for fecal incontinence, 821
Pinworm infections, pruritus ani in, 806
Plugs, fistula, for anal fistula, 781
Podofilox, for warts, 885–886
Polymerase chain reaction, herpes simplex virus, 883–884
Polyphenon E, for warts, 886
Pregnancy
  anal fissures in, 731
  pelvic girdle pain in, 792–793

Premalignant diseases, pruritus ani in, 806–807
Preparation H, for hemorrhoids, 763
Presacral fascia, anatomy of, 703
Procidentia. *See* Rectal prolapse.
Proctalgia, chronic, 792
Proctalgia fugax, 792
Proctectomy, for radiation proctitis, 921
Proctitis
    radiation, **913–925**
    sexually transmitted. *See* Sexually transmitted diseases.
Proctosigmoidectomy, for rectal prolapse, 845–847
Prolapse, rectal. *See* Rectal prolapse.
PROSPER trial, for rectal prolapse, 845
Prostatitis, chronic, 791
Pruritus ani, **801–813**
    definition of, 801
    etiology of, 802
    historical perspective of, 801–802
    primary (idiopathic) causes of, 808–810
    secondary causes of, 802–808
Psoriasis, 803
Puborectalis muscle
    function of, 710
    paradoxic, 869–870
Pudendal nerve terminal motor latency test, 716, 722–725
    for fecal incontinence, 819
    for rectal prolapse, 843–844

R

Radiation proctitis, **913–925**
    acute, 914–915
    chronic, 914–915
    classification of, 915
    clinical features of, 914–915
    definitions of, 914
    diagnosis of, 915
    histology of, 914–915
    prevention of, 915–916
    treatment of, 916–921
Radiofrequency ablation
    for fecal incontinence, 829–830
    for radiation proctitis, 920
Radiography
    in colonic transit studies, 716, 725–726
    in defecography, 708–709, 716, 720–721
Rapid reagin test, for syphilis, 881–882
Rectal outlet obstruction. *See* Pelvic outlet obstruction.
Rectal prolapse, **837–861**
    ancillary studies for, 841–844
    causes of, 838–839

classification of, 841
complications of, 839
definition of, 837–838
differential diagnosis of, 840–841
epidemiology of, 838
evaluation of, 839–840
in pediatric patients, 838
risk factors for, 839
treatment of, 844–852
Rectal veins, anatomy of, 703
Rectoanal inhibitory reflex, in fecal incontinence, 819
Rectoceles, 793, 871, 873
Rectopexy, for rectal prolapse, 847–848
Rectosigmoid junction, anatomy of, 702
Resection rectopexy, for rectal prolapse, 850
Ripstein procedure, for rectal prolapse, 847–849
Rome II criteria, for constipation, 864
Rotational flaps, for anal stenosis, 749, 751
Rubber band ligation, for hemorrhoids, 764–766

S

Sacral nerve stimulation
    for fecal incontinence, 824–826
    for interstitial cystitis, 791
    for pelvic dyssynergy, 869–870
Scabies, pruritus ani in, 806
Sclerotherapy, 766
Sealant glue, for anal fistula, 781
Seborrheic dermatitis, 804
Secca procedure, for fecal incontinence, 829–830
Sensory physiology, 709
Setons, for anal fistula, 781
Sexually transmitted diseases, 793, **877–892**
    chancroid, 882
    Chlamydia, 880–881
    chronic pelvic pain in, 793
    clinical presentation of, 878
    donovanosis, 882
    giant condyloma, 887
    gonorrhea, 879
    herpes simplex virus, 883–884
    human immunodeficiency virus infection, 879, 884–885, 894–895, 904–907
    human papillomavirus, 885–886, 894–895, 904–905
    molluscum contagiosum, 887–888
    prevention of, 878–879
    reporting of, 878
    syphilis, 881–882
    treatment of, 878
Short-chain fatty acid enemas, for radiation proctitis, 918
Short-segment Hirshsprung disease, 869

Sigmoidoceles, 871
Sigmoidoscopy, for radiation proctitis, 915
Sitz baths, for anal fissure, 732
Skin tags, pruritus ani in, 807–808
Sliding flaps, for anal stenosis, 749, 751
Spastic pelvic floor syndrome (pelvic dyssynergy), 869–870
Sphincteroplasty, for fecal incontinence, 821–823
Sphincterotomy
    for anal stenosis, 752
    lateral internal, for anal fissure, 732, 744, 746–747
Squamous intraepithelial neoplasia, **893–912**
    cytology of, 899–901
    epidemiology of, 894–895
    grading of, 895–896
    historical perspective of, 894
    human papillomavirus and, 894–897, 904–905
    identification of, 902–903
    incidence of, 893–895
    natural history of, 895
    nomenclature of, 895–896
    pathology of, 897–899
    progression to higher-grade pathology, 895
    pruritus ani in, 806–807
    surveillance of, 907
    treatment of, 901–902
        nonoperative, 903–905
        operative, 905–907
Stapled hemorrhoidectomy, 769–770
STARR (stapled transanal rectal resection) procedure
    for pelvic outlet obstruction, 872–873
    for rectal prolapse repair, 852
Stenosis, anal, 745, 748–752
Stomas
    for fecal incontinence, 831–832
    for pelvic outlet obstruction, 873
Stool softeners, for anal stenosis, 745
Streptococcal infections, pruritus ani in, 805–806
Stretta procedure, for fecal incontinence, 829–830
Stricturotomy, for anal stenosis, 750
Sucralfate, for radiation proctitis, 917
Suction litigators, for hemorrhoids, 764
Sulfasalazine, for radiation proctitis, 917
Supralevator anal abscess, 775–777
Syphilis, 881–882

T

Targeted destruction, for squamous intraepithelial neoplasia, 905–907
Tattooing treatment, for pruritus ani, 810
Thiersch procedure, for rectal prolapse, 845–847
Tibial nerve stimulation, for fecal incontinence, 829

—

Transanal devascularization, for hemorrhoids, 770
Treponemal tests, for syphilis, 881–882
Trichloroacetic acid, for warts, 886

U

Ulcers, in sexually transmitted diseases, 878
Ultrasonography, endorectal, 705–707, 716–719
    for fecal incontinence, 818
    for rectal prolapse, 842
Uremic pruritus, 806
Urethral syndrome, 791
Urologic disorders, chronic pelvic pain in, 791

V

Vaccination, for human papillomavirus, 886, 904–905
Vaginitis, 790–791
Valacyclovir, for herpes simplex virus, 884
Valsalva maneuver, for rectal prolapse, 840
Valves of Houston, anatomy of, 702–703
Vasculopathy, in radiation proctitis, 915
Vasoconstrictive medications, for hemorrhoids, 763–764
Venereal disease research laboratory test, for syphilis, 881–882
Ventral rectopexy, for rectal prolapse, 850–851
Vitamin A, for radiation proctitis, 918
Vulvar vestibulitis, 790–791
Vulvodynia, 790–791

W

Warts, anogenital, 885–886
Whitehead hemorrhoidectomy, 768

Z

Zinc-oxide ointment, for pruritus ani, 808

Perianal condylomatosis for hemorrhoids, 770
Nonmercurial meas. for syphilis, 661–662
Trichloroacetic acid for warts, 668

U

Ulcers – sexually transmitted disease, 679
Ultrasonography, endorectal, 700–701, 715, 716
   for fecal incontinence, 646
   for rectal prolapse, 842
   uterine pruritus, 809
Urethral lymphoma, 781
Urologic disorders, chronic pelvic pain in, 791

V

Vaccination, for human papillomavirus, 665, 664–665
Vaginitis, 780–781
Valacyclovir, for herpes simplex virus, 654
Valsalva maneuver, for rectal prolapse, 842
Valves of Houston, anatomy of, 702–703
Vasculopathy, in radiation proctitis, 915
Vasoconstrictive medications, for hemorrhoids, 763–764
Venereal disease research laboratory test, for syphilis, 661–662
Ventrorectopexy, for rectal prolapse, 850–851
Vitamin A, for radiation proctitis, 916
Vulvar vestibulitis, 790–791
Vulvodynia, 790–791

W

Warts, anogenital, 665–668
Whitehead hemorrhoidectomy, 768

Z

Zinc oxide ointment, for pruritus ani, 804

United States Postal Service

Statement of Ownership, Management, and Circulation
(All Periodicals Publications Except Requestor Publications)

1. Publication Title	2. Publication Number	3. Filing Date
Gastroenterology Clinics of North America	0 0 0 - 2 7 9	9/14/13

4. Issue Frequency	5. Number of Issues Published Annually	6. Annual Subscription Price
Mar, Jun, Sep, Dec	4	$305.00

7. Complete Mailing Address of Known Office of Publication (Not printer) (Street, city, county, state, and ZIP+4®)

Elsevier Inc.
360 Park Avenue South
New York, NY 10010-1710

Contact Person
Stephen R. Bushing

Telephone (Include area code)
215-239-3688

8. Complete Mailing Address of Headquarters or General Business Office of Publisher (Not printer)

Elsevier Inc., 360 Park Avenue South, New York, NY 10010-1710

9. Full Names and Complete Mailing Addresses of Publisher, Editor, and Managing Editor (Do not leave blank)

Publisher (Name and complete mailing address)

Linda Belfus, Elsevier, Inc., 1600 John F. Kennedy Blvd. Suite 1800, Philadelphia, PA 19103-2899

Editor (Name and complete mailing address)

Kerry Holland, Elsevier, Inc., 1600 John F. Kennedy Blvd. Suite 1800, Philadelphia, PA 19103-2899

Managing Editor (Name and complete mailing address)

Adrianne Brigido, Elsevier, Inc., 1600 John F. Kennedy Blvd. Suite 1800, Philadelphia, PA 19103-2899

10. Owner (Do not leave blank. If the publication is owned by a corporation, give the name and address of the corporation immediately followed by the names and addresses of all stockholders owning or holding 1 percent or more of the total amount of stock. If not owned by a corporation, give the names and addresses of the individual owners. If owned by a partnership or other unincorporated firm, give its name and address as well as those of each individual owner. If the publication is published by a nonprofit organization, give its name and address.)

Full Name	Complete Mailing Address
Wholly owned subsidiary of	1600 John F. Kennedy Blvd., Ste. 1800
Reed/Elsevier, US holdings	Philadelphia, PA 19103-2899

11. Known Bondholders, Mortgagees, and Other Security Holders Owning or Holding 1 Percent or More of Total Amount of Bonds, Mortgages, or Other Securities. If none, check box ☐ None

Full Name	Complete Mailing Address
N/A	

12. Tax Status (For completion by nonprofit organizations authorized to mail at nonprofit rates) (Check one)
The purpose, function, and nonprofit status of this organization and the exempt status for federal income tax purposes:
☐ Has Not Changed During Preceding 12 Months
☐ Has Changed During Preceding 12 Months (Publisher must submit explanation of change with this statement)

PS Form 3526, September 2007 (Page 1 of 3 (Instructions Page 3)) PSN 7530-01-000-9931 PRIVACY NOTICE: See our Privacy policy in www.usps.com

---

13. Publication Title	14. Issue Date for Circulation Data Below
Gastroenterology Clinics of North America	September 2013

15. Extent and Nature of Circulation		Average No. Copies Each Issue During Preceding 12 Months	No. Copies of Single Issue Published Nearest to Filing Date
a. Total Number of Copies (Net press run)		829	753
b. Paid Circulation (By Mail and Outside the Mail)	(1) Mailed Outside-County Paid Subscriptions Stated on PS Form 3541. (Include paid distribution above nominal rate, advertiser's proof copies, and exchange copies)	305	283
	(2) Mailed In-County Paid Subscriptions Stated on PS Form 3541 (Include paid distribution above nominal rate, advertiser's proof copies, and exchange copies)		
	(3) Paid Distribution Outside the Mails including Sales Through Dealers and Carriers, Street Vendors, Counter Sales, and Other Paid Distribution Outside USPS®	216	232
	(4) Paid Distribution by Other Classes Mailed Through the USPS (e.g. First-Class Mail®)		
c. Total Paid Distribution (Sum of 15b (1), (2), (3), and (4))	▶	521	515
d. Free or Nominal Rate Distribution (By Mail and Outside the Mail)	(1) Free or Nominal Rate Outside-County Copies Included on PS Form 3541	86	88
	(2) Free or Nominal Rate In-County Copies Included on PS Form 3541		
	(3) Free or Nominal Rate Copies Mailed at Other Classes Through the USPS (e.g. First-Class Mail)		
	(4) Free or Nominal Rate Distribution Outside the Mail (Carriers or other means)		
e. Total Free or Nominal Rate Distribution (Sum of 15d (1), (2), (3) and (4))	▶	86	88
f. Total Distribution (Sum of 15c and 15e)	▶	607	603
g. Copies not Distributed (See instructions to publishers #4 (page #3))	▶	222	150
h. Total (Sum of 15f and g)	▶	829	753
i. Percent Paid (15c divided by 15f times 100)		85.83%	85.41%

16. Publication of Statement of Ownership

☐ If the publication is a general publication, publication of this statement is required. Will be printed in the **December 2013** issue of this publication. ☐ Publication not required

17. Signature and Title of Editor, Publisher, Business Manager, or Owner	Date
Stephen R. Bushing – Inventory Distribution Coordinator	September 14, 2013

I certify that all information furnished on this form is true and complete. I understand that anyone who furnishes false or misleading information on this form or who omits material or information requested on the form may be subject to criminal sanctions (including fines and imprisonment) and/or civil sanctions (including civil penalties).

PS Form 3526, September 2007 (Page 2 of 3)

Moving?

Make sure your subscription moves with you!

To notify us of your new address, find your **Clinics Account Number** (located on your mailing label above your name), and contact customer service at:

Email: journalscustomerservice-usa@elsevier.com

800-654-2452 (subscribers in the U.S. & Canada)
314-447-8871 (subscribers outside of the U.S. & Canada)

Fax number: 314-447-8029

Elsevier Health Sciences Division
Subscription Customer Service
3251 Riverport Lane
Maryland Heights, MO 63043

*To ensure uninterrupted delivery of your subscription, please notify us at least 4 weeks in advance of move.

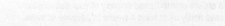

Printed and bound by CPI Group (UK) Ltd, Croydon, CR0 4YY

03/10/2024

01040493-0006